Histopath

Springer

London
Berlin
Heidelberg
New York
Barcelona
Hong Kong
Milan
Paris
Singapore
Tokyo

Derek C. Allen

Histopathology Reporting

Guidelines for Surgical Cancer

With 143 Figures

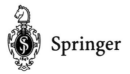

Springer

Derek C. Allen, MD, FRCPATH
Honorary Senior Lecturer and Consultant in
Histopathology and Cytopathology
Histopathology Laboratory, Belfast City Hospital,
Belfast BT9 7AD, UK

ISBN 1-85233-185-2 Springer-Verlag London Berlin Heidelberg

British Library Cataloguing in Publication Data
Allen, Derek C. (Derek Creswell)
    Histopathology reporting: guidelines for surgical cancer
    1. Cancer – Surgery 2. Cancer – Histopathology
    I. Title
    616.9′94′059
ISBN 1852331852

Library of Congress Cataloging-in-Publication Data
Allen, Derek C.
    Histopathology reporting: guidelines for surgical cancer/Derek
    C. Allen.
        p.;cm.
    Includes biographical references and index
    ISBN 1-85233-185-2 (alk. paper)
    1. Cancer–Histopathology–reporting. I. Title: Guidelines for
surgical cancer. II. Title.
    [DNLM: 1. Neoplasms–diagnosis. 2. Histological Techniques.
3. Medical Records–standards. 4. Neoplasms–pathology.
5. Neoplasms–surgery. 6. Pathology, Surgical–standards.
QZ 241 A425h 2000]
RC270.3.H56 A54 2000
616.99′407583–dc21   99-054065

Typeset by Florence Production Ltd, Stoodleigh, Devon
Printed at the Athenæum Press Ltd, Gateshead, Tyne & Wear
28/3830-543210 Printed on acid-free paper SPIN 10735592

To Alison, Katie, Rebecca and Amy

Preface

Current reorganisation of cancer services has emphasised the need for higher quality standardised
histopathology reports on surgical cancer specimens.
Increasing clinical subspecialisation is demanding
detailed histopathology reports which are inclusive of
multiple diagnostic and prognostic data directly relevant to the clinical management of each cancer type
in individual patients. It is increasingly difficult for the
consultant or trainee pathologist, surgeon or oncologist to recall those facts most salient to each cancer
type particularly if they are practising across a number
of subspecialties and are generalist in remit. From this
has arisen standardised or minimum dataset reports
as a practical educative and reporting aid for surgical
histopathology specimens. This approach is being
actively pursued by various national bodies such as the
Royal College of Pathologists (UK) and the Association
of Directors of Anatomic and Surgical Pathology
(USA). This book aims to supplement and complement
this trend by acting as an educative and practical tool
for both trainees and consultants. It provides an easily
understood and memorised framework for standardised histopathology reports in surgical cancer. It notes
the gross description, histological classification,
tumour differentiation, extent of local tumour spread,
involvement of lymphovascular channels, lymph nodes
and excision margins of the common carcinomas and
summarises non-carcinomatous malignancies. It incor-
porates the fifth edition TNM classification of cancer
spread, comments on any associated pathology and
gives diagnostic clues and prognostic criteria. The
staging information is supplemented visually by line
diagrams. It emphasises those features of a particular
cancer that are relevant to clinical management and
prognosis. It aims to give the reader a more systematic
and analytical approach to the description of surgical

pathology specimens resulting in reports that are consistent and inclusive of the data necessary for the surgical and oncological management of patients. Its format acts as an aide-memoire for routine reporting of the common cancers but it also lists diagnostic options and summary features of rarer cancers as a pointer to their diagnosis and consultation of specialist texts, as listed in the bibliography. Reports inclusive of the data herein should also facilitate demographic, research, quality control and audit procedures. I hope that you find the information in this book to be interesting, relevant and of practical use.

The author gratefully acknowledges the use of illustrations from Hermanek P, Hutter RVP, Sobin LH, Wagner G, Wittekind Ch (eds) *TNM Atlas: Illustrated Guide to the TNM/pTNM Classification of Malignant Tumours.* 4th edn. Berlin Heidelberg New York: Springer 1997.

I would like to express my grateful appreciation to Nick Mowat, Phil Bishop, Nick Wilson and the staff at Springer, my colleagues at the Belfast City Hospital Histopathology Laboratory and Mrs Debbie Green and Miss Kim Turkington for their secretarial expertise. Thanks also to my wife Alison and our girls, Katie, Rebecca and Amy who often kept quiet when "Mr Grumpy" wanted them to.

Derek Allen
Belfast

Histopathology Reporting

Contents

Respiratory and Mediastinal Cancer

Skin Cancer

Breast cancer

Gynaecological Cancer

Urological Cancer

Lymph Node Cancer

Bone and Soft Tissue Cancer

Ophthalmic Cancer

Introduction

Histopathology reports on surgical cancer specimens are becoming increasingly complex for many reasons. With closer clinicopathological correlation and the use of novel immunocytochemical and molecular techniques new entities and classifications of tumour emerge that are linked to prognosis and response to various treatment modalities. Increasingly the surgical oncologist wants tissue biopsy proof of cancer diagnoses so that patients may be recruited to suitable treatment protocols. No longer is it sufficient to simply say what it is but this must be qualified by assessment of prognostic indicators such as tumour grade, extent of spread, relationship to primary excision margins, lymph node and vascular spread. Accurate classification and information on tumour stage and prognosis requires increased time and detail on surgical pathology dissection and reporting. These necessary, but stringent demands are met by diagnostic surgical pathologists with varying degrees of success and standards of reporting. For example, an audit of colorectal cancer pathology reports in one National Health Service region of the United Kingdom showed that only 78% of colonic cancer reports and 47% of rectal cancer reports met previously agreed criteria in providing the prognostically important information.

From this has arisen a trend towards set format reports or minimum data sets for the common cancers. In the United Kingdom this is sponsored by the Royal College of Pathologists allied to other interested parties, such as the Association of Clinical Pathologists and the UK Association of Cancer Registries. They do not work in isolation but in co-operation with other bodies specifically active in individual cancer types, e.g. breast cancer: NHS Breast Screening Programme, European Commission Working Group on Breast Screening Pathology and the British Breast Group.

These new standards mirror changes in the organisation and provision of cancer services in the United Kingdom reflected in the Calman–Hine Report "A Policy Framework for Commissioning Cancer Services". Similar standards for pathologists are also set in the United States by the Association of Directors of Anatomic and Surgical Pathology and published regularly in the journal *Human Pathology*. Parallel initiatives have been published in *Archives of Pathology and Laboratory Medicine* by the College of American Pathologists. From the pathologist's point of view standard reports act as an important aide-memoire for the inclusion of necessary data and audit shows that quality standards of information increase accordingly. Also, once the pathologist is familiarised with them such reports are relatively time-efficient to dictate and transcribe. The clinician (surgeon or oncologist) can extract from them the relevant data with ease and cancer registries can be facilitated – supplemented by automated download if the database is suitably computerised.

The approach taken herein is aimed at fostering the use of standard format reports in surgical cancer. The headings used are common to all cancers, and can be preset onto a computer field or, if this is not available, easily memorised, dictated and typed in a listed format. The end product is concise, clear and relevant to patient management. The format is:

1. Gross description
   Specimen: description
   Tumour:
   > Site
   > Size
   > Appearance
   > Edge
2. Histological type
3. Differentiation/grade
4. Extent of local tumour spread
5. Lymphovascular invasion
6. Lymph nodes
7. Excision margins
8. Other pathology
9. Other malignancy

These criteria are chosen for the following reasons:

1. Gross description

Specimen

Specimen type; biopsy or resection. Full standard format reports are most relevant to resection specimens although the principles and abridged forms are applicable to biopsies. Biopsy reports should at least comment on the following (if the data are available): tumour point of origin, type of cancer, differentiation or grade, extent of mucosal or submucosal spread, adjacent dysplasia and involvement of lymphovascular channels. The proportion of tissue involved by tumour can be useful, e.g. prostate cancer. It is important epidemiologically that cancer registries can distinguish between biopsy and resection specimens to avoid duplication of statistical data leading to overestimates of cancer incidence and prevalence. This can be achieved by unique patient identification and careful indexing of SNOMED T (topography) and P (procedure) codes – this also facilitates audit of biopsy and resection-proven cancer numbers and correlation with other techniques such as exfoliative or fine needle aspiration cytology, radiological imaging and serum marker levels (e.g. prostate specific antigen, PSA).

Specimen type also has implications for excision margins and clinical adjuvant treatment and follow-up, e.g. breast-sparing excision biopsy versus mastectomy, diathermy snare polypectomy versus colonic resection.

Specimen weight and size. This may also be an indicator of the underlying pathology, e.g. primary adrenal cortical lesions > 50 g are usually carcinoma rather than adenoma, and abundant vesicular uterine curettings up to 100 g suggests complete hydatidiform mole with subsequent potential for persistent trophoblastic disease and choriocarcinoma.

Tumour

Site
Location of tumour within the mucous membrane or wall can often give clues as to its nature. Mucous membrane lesions are often primary and epithelial or lymphoid in character. Mural lesions may be primary and mesenchymal or, similar to serosal disease, secondary and extrinsic. Site dictates which adjacent tissues are involved by direct spread (e.g. cervix carcinoma–ureter) and can indicate variable tumour differentiation and prognosis within a given structure (e.g. adenocarcinoma of the hilum versus the distal third of the extrahepatic bile ducts). It can also be used as an audit tool to monitor resection rates as in anterior resection versus abdominoperineal resection for rectal carcinoma. It can influence the diagnosis, e.g. epiphyseal versus diaphyseal bone tumours, renal pelvis (transitional cell) carcinoma versus renal cortical (clear cell) carcinoma. Laterality (right or left) is obviously extremely important in patient management. Some cancers also have a tendency for multifocal growth, e.g. transitional cell carcinoma of the urinary tract, thyroid papillary carcinoma.

Size
Size influences the diagnosis (gastrointestinal stromal tumours > 5 cm are more likely to be malignant) and the prognosis (renal cell carcinoma: ≤ 7 cm = pT1, > 7 cm = pT2; sarcoma: prognosis relates to tumour grade, size and adequacy of excision; breast carcinoma: Nottingham Prognostic Index = $0.2 \times$ size (cm) + grade + lymph node stage). Gross measurements should ideally be made on the fresh tissue and checked against the histological slide allowing for tissue shrinkage with fixation and processing (say 15%). Small measurements are done with the stage micrometer or an eyepiece graticule. Guidelines are given

(National Health Service Breast Screening Programme) to distinguish between size of invasive tumour from whole size (+ in-situ change) tumour measurements and a radiological performance indicator is the percentage yield of invasive tumours<1.5 cm in diameter.

Appearance
Luminal and polypoid
— oesophageal spindle cell carcinoma.
— uterine malignant mixed mesodermal tumour (carcinosarcoma).
— multiple lymphomatous polyposis or familial adenomatous polyposis coli.

Nodular
— carcinoid tumour of bronchus.
— malignant melanoma.

Sessile/plaque
— early gastrointestinal carcinoma (stomach, oesophagus, colorectum).
— lymphoma of gut.
— high-grade bladder carcinoma.

Ulcerated
— usual carcinoma morphology.

Fleshy
— malignant lymphoma.

Pigmented
— malignant melanoma.

Haemorrhagic
— choriocarcinoma (gestational or testicular).

Cystic
— ovarian carcinoma.
— renal carcinoma.
— thyroid papillary carcinoma.
— secondary squamous carcinoma of head and neck.

Edge
Circumscribed
— mucinous carcinoma, medullary carcinoma and phyllodes tumour of breast, pancreatic endocrine tumours, some gut cancers.

Irregular
— infiltrating carcinoma.

2. Histological type

For the most part this mirrors the World Health Organization (WHO) International Classification of Tumours but draws on other classifications where appropriate, e.g. REAL – Revised European American Lymphoma classification. The classifications have also been partially edited to reflect those diagnoses that are more commonly encountered or discussed as differential diagnoses.

Histological type influences:

1. Prognosis – breast carcinoma
— excellent: tubular, cribriform, mucinous.
— good: tubular mixed, alveolar lobular.
— intermediate: classical lobular, invasive papillary, medullary.
— poor: ductal (no special type), mixed ductal and lobular, solid lobular.

2. Management – lung carcinoma
— non-small cell carcinoma: surgery ± radiotherapy depending on stage.
— small cell carcinoma: chemo-/radiotherapy.

3. Tumour distribution
— thyroid papillary carcinoma: potentially multifocal.
— ovarian epithelial borderline tumours: bilaterality, peritoneal implants, pseudomyxoma peritonei, appendiceal neoplasia.

4. Associated conditions
— thyroid medullary carcinoma: multiple endocrine neoplasia syndromes (MEN).
— duodenal periampullary carcinoma: familial adenomatous polyposis coli.

3. Differentiation/grade

Three-tier systems (well/moderate/poor differentiation, bladder carcinoma WHO I/II/III) have traditionally been used based on subjective assessment of similarity to the ancestral tissue of origin, cellular pleomorphism,[1] mitoses[2] and necrosis.[3] This is strengthened when the individual criteria are formally evalu-

---

[1]Cellular pleomorphism: This largely relates to nuclear alterations in size, shape, polarity, chromasia, crowding and nucleolar prominence. Cytoplasmic differentiation may also be taken into account (e.g. breast carcinoma – tubule formation).

[2]Mitoses: The assessment of mitotic activity either as a stand-alone mitotic activity index or as part of a grading system is a strong prognostic factor as in breast carcinoma. However, care must be taken: (a) Delayed fixation may significantly alter numbers of mitoses but also makes them more difficult to identify. (b) Hyperchromatic, pyknotic, apoptotic bodies should be ignored and only clearly defined mitotic figures counted. Strict criteria should be used such as absence of the nuclear membrane and clear hairy extension of nuclear material ± increased basophilia of the cell cytoplasm. (c) Counts should be related to a fixed field area against which various high-power microscope objectives can be calibrated. In general a ×40 objective is used.

ated and assimilated into a score that gives strong prognostic information (breast carcinoma, sarcoma). However a subjective three-tier system is not advantageous when the majority of lesions fall into one category (e.g. colorectal carcinoma is predominantly moderately differentiated) and there is a lack of prognostic stratification. It is also compounded by poor reproducibility and tumour heterogeneity. This has resulted in emergence of two-tier systems to identify prognostically adverse cancers (poorly differentiated versus others in colorectal carcinoma; low-grade/high-grade in non-Hodgkin's lymphoma and soft tissue sarcoma). In addition specific grading systems exist, e.g. Fuhrman nuclear grade in renal cell carcinoma.

4. Extent of local tumour spread

Blocks
Due to tumour heterogeneity and variation in direct extension multiple blocks of tumour and adjacent structures should be taken to ensure a representative sample. A useful general principle is one block per centimetre diameter of tumour mass with targeting of specific areas, e.g. solid foci in ovarian tumours, haemorrhagic foci in testicular tumours (choriocarcinoma).

Colorectal carcinoma: 4 or 5 to show the tumour in relation to mucosa, wall, serosa and mesentery

Thyroid nodule: 8 to 10 including the capsule to distinguish follicular adenoma from minimally invasive follicular carcinoma

Ovarian tumours: 1 block/centimetre diameter to account for the spectrum of benign, borderline and malignant changes in one lesion, particularly mucinous tumours.

Border
Pushing/infiltrative.

Lymphocytic reaction
Prominent/sparse.

Carcinomas with a pushing border and prominent lymphocytic reaction are regarded as having a better prognosis than those with a diffusely irregular infiltrating margin and sparse lymphocytic reaction, e.g. colorectal carcinoma, head and neck carcinoma, malignant melanoma, medullary carcinoma of breast, advanced gastric carcinoma.

Perineural spread
Carcinoma prostate, gall bladder and extrahepatic bile duct, pancreas and adenoid cystic carcinoma. In prostatic cancer there is some evidence that perineural invasion relates to the presence of extracapsular spread of disease and in other cancers it increases the likelihood of local recurrence.

Breslow depth/Clark level

---

[3]Tumour necrosis: Apoptotic (single cell) or coagulative (confluent).

Malignant melanoma. Direct linear measurement (mm) and anatomical level of invasion of the vertical component are strong prognostic indicators.

TNM (Tumour Nodes Metastases) classification

The TNM classification is an international gold standard for the assessment of spread of cancer and the revised 5th edition has been published by the UICC (International Union Against Cancer) taking into account new prognostic information, investigations and treatments. The system has evolved over 50 years as a tool for the careful collection of accurate data pertaining to cancer spread which can then be consistently related to planning of treatment, prognosis, evaluation of treatment and exchange of information between clinicians and centres. Virtues are that it translates into hard data some of the subjective language used in descriptive pathology reports and also encourages the pathologist to be more analytical in approach. It also improves pathologist-to-clinician communication. The post-surgical histopathological classification is designated pTNM and is based on pre-treatment, surgical and pathological information.

pT   requires resection of the primary tumour or biopsy adequate for evaluation of the highest pT category or extent of local tumour spread

pN   requires removal of nodes sufficient to evaluate the absence of regional node metastasis (pN0) and also the highest pN category

pM   requires microscopic examination of distant metastases which is often not available to the pathologist and therefore designated on clinical or radiological grounds. If available the TNM categories can be stratified into clinical stage groupings which are used to select and evaluate therapy, e.g. carcinoma in-situ is stage 0 while distant metastases is stage IV. However for the most part the pathologist concentrates on pT and pN which gives reasonably precise data to estimate prognosis and calculate end results.

Multiple synchronous tumours: classify the tumour with the highest pT category and indicate the number of tumours in brackets, e.g. pT2 (4).

pT	primary tumour
pTX	primary tumour cannot be assessed histologically
pT0	no histological evidence of primary tumour
pTis	carcinoma in-situ
pT1, pT2, pT3, pT4	increasing size and/or local extent of the primary tumour histologically.
pN	regional lymph nodes
pNX	regional lymph nodes cannot be assessed histologically
pN0	no regional lymph node metastasis histologically
pN1, pN2, pN3	increasing involvement of regional lymph nodes histologically.

Main categories can be subdivided for further specificity, e.g. pT1a or pT1b to signify unifocality or multifocality.

The TNM classification is applied to carcinoma only in the majority of tissues. Other qualifying malignant tumours are malignant mesothelioma, malignant melanoma, gestational trophoblastic tumours, germ cell tumours and retinoblastoma.

TNM optional descriptors

L lymphatic invasion
    LX   cannot be assessed
    L0   not present
    L1   present
V venous invasion
    VX   cannot be assessed
    V0   not present
    V1   microscopic
    V2   macroscopic

Prefix

y tumour is classified during or after initial multimodality therapy
r recurrent tumour, staged after a disease free interval
a classification first determined at autopsy

Suffix

m multiple primary tumours at a single site

Where appropriate other internationally recognised staging systems are also given, e.g.

malignant lymphoma	Ann Arbor
gynaecological cancers	International Federation of Gynaecology and Obstetrics (FIGO)

5. Lymphovascular invasion (LVI)

Definition

LVI usually relates to microscopic tumour emboli within small thin-walled channels in which distinction between venule and lymphatic channel is not possible – hence the general term LVI is used. It is important to identify an endothelial lining to differentiate from retraction space artefact, which often comprises a rounded aggregate of tumour sited centrally and free within a tissue space. Other helpful features of LVI are the presence of red blood cells, thrombosis and a point of attachment to the endothelium. In difficult cases endothelial markers (Factor VIII antigen, *Ulex europaeus*, CD 31) may be helpful, but in general adherence to strict morphological criteria is recommended.

Significance

There is controversy as to the significance of LVI but in practice most pathologists view tumours with prominent LVI as those that are most likely to show longitudinal submucosal spread/satellite lesions and lymph node involvement. Extratumoural LVI is regarded as more significant than intratumoural LVI and is most frequently encountered at the invasive edge of the tumour. LVI in tissue well away from the tumour is a strong marker of local and nodal recurrence in breast carcinoma, and is a criterion indicating the need for postoperative adjuvant therapy. When present in the overlying skin it denotes the specific clinicopathological entity of inflammatory breast carcinoma which is staged pT4. LVI is also a strong determinant of adjuvant chemotherapy in testicular germ cell tumours.

Vascular involvement

Some tumours (hepatocellular carcinoma, renal cell carcinoma) have a propensity for vascular involvement and care should be taken to identify this on specimen dissection and microscopy as it also alters the tumour stage. Extramural vascular invasion is a significant adverse prognostic factor in colorectal carcinoma but can be difficult to define. Sometimes one is reliant on circumstantial evidence of a tumour-filled longitudinal structure with a wall partly formed of smooth muscle, lying at right angles to the muscularis propria and adjacent to an arteriole. Widowed arteries can be a useful indicator of venular involvement in a number of situations. The significance of vessel wall infiltration without luminal disease is uncertain but probably indicates potential access to the circulation.

6. Lymph nodes

As discussed above the assessment of regional lymph nodes in a surgical cancer resection requires sufficient numbers to be able to comment on the absence of regional metastases and also the highest pN category, i.e. the total node yield and the number involved are important. In gastric carcinoma this means sampling and examining up to 15 regional nodes. Thus node yields can be used to audit both care of dissection by the pathologist, adequacy of resection by the surgeon and the choice of operation, e.g. axillary node sampling versus clearance. All nodes in the specimen should be sampled and although ancillary techniques exist (e.g. xylene clearance, revealing solutions) there is no substitute for time spent at careful dissection. Care should be taken not to double-count the same node. Sometimes minimum target yields can be used – 8 nodes will detect the vast majority of Dukes' C colorectal carcinomas. The pathologist should also remember to count those nodes in the histological slides that are immediately adjacent to the tumour as they are sometimes ignored yet more likely to be involved.

What is a node?

— a lymphoid aggregate ≥ 1 mm diameter with an identifiable subcapsular sinus.
— direct extension of the primary tumour into lymph nodes is classified as a lymph node metastasis (TNM rule).
— a tumour nodule > 3 mm in the connective tissue of a lymph drainage area (e.g. mesorectum) without histological evidence of residual lymph node is classified in the pN category as a regional lymph node metastasis. A tumour nodule up to 3 mm is classified in the pT category as discontinuous extension (TNM rule).

When size is a criterion for pN classification, e.g. breast carcinoma, measurement is of the metastasis, not the entire node (TNM rule).

Micrometastases

The significance of nodal micrometastases ≤ 2 mm and single cells demonstrated by immunohistochemistry is not resolved. In practical terms an accommodation within available resources must be made. Most busy general laboratories will submit small nodes (< 5 mm) intact or bisected, and a mid-slice of larger ones; additional slices may be processed as required if the histology warrants it. Sometimes there is circumstantial evidence of occult metastases, e.g. a granulomatous response that will promote the use of immunohistochemistry in the search for single cell spread. The prognostic significance of micrometastases has yet to be clarified for the majority of cancers, e.g. a search for micrometastases is advocated in breast and colorectal carcinoma but considered to be of equivocal significance in oesophageal carcinoma. This area needs further clarification from large international trials which examine clinical outcome related to the immunohistochemical and molecular (RT-PCR) detection of minimal residual disease in lymph nodes and bone marrow samples considered tumour-negative on routine examination.

Limit node

The limit node is the nearest node(s) to the longitudinal and/or apical resection limits and suture ties. Some specimens, e.g. transverse colon, will have more than one and they should be identified as such.

Extracapsular spread

Anecdotally extracapsular spread is an adverse prognostic sign and an indicator for potential local recurrence, particularly if the spread is near to or impinges upon a resection margin, e.g. axillary clearance in breast carcinoma.

7. Excision margins

The clearance of excision margins has important implications for patient follow-up, adjuvant therapy and local recurrence of tumour. Positive resection margins in a breast cancer may mean further local excision, conversion to a total mastectomy and/or radiotherapy to the affected area. Measurements should be made on the gross specimen, checked against the histological slide and verified using the stage micrometer or eyepiece graticule. Painting of the margins by ink supplemented by labelling of the blocks is important. Paint adheres well to fresh specimens but also works on formalin-fixed tissue. India ink or alcian blue are commonly used. Commercially available multi-coloured inks are more satisfactory, particularly if there are multiple margins as in breast carcinoma. The relevance of particular margins varies according to specimen and cancer type.

1. *Longitudinal margins.* Involvement can be by several mechanisms:

    (a) *Direct spread.* In rectal carcinoma the longitudinal margin in an anterior resection is considered satisfactory if the anastomosis is 2–3 cm beyond the macroscopic edge of the tumour, i.e. direct longitudinal spread is minimal. However, there may be involvement if the tumour is extensively infiltrative, poorly differentiated or of signet ring cell type, or shows prominent LVI. Appropriate limit blocks should be taken. In addition to the resection specimen limits separate anastomotic rings are also usually submitted.

    (b) *Discontinuous spread.* In oesophageal and gastric carcinoma there is a propensity for discontinuous lymphovascular submucosal and mural spread, and margins should be checked microscopically even if some distance from the primary tumour.

    (c) *Multifocal spread.* In transitional cell carcinoma of the urinary tract, malignant lymphoma of the bowel and papillary carcinoma of the thyroid potential multifocality must be borne in mind.

2. *Circumferential radial margin (CRM).* An often ignored measurement these margins are assuming increasing importance in relation to local recurrence and morbidity, e.g. mesorectal CRM and rectal carcinoma. It is recommended practice to measure how far the carcinoma has spread beyond the organ wall and how far it is from the CRM. Other examples are: oesophageal carcinoma and the adventitial margin, cervical carcinoma and the parametrial margin, renal carcinoma and the perinephric fat/fascial margin. Lymph node mestastasis at a CRM is also considered positive. The significance of some other examples is uncertain but comment should be made, e.g. the mesenteric edge in colonic carcinoma.

3. *Quadrant margins.* Examples are a skin ellipse for carcinoma or malignant melanoma. Usually the longitudinal axis margins are well clear and the nearest to the tumour are the transverse axis and deep aspects. It is important to check clearance not only of the infiltrating tumour but also adjacent field change, e.g. epidermal dysplasia or radial spread of a malignant melanoma. Actual measurement of margin clearance can be important in assessing the need for further local excision, e.g. malignant melanoma.

4. *Serosa or peritoneum.* This is a visceral margin and breech of it allows carcinoma to access the abdominal and pelvic cavities. Its importance has recently been re-emphasised, as for example at the upper anterior aspect of the rectum where there is potential for peritoneal disease as well as local mesorectal recurrence posterolaterally. Standard practice should involve measuring the distance from the serosa to the invasive edge of the tumour, e.g. uterine adenocarcinoma.

5. *Multiple margins.* As in breast carcinoma (lateral/medial, superior/inferior, superficial/deep) this requires differential painting and block labelling, according to a previously agreed protocol for specimen orientation markers, e.g. surgical sutures.

6. *Involvement.* Inadequate clearance of excision margins varies according to the tissues and tumours concerned:

   Breast carcinoma: invasive,<5 mm; in-situ (ductal),<10 mm

   Rectal carcinoma: mesorectum; ≤ 1 mm (either by direct extension or discontinuous in a node or lymphovascular channel)

   Colonic carcinoma: serosa; prognostic distinction is made between carcinoma in a subserosal inflammatory fibrous reaction and carcinoma being at and ulcerating the serosal surface.

TNM resection classification

R   residual tumour

Rx   presence of residual tumour cannot be assessed

R0   no residual tumour

R1   microscopic residual tumour (proven by tumour bed biopsy or cytology) and in effect if tumour involves (to within ≤ 1 mm) the resection margin

R2   macroscopic residual tumour.

8. Other pathology

This heading reminds the pathologist to look for and comment on relevant predisposing and concurrent lesions, associated conditions and useful markers.

Some examples are:

— gastric carcinoma, incomplete (type IIb) intestinal metaplasia, gastric atrophy, dysplasia, synchronous MALToma, *Helicobacter pylorii.*

— colorectal carcinoma, adenomatous polyps, familial adenomatous polyposis coli, periampullary carcinoma and duodenal adenoma.

— thyroid medullary carcinoma, multiple endocrine neoplasia (MEN) syndromes.

— hepatocellular carcinoma, hepatitis B/C infection, cirrhosis, Budd–Chiari syndrome, varices.

Other general comments are included such as diagnostic criteria, prognostic indicators, clinical and treatment parameters. Local recurrence and survival rates are both specific to individual sources and broadly indicative of the data available in the bibliography references.

9. Other malignancy

The TNM classification is targeted primarily at carcinoma but also includes malignant mesothelioma, malignant melanoma, gestational trophoblastic tumours, germ cell tumours and retinoblastoma. This section notes the commoner non-carcinomatous cancers such as uterine and gastrointestinal smooth muscle/stromal tumours, lymphoma/leukaemia and sarcoma. Summary diagnostic and prognostic criteria are given where relevant.

Ancillary techniques

Various ancillary techniques can be useful in the histopathology of surgical cancer and should be employed as appropriate. Some of these are commented on at various points in the protocols, e.g. under sections "2. Histological type" and "8. Other pathology".

Cytology

Fine needle aspiration cytology (FNAC) has become the first-order investigation in many cancers due to its speed, cost-effectiveness, proficiency and convenience for both clinician and patient. It can not only provide specific inflammatory (e.g. Hashimoto's thyroiditis) and malignant diagnoses (e.g. thyroid papillary carcinoma) but can sort patients into various management groups: viz., inflammatory and treat, benign and reassure, atypical and further investigation (by core/open biopsy or excision) or malignant with specific therapy (surgery, chemotherapy, radiotherapy). It can be used to refute or confirm recurrence in patients with a known previous diagnosis of malignancy and to monitor response to therapy or change in grade of disease. It provides a tissue diagnosis of cancer in patients unfit for more invasive investigations or when the lesion is relatively inaccessible, e.g. in the lung periphery, mediastinum, abdomen, pelvis and retroperitoneum. It must be integrated with the clinical features and investigations (serology, radiology) and can be complemented by other techniques, e.g. core biopsy. It potentially provides material for routine morphology, histochemical and immunohistochemical techniques, electron microscopy, cell culture and flow cytometry. The direct smear and cytospin preparations can be augmented by formalin-fixed paraffin-processed cell blocks of cell sediments and needle core fragments (mini-biopsies) which can combine good morphology (the cores providing a tissue pattern) and robust immunohistochemistry. It can be applied to many organs: salivary gland, thyroid gland, palpable lymphadenopathy, breast, skin, prostate, subcutaneous tissues and deep connective tissues. Radiologically guided FNAC is useful for non-central respiratory cancers and tumours in the mediastinum, liver, pancreas, kidney, retroperitoneum, abdomen and pelvis. Endoscopic FNAC is also being used more frequently, e.g. transbronchial, transrectal, transduodenal and transgastric/transoesophageal for lymph node staging or tumours covered by intact mucosa. Body cavity fluid cytology (both aspirates of free pleural, pericardial and peritoneal fluid and peritoneal/pelvic washings) continues to play an active role in the diagnosis, staging and monitoring of cancer. Yield of information is maximised by a combination of morphology and immunohistochemistry on direct smear/cytospin preparations (using air-dried Giemsa and wet-fixed Papanicolaou/H and E stains) and cell blocks (cell sediments and fragments).

Exfoliative cytology along with cytological brushings and washings is also pivotal in the assessment of various cancers, e.g. lung cancer, where the information obtained is complementary to that derived from direct biopsy and aspiration cytology. It can provide diagnostic cells not present in the biopsy specimen (for reasons of sampling error, tumour type or accessibility), correlate with it or allow subtyping that is otherwise obscured in artefacted biopsy material. Common sites of application are bronchus, mouth, oesophagus, stomach, bile duct, large intestine, bladder, renal pelvis and ureter.

Frozen sections

There has been a dramatic reduction in breast pathology due to the triple approach of clinical, radiological and cytological examination (supplemented by wide bore needle biopsy) resulting in preoperative diagnosis and appropriate planning of treatment. Frozen section is contraindicated in impalpable screen-detected lesions. Other uses are:

— check excision of parathyroid glands versus thyroid nodules or lymph nodes in hyperparathyroidism.
— operative margins in gastric carcinoma, partial hepatectomy, head and neck and urinary cancers.
— cancer versus inflammatory lesions at laparotomy.
— lymph node metastases in head and neck, urological, and gynaecological cancers prior to radical dissection.
— Mohs' micrographical surgery in resection of basal cell carcinoma of the face.
— frozen sections should be used sparingly due to problems of interpretation and sampling in the following cancers: malignant lymphoma, ovarian carcinoma, minimally invasive thyroid carcinoma, pancreas and extrahepatic bile duct carcinoma.

Histochemical stains

Histochemical stains are appropriately mentioned and can be valuable, examples being: PAS ± diastase or mucicarmine for adenocarcinomatous differentiation, PAS-positive inclusion bodies in malignant rhabdoid tumours and alveolar soft part sarcoma, PAS-positive glycogen in renal cell carcinoma.

Immunohistochemistry

Immunohistochemistry has become the surgical pathologist's "second H and E" and is invaluable in assessing tumour type, prognosis and treatment.

Tumour type

Carcinoma:	cytokeratins (low and high molecular weights), EMA, BerEP4, LeuM1 (CD 15), CEA, etc.
Melanoma:	S100, HMB-45, melan-A.
Germ cell tumours:	HCG, AFP, PLAP, HPL; human chorionic gonadotrophin; alphafetoprotein; placental alkaline phospatase; human placental lactogen.
Lymphoma:	CLA (CD 45), L26 (CD 20), CD 3, UCHL1 (CD 45R0), κ/λ light chain restriction, CD 15, CD 30, bcl-2/bcl-1, CD 5, CD 10, tdt.
Sarcoma:	vimentin, desmin, S100; sarcomeric and smooth muscle actin.
Mesothelioma:	HBME-1, thrombomodulin, cytokeratins, EMA

Metastatic adenocarcinoma of unknown origin:

1. specific
— thyroglobulin (papillary/follicular carcinoma thyroid)
— CEA, chromogranin and calcitonin (medullary carcinoma thyroid)
— surfactant (PE10) antibody (bronchioloalveolar and other lung carcinomas)
— PSA/PSAP (prostate carcinoma)
— CA125 (ovarian serous carcinoma)
2. helpful
— gross cystic disease fluid protein 15 (GCDFP-15), oestrogen and progesterone receptors (breast carcinoma)
— AFP and canalicular polyclonal CEA (hepatocellular carcinoma)
— CA19-9 and CEA (pancreatic and gastrointestinal carcinoma)
— differential cytokeratin expression, e.g. gut carcinoma is cytokeratin 20 positive/cytokeratin 7 negative whereas lung, breast and gynae carcinomas are often cytokeratin 20 negative/cytokeratin 7 positive.

Prognosis

— progesterone receptors, c-erbB2, p53 oncogene expression, Ki-67 (MIB-1) proliferation index.

Treatment

— oestrogen/androgen receptors and hormonal response in breast and prostate cancer.

Antibodies should not be used in isolation but a panel employed with positive and negative in-built and external controls. This is due to a spectrum of co-expression seen with a number of antibodies, e.g. EMA (carcinoma, plasmacytoma, Hodgkin's disease and anaplastic large cell lymphoma) and CD 15 (Hodgkin's disease and lung adenocarcinoma). Interpretation should also be closely correlated with the morphology. The above are only part of a rapidly enlarging spectrum of new generation, robust antibodies that can be used with formalin-fixed, paraffin-embedded tissues and show enhanced demonstration of expression by retrieval techniques such as microwaving and pressure cooking.

Electron microscopy

Electron microscopy has a diagnostic role to play where morphology and immunochemistry are inconclusive. Specific features can be sought in:

— carcinoma (tight junctions, short microvilli, secretory vacuoles, intermediate filaments).
— melanoma (pre-/melanosomes).
— vascular tumours (intra-cytoplasmic lumina, Weibel-Palade bodies).
— neuroendocrine carcinoma (neurosecretory granules).
— mesothelioma (long microvilli).
— smooth muscle/myofibroblastic tumours (longitudinal myofilaments with focal dense bodies).
— rhabdomyosarcoma (basal lamina, sarcomere Z line formation).
— perineural/meningeal lesions (elaborate complex cytoplasmic processes).

Molecular and chromosomal studies

Evolving areas of diagnostic use of molecular and chromosomal studies are clonal immunoglobulin heavy chain and T cell receptor gene rearrangements in the confirmation of lymphoma, and the characterisation of various cancers (particularly lymphoma, sarcoma and some carcinomas, e.g. renal) by specific chromosomal changes. Gene rearrangement studies can be carried out on formalin-fixed paraffin-embedded material but fresh tissue put into suitable transport medium is required for chromosomal analysis – although reverse transcriptase polymerase chain reaction (RT-PCR) methods are being developed for paraffin material. Genotypic subtypes of various malignancies, e.g. rhabdomyosarcoma, have been defined with differing clinical presentation, prognosis and response to therapy. Some examples are:

follicle centre lymphoma, follicular	t (14 ; 18)
mantle cell lymphoma	t (11 ; 14)
synovial sarcoma	t (X : 18) (p 11.2; q 11.2)
myxoid liposarcoma	t (12 ; 16) (q 13 ; p 11)

Quantitative methods

There is an expanding literature regarding the use of quantitative methods as diagnostic aids. These include stereology, morphometry, automated image analysis, DNA cytophotometry and flow cytometry. In general adverse prognosis is related to alterations in tumour cell nuclear size, shape, chromasia, texture, loss of polarity, mitotic activity index, proliferation index (Ki-67 or S-phase fraction on flow cytometry), DNA aneuploidy and spatial density. Most of these techniques show good correlation with carefully assessed basic histopathological criteria and, rather than replacing the pathologist and microscope, serve to emphasise the importance of various parameters and sound morphological technique. Areas of incorporation into pathological practice are:

— morphometric measurement of Breslow depth of melanoma invasion, osteoid seams in osteomalacia and muscle fibre type and diameter in myopathy.
— mitotic activity index in breast carcinoma.
— DNA ploidy in borderline versus malignant ovarian epithelial tumours.

With the advent of more sophisticated computers and machine-driven technology artificial intelligence and automated tissue analysis are being explored:

— automated cervical cytology.
— inference and neural networks in prostatic cancer and colonic polyps.
— Bayesian belief networks and decision support systems in breast cytology.
— MACs (malignancy associated changes) in prostate cancer based on alterations in nuclear texture.

This whole area is rapidly developing and evolving and it remains to be resolved as to which facets will eventually be incorporated into routine practice.

Gastrointestinal Cancer

- Oesophageal Carcinoma

- Gastric Carcinoma

- Ampulla of Vater and Head of Pancreas Carcinoma

- Small Intestinal Carcinoma

- Colorectal Carcinoma

- Vermiform Appendix Tumours

- Anal Canal Carcinoma

- Gall Bladder Carcinoma

- Extrahepatic Bile Duct Carcinoma

- Liver Carcinoma

Oesophageal Carcinoma

1. Gross description

Specimen:

— biopsy/partial oesophagectomy/oesophagogastrectomy/lymphadenectomy ± omentectomy.
— number of fragments/length of oesophagus and proximal stomach (cm).

Tumour:

Site

— mid/lower oesophagus/oesophagogastric junction/cardia. Tumour is considered oesophageal if > 50% of its mucosal bulk is above the oesophagogastric junction as defined by internal or external landmarks. Equally, adjacent oesophageal mucosal dysplasia indicates an oesophageal lesion, and gastric mucosal dysplasia a gastric tumour.
— distances (cm) to the proximal and distal resection limits and the oesophagogastric junction. The junction can vary in location or be obscured by tumour and anatomically distal oesophagus has an external layer of adventitia whereas proximal stomach is orientated to serosa (distinction is important as the TNM staging and mode of spread differs).

Size

— length × width × depth (cm) or maximum dimension (cm).
— superficial carcinoma is often small (< 2–3 cm long): advanced carcinoma frequently involves long segments of oesophagus.

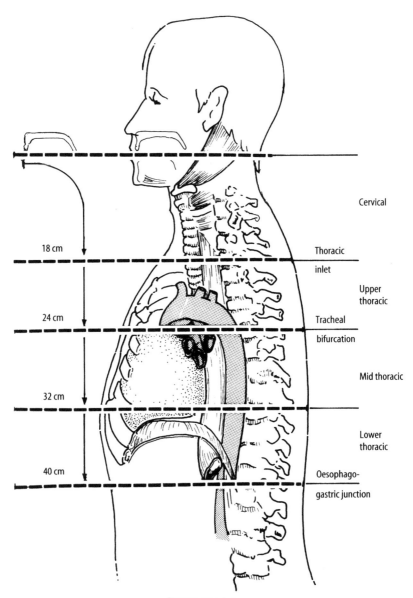

Cervical

18 cm — Thoracic inlet

Upper thoracic

24 cm — Tracheal bifurcation

Mid thoracic

32 cm

Lower thoracic

40 cm — Oesophago-gastric junction

Figure 1. Oesophagus.

Appearance

— polypoid: spindle cell carcinoma; good prognosis.

— warty/verrucous: verrucous carcinoma.

— nodular/plaque: superficial carcinoma (the gross and endoscopic appearances may be classified similar to that of early gastric cancer; see Chapter 2).

— fungating/stricture/ulcerated/infiltrative: usual type.

— multifocal.

Edge

— circumscribed/irregular.

Other pathology

— diverticulum.

— achalasia.

— Barrett's metaplasia.

— male preponderance (3:1).

2. Histological type

Adenocarcinoma

— 50–60% of cases.

— distal oesophagus/oesophagogastric junction on the basis of specialised enteric type Barrett's metaplasia and dysplasia. The incidence of this tumour has greatly increased (×3–5 in the last 20 years). Various suggested factors are improved socio-economic conditions with a Western diet rich in processed foods, antibiotic eradication of acid-suppressing pangastric cag-A (cytotoxin associated gene product) positive *Helicobacter pylorii* with restoration of gastric acidity and increased gastro-oesophogeal reflux disease, proton pump inhibitor therapy and bile reflux. Most are tubular or papillary and of intestinal type, some are signet ring cell or mucinous. Prognosis is poor as presentation is at a late stage, typically with perineural invasion.

Squamous cell carcinoma

— 30–40% of cases.

— mid-oesophagus, old age.

— large cell/small cell; keratinising/non-keratinising; usually moderately differentiated keratinising.

— verrucous: exophytic and keratotic with a pushing deep margin of cytologically bland bulbous processes. Slow growing but may become more aggressive especially after radiation.

— basaloid: poor prognosis, aggressive, deeply invasive nested pattern of basaloid cells with central necrosis, atypia and mitoses.

Spindle cell carcinoma (polypoid carcinoma/carcinosarcoma)
— probably a spindle cell carcinoma that undergoes varying degrees of stromal metaplasia and mesenchymal maturation.
— men, sixth decade.

Adenosquamous carcinoma
— mixed differentiation, aggressive.

Mucoepidermoid/adenoid cystic carcinoma
— of oesophageal submucosal duct origin. Tendency to local recurrence and metastases in 50%.

Small cell carcinoma
— primary or secondary from lung, or as part of a mixed differentiation oesophageal cancer. Poor prognosis. Distinguish from poorly differentiated squamous/adenocarcinoma by chromogranin expression and paranuclear dot CAM 5.2 expression.

Malignant melanoma
— primary or secondary. Primary requires adjacent mucosal junctional atypia. Comprises 0.1% of oesophageal malignancy – polypoid, ulcerated, satellite nodules, pigment, poor prognosis.

Metastatic carcinoma
— direct spread – stomach, thyroid, hypopharynx, bronchus and lung
— distant spread – breast, malignant melanoma.

3. Differentiation

Well/moderate/poor.
— influence on prognosis is uncertain unless the tumour is anaplastic.
— heterogeneity of differentiation within individual tumours is not uncommon.

4. Extent of local tumour spread

Border: pushing/infiltrative.
Lymphocytic reaction: prominent/sparse.
Depth (cm) and distance (mm) to the nearest painted perioesophageal circumferential resection margin.

Superficial or "early" squamous carcinoma of the oesophagus is defined as intraepithelial or invasive squamous carcinoma confined to the mucosa or submucosa, with or without lymph node spread (pTis, pT1) and is of more favourable prognosis than deep or "advanced" carcinoma (60–90% 5 year survival rates versus 5–10%). Carcinoma invading submucosa does less well (35% nodal

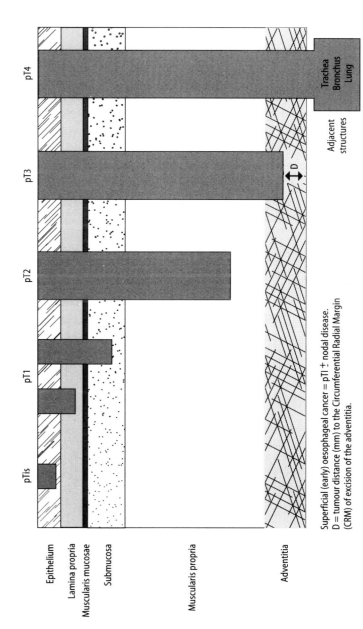

Superficial (early) oesophageal cancer = pT1 + nodal disease.
D = tumour distance (mm) to the Circumferential Radial Margin
(CRM) of excision of the adventitia.

Figure 2. Oesophageal carcinoma.

metastases, 55% 5 year survival) than that confined to the mucosa alone (88% 5 year survival irrespective of nodal status). Depth of invasion is the most important prognostic indicator on multivariate analysis and requires histological assessment as there is variable correlation with gross and endoscopic appearances. Note that on biopsy distinction between dysplastic glands and epithelium abutting an irregular muscularis mucosae and true invasion can be difficult: look for single cells and nests of infiltration (± a desmoplastic stromal reaction).

pTis carcinoma in-situ
pT1 tumour invades lamina propria or submucosa
pT2 tumour invades muscularis propria
pT3 tumour invades adventitia
pT4 tumour invades adjacent structures.

Note that the gastric component of a junctional tumour may show serosal involvement and this should be noted separately. About 50% of distal oesophageal carcinomas spread into the proximal stomach.

5. Lymphovascular invasion

Present/absent.
Intra-/extratumoural.

The presence of lymphovascular invasion (LVI) is a strong prognostic indicator. In advanced carcinoma lamina propria and submucosal LVI are not infrequent, resulting in carcinomatous emboli several centimetres beyond the gross tumour edge. Perineural invasion is also characteristic.

6. Lymph nodes

The significance of nodal micrometastases (< 2 mm diameter) is uncertain but involvement of lymph nodes, particularly if multiple, is a strong prognostic indicator. Nodal metastases occur early in the disease course and are the commonest cause of treatment failure. Involvement of stomach and later liver, lungs and adrenal gland is not infrequent.

Site/number/size/number involved/limit node/extracapsular spread.
Regional nodes: cervical oesophagus – cervical/supraclavicular; intrathoracic oesophagus – mediastinal/perigastric excluding coeliac

pN0 no regional lymph nodes involved
pN1 metastasis in regional lymph node(s)
pM1 distant metastasis
        commonest sites are mediastinum, lung and liver
        tumour thoracic oesophagus
                lower   M1a coeliac nodes
                          M1b other distant metastasis

The regional lymph nodes are, for the cervical oesophagus, the cervical nodes including supraclavicular nodes and, for the intrathoracic oesophagus, the mediastinal and perigastric nodes, excluding the coeliac nodes

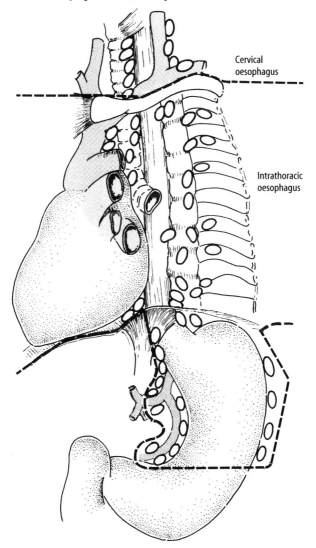

Cervical oesophagus

Intrathoracic oesophagus

Figure 3. Oesophagus: regional lymph nodes.

upper	M1a cervical nodes
	M1b other distant metastasis
mid	M1b distant metastasis
	including non-regional nodes.

7. Excision margins

Distances (cm) to the proximal and distal limits of excision.

Distance (mm) to the painted perioesophageal circumferential radial margin. Involvement (tumour present to within 1 mm) is an index of the degree of tumour spread and extent of surgical resection with potential for local recurrence or residual mediastinal disease.

Oesophageal carcinoma may show multifocality (10–25%), direct or discontinuous submucosal and lymphovascular spread and intramural metastasis (15%). This has obvious implications for examination of resection margins and potential for local recurrence.

8. Other pathology

Diverticula, achalasia and Plummer-Vincent syndrome have an increased incidence of oesophageal carcinoma.

Barrett's metaplasia: defined as replacement of the lower oesophageal squamous mucosa by metaplastic glandular epithelium due to gastro-oesophageal reflux disease. The Barrett's segment can be classical (> 3 cm long), short (< 3 cm long) or ultra-short (cardia/junctional) each of which has an increased risk of malignancy. An approximate guide is that 10% of patients with hiatus hernia and/or gastro-oesophageal reflux develop Barrett's metaplasia and that 10% of these subsequently have dysplasia or adenocarcinoma with a ×30–40 risk that of the general population. The specialised intestinal or enteric variant of Barrett's metaplasia is the usual precursor to dysplasia rather than the atrophic gastric fundic or non-specialised cardia types. The biological behaviour of low-grade dysplasia is uncertain with potential for regression or progression; it requires reassessment and endoscopic surveillance. There is a strong (40–60%) association between high-grade dysplasia and concurrent or subsequent adenocarcinoma, indicating the need for immediate clinicopathological reassessment, short-term follow-up and consideration of surgery. The recognition of significant dysplasia requires confirmation by a second experienced pathologist or positive repeat biopsy. Useful clues to the presence of dysplasia are mucosal villousity and persistence of cytological dysmaturation into the surface epithelium. Observer agreement rates are reasonably high for high-grade dysplasia. However, it is important to distinguish florid regenerative changes in oesophageal squamous and glandular mucosae from dysplasia taking into account erosion, ulceration and the degree of inflammation that is present as well as cytoarchitectural changes, e.g. nuclear enlargement with nucleolar prominence and basal cell hyperplasia. Squamous epithelial regrowth with antireflux, laser or photodynamic ablative therapy can produce variably bland metaplastic-type epithelium to quite alarming cellular changes, as does chemo-/radiation therapy. Maturation towards the epithelial surface is reassuring. Overexpression of p53 antibody and Ki-67 proliferation index may help to confirm mucosal dysplasia and its potential for progression to carcinoma in dysplastic Barrett's mucosa, although they are not routinely applicable. It should be noted that the primary diagnosis of Barrett's metaplasia is heavily dependent on the endoscopic findings and site of biopsy. Pathognmonic histological features are metaplastic glandular epithelium associated with native oesophageal structures, e.g. submucosal glands or ducts. Glandular mucosa with squamous epithelial islands is also a useful clue. Specialised enteric differentiation is reasonably distinctive whereas fundic gastric mucosa is more often associated with hiatus hernia. Surveillance for dysplasia in Barrett's mucosa is somewhat empirical with varying guidelines; the most active advocates suggest annual endoscopy with quadrantic, segmental (every 2 cm) biopsies and target biopsy of any gross lesion (ulcers, nodules, plaques, strictures).

Field change dysplasia/carcinoma in-situ: may be encountered adjacent to or overlying squamous cell carcinoma. A precancerous phase and the biological course of these premalignant changes is uncertain but better established in countries such as China and Japan where the incidence of oesophageal carcinoma is greater. This has led to the establishment of endoscopic and cytological screening programmes targeted at the early detection of lesions. As with glandular dysplasia a two-tiered system of low- and high-grade dysplasia is used. Dysplasia is found more frequently overlying and adjacent to superficial than advanced squamous cell carcinoma.

Concurrent squamous cell carcinoma of bronchus and oropharyngolaryngeal ring has an incidence of 10–15%.

Radio-/chemotherapy necrosis and tumour regression: cell apoptosis, vacuolation and degeneration, necrosis, inflammation, fibrosis, residual aggregates of keratin with a giant cell reaction and perforation may all be seen leaving only residual microscopic tumour. Radiotherapy is the main treatment for carcinoma of the middle third of the oesophagus and surgery for the distal third. Preoperative chemo-/radiotherapy are being increasingly used in an attempt to downstage the tumour and achieve better operative resectability. It is estimated that some 50–60% of tumours show quite marked morphological changes of regression, with squamous carcinoma probably being more responsive than adenocarcinoma. More sophisticated preoperative staging (e.g. CT scan and endoluminal ultrasound with fine needle aspiration cytology) is being assessed as a means of predicting those patients likely to benefit from preoperative adjuvant therapy and in selecting patients for resection (e.g. positive or negative supraclavicular lymph nodes).

Cytokeratin and mesenchymal markers (vimentin, desmin, actin) are helpful in spindle cell carcinoma (syn. carcinosarcoma). These tumours show a biphasic spectrum of malignant epithelial (squamous) and mesenchymal (usually sarcoma not otherwise specified, sometimes cartilage, bone, striated muscle) differentiation with either intimate intermingling or juxtaposition of the components which are present in variable amounts (the epithelial component may be microscopic or in-situ). Prognosis is intermediate to good because they are exophytic intraluminal lesions which present early at a relatively early stage despite their size (50% 5 year survival).

Squamous cell carcinoma is common in the mid-thoracic oesophagus while Barrett's-related adenocarcinoma is commoner, being the most frequent malignant tumour of the distal oesophagus. The incidence of Barrett's-related adenocarcinoma is markedly increasing along with that of oesophagogastric junctional lesions.

Prognosis

Prognosis of oesophageal cancer is poor (5 year survival 5–10% in the Western Hemisphere) and relates to tumour type (small cell carcinoma, basaloid carcinoma are adverse), grade (equivocal), diameter (in superficial carcinoma) but most importantly depth of invasion and stage. Nodal status and whether the longitudinal and circumferential radial margins are positive (55% recurrence rate, 25% 5 year survival) or negative (13% recurrence rate, 47% 5 year survival in one series) are important independent prognostic variables. Early oesophageal squamous cell carcinoma does significantly better than advanced disease. Early (pT1) adenocarcinoma may show less recurrence than equivalent squamous lesions but, for the majority of cases, although adenocarcinoma may have slightly better overall 5 year survival (25%), the two main pathological types have little differential influence on prognosis.

9. Other malignancy

Lymphoma/leukaemia
— rare. More usually secondary to systemic/nodal disease.
— primary lymphoma is large B cell in type.
— consequences of immunosuppression due to the tumour or its treatment may be seen, e.g. CMV, herpetic or fungal oesophagitis.

Leiomyoma/ leiomyosarcoma
— leiomyomas greatly outnumber leiomyosarcomas (malignancy: > 5 cm diameter, necrosis, mitoses > 5/50 high-power fields, cellular atypia, infiltrative margins). Most are small, identified by endoscopy and arise from the muscularis mucosae or inner muscularis propria. They can be multiple, intraluminal or intramural.

Sarcoma
— rare. Ninety percent are leiomyosarcoma.
— embryonal rhabdomyosarcoma (childhood).
— Kaposi's sarcoma (AIDS).
— synovial sarcoma.
— exclude the more common possibility of a spindle cell carcinoma (polypoid carcinoma/carcinosarcoma) with cytokeratin-positive spindle cells and varying degrees of homologous or heterologous mesenchymal differentiation.

Gastric Carcinoma

1. Gross description

Specimen

— cytological brushing, washing or aspirate/biopsy/ partial or total gastrectomy/ oesophagogastrectomy/lymphadenectomy ± omentectomy.
— length (cm) along greater curvature.
— length (cm) of oesophagus and duodenum.

Tumour

Site

— distal oesophagus/cardia/fundus/antrum/ duodenum.
— lesser curve/greater curve.
— anterior/posterior.

Antrum (50%) and lesser curve (15%) are traditionally the most frequent sites. However, the incidence of distal gastric carcinoma is decreasing while that of the proximal stomach and cardia is markedly increasing. It is associated with junctional/short segment Barrett's metaplasia and presents at a more advanced stage than equivalent-size distal lesions with similarities in behaviour to distal oesophageal adenocarcinoma.

— multifocal 6%.

Size

— length × width × depth (cm) or maximum dimension (cm).

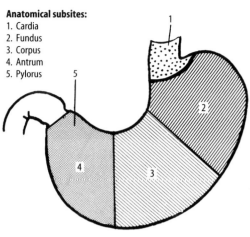

Anatomical subsites:
1. Cardia
2. Fundus
3. Corpus
4. Antrum
5. Pylorus

Figure 4. Stomach.

Appearance
— polypoid/plaque/ulcerated/infiltrative/mucoid/linitis plastica/scirrhous/fleshy.

Edge
— circumscribed/irregular.

2. Histological type

Adenocarcinoma

intestinal	50%	antrum
diffuse	20%	body of stomach, young patients
mixed	25%	

Intestinal carcinomas have tubular, papillary or mucinous (colloid) patterns, form polypoid or ulcerative lesions with expansile margins and are associated with atrophic gastritis, intestinal metaplasia and dysplasia.

Diffuse carcinomas comprise single cells with signet ring or granular cytoplasmic appearances and form linitis plastica with infiltrating margins. A point of origin from dysplasia is often difficult to demonstrate and the tumour emanates from the mid-mucosal proliferative zone (from non-metaplastic foveolar or mucous neck cells), or, deep lamina propria invading submucosa, muscularis, serosa and into the peritoneal cavity.

Adenocarcinoma variants, e.g.
Hepatoid carcinoma: glandular and hepatocellular differentiation, marked vascular invasion; poor prognosis. ± AFP immunoexpression, polyclonal CEA positive.

Parietal cell carcinoma: rare. Solid sheets of cells with eosinophilic granular cytoplasm.

Medullary carcinoma (syn. lymphoepithelial carcinoma): circumscribed, dense lymphoplasmacytic infiltrate, regular, vesicular nuclei, small nucleoli.
77% 5 year survival and associated with EBV infection.

Adenosquamous carcinoma and squamous cell carcinoma
— need keratinisation and intercellular bridges. Vascular invasion, aggressive.

Neuroendocrine carcinoma
— carcinoid, small cell/large cell carcinoma.

Lymphoma
— low/high-grade MALToma.

Metastatic carcinoma
— direct spread: pancreas, oesophagus.
— distant spread: small cell carcinoma lung, malignant melanoma, breast, kidney, choriocarcinoma (1° or 2°), ovary.
— metastatic infiltrating lobular carcinoma of breast can mimic signet ring cell carcinoma of stomach; a known clinical history of a previous breast primary is crucial to the diagnosis. Breast cancer may also be ER/PR/cytokeratin 7 positive and cytokeratin 20 negative.

3. Differentiation

Well/moderate/poor/undifferentiated (solid sheets of tumour cells with no structural or functional differentiation).
Undifferentiated gastric carcinoma requires positive cytokeratin stains to distinguish it from lymphoma or sarcoma.
Goseki grade – based on mucin secretion and tubule formation:

I   tubules well differentiated, mucin-poor
II   tubules well differentiated, mucin-rich
III   tubules poorly differentiated, mucin-poor
IV   tubules poorly differentiated, mucin-rich.

Well-differentiated mucin-poor cancers have better (50–80%) 5 year survival rates than moderately or poorly differentiated mucin-rich tumours (18–46%).

4. Extent of local tumour spread

Border: pushing/infiltrative.
Well circumscribed tumours have longer patient survival than infiltrating cancers (except in early gastric cancer).

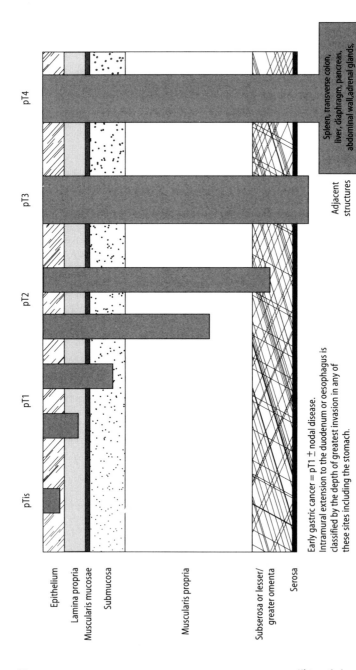

Figure 5. Gastric carcinoma.

Early gastric cancer = pT1 ± nodal disease.
Intramural extension to the duodenum or oesophagus is classified by the depth of greatest invasion in any of these sites including the stomach.

pTis pT1 pT2 pT3 pT4

Adjacent structures

Spleen, transverse colon, liver, diaphragm, pancreas, abdominal wall, adrenal glands, kidney, bowel, retroperitoneum

Epithelium
Lamina propria
Muscularis mucosae
Submucosa

Muscularis propria

Subserosa or lesser/ greater omenta
Serosa

Lymphocytic reaction: prominent/sparse.
Gastric cancer is considered as either early (pT1) or advanced (pT2) as there is prognostic discrepancy between these two levels of invasion.

pTis   carcinoma in-situ: intraepithelial tumour without invasion of the lamina propria
pT1   tumour invades lamina propria or submucosa (early gastric cancer EGC)
pT2   tumour invades muscularis propria or subserosa or lesser/greater omenta
pT3   tumour penetrates serosa (visceral peritoneum) without invasion of adjacent structures
pT4   tumour invades adjacent structures (spleen, transverse colon, liver, diaphragm, pancreas, abdominal wall, adrenal gland, kidney, small intestine, retroperitoneum).

Intramural extension to the oesophagus or duodenum is classified by the depth of greatest invasion in any of these sites.

Diffuse gastric carcinoma may not elicit a desmoplastic stroma and the depth of mural invasion, which is often extensive and can be characterised by small, inapparent non-mucinous tumour cells in the muscularis propria and adventitia, may be underestimated. Stains (PAS ± diastase, cytokeratins, CEA, EMA) should be used to show its full extent and also to distinguish tumour cells from histiocytes in both the mucosa and lymph node sinus network.

5. Lymphovascular invasion

Present/absent.
Intra-/extratumoural.

Intestinal gastric adenocarcinoma tends to venous invasion with spread to liver, lung, adrenal and bone whereas diffuse gastric carcinoma favours lymphatic and direct peritoneal spread. Bilateral ovarian metastases comprise the majority of Krukenberg tumours. Uterine body and cervix can also be involved.

6. Lymph nodes

Site/number/size/number involved/limit node/extracapsular spread.
Regional nodes: perigastric, hepatoduodenal, nodes along the left gastric, common hepatic, splenic and coeliac arteries. Other intra-abdominal lymph nodes are distant metastases (pM1).

pN0   no regional lymph node metastasis
pN1   1 to 6 involved regional nodes
pN2   7 to 15 involved regional nodes
pN3   more than 15 involved regional nodes.

The regional lymph nodes are the perigastric nodes along the lesser (*1, 3, 5*) and greater (*2, 4a, 4b, 6*) curvatures, the nodes located along the left gastric (*7*), common hepatic (*8*), splenic (*10, 11*) and coeliac arteries (*9*) and the hepatoduodenal nodes (*12*). Involvement of other intra-abdominal lymph nodes such as the retropancreatic, mesenteric and para-aortic is classified as distant metastasis.

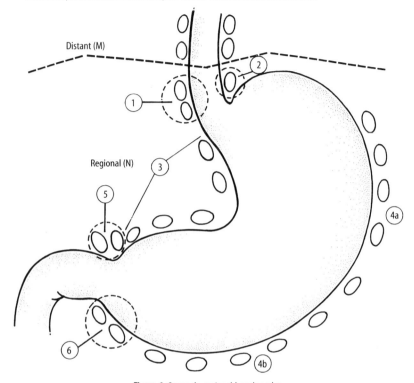

Figure 6. Stomach: regional lymph nodes.

7. Excision margins

Distances (mm) to the proximal and distal limits of excision and serosa.

Gastric carcinoma (especially diffuse signet ring cell) may show multifocality and submucosal skip lesions; margins need to be checked histologically even if well away from the main tumour mass on gross examination. Diffuse carcinoma present to within 5 cm of the resection margin has an adverse prognosis. Distal cancers tend to stop at the pylorus while proximal (cardia) tumours often involve distal oesophagus.

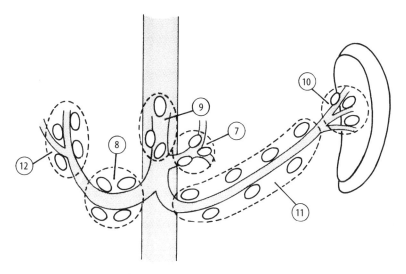

Figure 7. Stomach: regional lymph nodes.

8. Other pathology

Early gastric cancer (EGC)

Limited to the mucosa ± submucosa ± lymph node involvement. The 5 year survival is 85–95% compared with 20–35% for advanced gastric cancer. Designation as EGC is on a resection specimen as endoscopic biopsies are constrained by sampling limitations.

Macroscopic/endoscopic classification of EGC

Type I	protruded	10%
Type IIa	raised	
Type IIb	flat	superficial 80%
Type IIc	depressed	
Type III	excavated	10%

Mixed types are common. Types I and IIa tend to be well differentiated whereas types IIb, IIc and III also include poorly differentiated and signet ring tumours, although there is considerable overlap between macroscopic and microscopic appearances.

Lesser curve is the commonest site ; 10% are multifocal and require mapping of the resection specimen.

Tumours with lymph node metastases do worse than those without and tend to be large (> 5 cm – 80% positive nodes) or show submucosal invasion (20% positive nodes) rather than being confined to the mucosa (4% positive nodes).

Two prognostic paradoxes contrast with advanced gastric carcinoma:

1. diffuse-type EGC has a better prognosis than intestinal-type EGC due to vascular spread in the latter, and

2. EGC with a broad, expansile deep margin destroying muscularis mucosae (pen A) is more aggressive than EGC with an irregular infiltrating margin fenestrating the muscle (pen B). The tendency for pen A tumours to progress to advanced carcinoma is thought to relate to higher DNA aneuploidy rates. Pen A tumours form a minority (10%) of EGC but have higher rates of lymphovascular invasion, lymph node metastases (25%) and lower 10 year survival rates (65%),

3. i.e. well-differentiated cancers with a pushing margin do worse than poorly differentiated tumours with an infiltrating margin.

Treatment is usually by partial gastrectomy but local excision by endoscopic resection is possible. Risk factors predictive of nodal metastases and the need for further surgery are: surface ulceration (> 50% of the area), submucosal invasion, lymphovascular invasion and incomplete excision.

Predisposing lesions

Gastritis: [1] ± *Helicobacter pylorii* (HP): (cresyl violet, Giemsa, Warthin-Starry stains; can assume a coccoid rather than spiral form in resections). HP positive patients have a ×3–6 increased cancer risk especially those with the cytotoxic (cag-A) genotype of HP.

Intestinal metaplasia: [1] type IIb/III (sulphomucin rich) – high iron diamine alcian blue or Gomori's aldehyde fuchsin alcian blue stains – the large intestinal variant of metaplasia, is more strongly associated with mucosal dysplasia and intestinal pattern gastric adenocarcinoma. Mucin subtyping is not routinely done as it is not considered a sufficiently strong predictive factor.

Atrophy: [1] ± pernicious anaemia with gastric parietal cell and intrinsic factor antibodies. 10–20% develop carcinoma.

Dysplasia: low/high-grade; either in flat (commonest), sessile or polypoid mucosa, and in metaplastic (intestinal) or non-metaplastic (gastric foveolar) mucosa.

There is a strong (30–80%) association between high-grade dysplasia and adenocarcinoma either concurrently or within 1–2 years of diagnosis. Distinction between high-grade dysplasia/carcinoma in-situ and lamina propria invasion can be difficult. In Europe there needs to be invasion of the lamina propria before the term (intramucosal) carcinoma is used, i.e. both cytological and architectural derangement. Diagnosis of dysplasia in a biopsy should be followed by reassessment with multiple biopsies to exclude concurrent carcinoma. If this is

---

[1]Classified and semi-quantitatively graded (none/mild/moderate/marked) using the Sydney classification.

absent low-grade dysplasia may be monitored endoscopically while high-grade dysplasia in flat or polypoid mucosa should be considered for resection. Distinguish dysplasia from regenerative change in inflammation and ulceration and reactive gastropathy, e.g. foveolar hyperplasia in bile reflux and drug ingestion (NSAIDs, aspirin).

Polyps

— hyperplastic: usual type; 1–3% risk of malignancy[2] particularly if large (> 2 cm) and multiple.
— fundic gland cyst: increasing incidence; association with colorectal pathology of various types (rare), familial adenomatous polyposis coli and proton pump inhibitor therapy (due to parietal cell hyperplasia secondary to hypergastrinaemia); rarely dysplastic (FAPC).
— adenomatous: 8% of cases; a 30–40% risk of malignancy[2] related to size, villous architecture and grade of dysplasia.

Ménétrier's disease and lymphocytic gastritis: hyperplastic gastropathy can be associated with adenocarcinoma.

Barrett's metaplasia for oesophagogastric junction lesions: the aetiology of the increasing incidence of oesophagogastric junctional adenocarcinoma is not resolved but may be contributed to by *Helicobacter* eradication and proton pump inhibitor therapy. It may arise in metaplastic cardia-type gastric mucosa or short (< 3 cm) segment Barrett's metaplasia with dysplasia.

Synchronous gastric lymphoma of mucosa associated lymphoid tissue (MALToma): also *Helicobacter* related.

Tumours covered by intact mucosa, such as diffuse gastric carcinoma (signet ring cell) or stromal tumours, can be difficult to demonstrate by routine biopsy; cytological brushings and washings or endoscopic fine needle aspiration cytology may be helpful. Multiple (5 or 6) biopsies should be taken from ulcerated carcinomas including the ulcer base and mucosal edges. Distinction must be drawn between carcinoma and pseudomalignant changes in glandular epithelium, endothelial cells and stromal cells in erosions and ulcer base tissue. Gastric xanthoma (CD 68 positive, cytokeratin and mucin negative) can also mimic diffuse gastric carcinoma and immune markers are helpful in these situations.

Gastric carcinoma is variably neutral and acidic mucin positive (PAS-AB, mucicarmine), cytokeratin (CAM 5.2, cytokeratin 7/20), EMA and CEA positive.

Prognosis

Prognosis of gastric cancer is poor, the majority of cases presenting with advanced disease, and it relates to histological type, grade and stage. Intestinal

---

[2]Either within the polyp or elsewhere in the stomach.

gastric carcinoma has higher 5 year survival rates than diffuse gastric carcinoma, e.g. for pT3 lesions 42% versus 17%. Intestinal gastric carcinoma may be considered for partial gastrectomy because of its expanding margins whereas total gastrectomy is advised for diffuse carcinoma. Additional important prognostic indicators are nodal status, lymphovascular invasion, resection line involvement and an infiltrative versus an expansive tumour margin. These factors tend to outweigh other parameters such as the Lauren and Ming classification or Goseki grade. EGC does considerably better (see above).

9. Other malignancy

Carcinoid tumour
NSE, chromogranin, synaptophysin, PGP 9.5 positive.

1. *Multiple* (benign): Commonly associated with autoimmune atrophic gastritis and endocrine cell hyperplasia (rarely Zollinger Ellison syndrome): gastric atrophy → hypochlorhydria → hypergastrinaemia → ECL (enterochromaffin-like cell) hyperplasia → microcarcinoidosis (multiple, mucosal, 1–3 mm).Can be monitored by endoscopy with biopsy excision of small polyps up to 1 cm diameter; polyps 1–2 cm in size are treated by polypectomy or local resection as they are of malignant potential.

2. *Single* (aggressive). If the lesion is large (> 2 cm) or ulcerated consider definitive resection.

   Malignancy relates to:
   — any functioning tumour
   — angio-invasion
   — non-functioning tumour ≥2cm diameter and with invasion beyond the submucosa
   — atypical features (atypia, necrosis, mitoses)
   — 5 year survival 70-80%
   — Indolent growth with spread to nodes, liver, bone and skin.

Gastrointestinal mesenchymal or stromal tumours(GISTs)
Myogenic: 20% – desmin/smooth muscle actin positive.

Neural: 15% – S100 positive.

Stromal: CD 34 and CD 117 (c-*kit*: tyrosine kinase receptor) positive and absent or incomplete myogenic/neural differentiation; putative precursors are the interstitial cells of Cajal, which are gut pacemaker cells located in the deep submucosa and myenteric plexus.

Note that there can be marked heterogeneity and focal expression of antigens. Malignancy, which is less frequent than in small intestinal stromal tumours, cannot be accurately predicted from the histology. However, some indicators are:

— size (> 5 cm)
— cellularity (cell density increases in sarcoma)
— atypia

- cell type (epithelioid is worse than spindle cell)
- necrosis (coagulative in type)
- margins (circumscribed versus infiltrative, e.g. invasion into mucosal lamina propria)
- mitoses > 5/50 high-power fields (Emory, et al. 1999)
- loss of CD 34 or CD 117 expression.

Histological grading of established sarcoma is contentious and tumour size is a suggested index of metastatic risk.

Biopsy proof can be difficult as GISTs are extramucosal lesions (submucosal and mural) often with surface ulceration; fine needle aspiration cytology at endoscopy may be helpful in establishing a diagnosis of a spindle cell lesion. The biopsy forceps may also be directed to the base of the ulcer where there is already mucosal loss.

See Chapter 4, Section 9.

Malignant lymphoma

- secondary to systemic/nodal disease or primary (commoner) in the stomach it is the commonest site for extranodal non-Hodgkin's lymphoma. Primary disease bulk is centred on the stomach and its regional nodes.

It can present as single or multiple lesions, a sessile plaque or thickened folds found incidentally at endoscopy, an ulcerated tumour or a thickened non-expansile stomach. The majority are of B cell MALT (mucosa associated lymphoid tissue) type, the low-grade variant being characterised by a proliferation of centrocyte-like cells, destructive lymphoepithelial lesions, monotypic immunoglobulin expression in surface plasma cells, and invasion between or into reactive follicles (follicular colonisation) and/or immunoglobulin gene rearrangements on PCR. There is evidence that some of these localised (i.e. without deep submucosal or muscle invasion) low-grade lesions may regress on anti-*Helicobacter* medication and they usually pursue an indolent time course with potential metastases to other extranodal sites, e.g. gastrointestinal tract and Waldeyer's ring. They may also transform to or present as high-grade lesions necessitating surgery and adjuvant therapy; this is also applicable to extensive low-grade disease. The cytological composition of MALToma can be heterogeneous and clear distinction between a mucosal or nodal origin can be arbitrary, especially in high-grade disease. From a practical point of view establishing a B cell phenotype, low- or high-grade character and full clinicopathological staging are the salient features relevant to management. Immunohistochemistry may also be helpful in establishing monoclonality (κ, λ light chain restriction), demonstrating lymphoepithelial lesions (cytokeratins) and lymphoma subtype (e.g. low-grade MALToma is CD 45/CD 20 positive but CD 5, CD 10, CD 23 and bcl-2 negative, separating it from other low-grade B cell lymphomas). Cytokeratins and common lymphoid antigen (CD 45) are also necessary to distinguish high-grade lymphoma from undifferentiated carcinoma and signet ring or plasmacytoid change in lymphoma from signet ring cell gastric carcinoma. Low- and high-grade areas may coexist in gastric lymphoma and there can be adjacent synchronous or metachronous (up to several years later) adenocarcinoma associated with MALToma. Forty to sixty per cent of gastric lymphomas are of high-grade large B cell type and diagnosis is usually straightforward (cytological atypia/monomorphous infiltrate) with confirmatory immunohistochemistry for lymphoid markers and negative epithelial markers. Distinction between low-grade lymphoma and lymphoid hyperplasia, as in *Helicobacter pylorii* gastritis or peptic ulcer, can be problematic and diagnosis depends on the density of the lymphoid infiltrate and degree of gland distortion and loss. Immunoglobulin gene rearrangements provide supportive evidence although monoclonality does not always correlate with potential for progression to malignancy. Sometimes designation of low-grade lymphoma is only attained after several biopsy episodes and when there is a lack of response of the lymphoid infiltrate to eradication of *Helicobacter pylorii*.

Overall prognosis is reasonably good (40–60% 5 year survival), low-grade lymphomas following an indolent course (65–95% 5 year survival) but with about 50% of high-grade lymphomas being aggressive with spread beyond the stomach (40–55% 5 year survival). Prognosis relates to both grade and stage of disease at the time of presentation. Treatment of extensive low-grade and high-grade disease is with surgery followed by radiotherapy and/or chemotherapy.

Other forms of lymphoma are rare in the stomach, e.g. follicular lymphoma, centrocytic lymphoma, Burkitt's lymphoma, anaplastic large cell lymphoma and T cell lymphoma.

Leukaemia

— stomach can be involved in up to 25% of cases.
— CD 68/chloroacetate esterase positive cells (granulocytic sarcoma).

Miscellaneous rare malignancy

— Kaposi's sarcoma: visceral involvement can be present in 30–60% of AIDS patients.
— angiosarcoma, rhabdomyosarcoma, alveolar soft part sarcoma, teratoma, choriocarcinoma, yolk sac tumour.

Ampulla of Vater and Head of Pancreas Carcinoma

1. Gross description

Specimen

— endoscopic/transduodenal core biopsy/transduodenal or percutaneous fine needle aspirate.
— Whipple's procedure (partial gastrectomy, duodenectomy and partial pancreatectomy).
— total pancreatectomy (partial gastrectomy, duodenectomy, total pancreatectomy and splenectomy).
— weight (g) and size/length (cm), number of fragments.

Tumour

Site

— non-ampullary duodenal mucosa/ampullary mucous membrane/muscularis/pancreatic head (60–70% of pancreatic carcinomas)/terminal common bile duct/multifocal.

Size

— length × width × depth (cm) or maximum dimension (cm).

Appearance

— polypoid/nodular/diffuse/ulcerated: ampullary tumours.
— scirrhous/mucoid/cystic: pancreatic exocrine tumours.
— circumscribed/pale: pancreatic endocrine tumours.

Edge

— circumscribed/irregular.

2. Histological type

Ampulla

— adenocarcinoma. Eighty per cent of cases usually well to moderately differentiated intestinal pattern arising from adenomatous dysplasia in the peri-/intraampullary mucosa.
— mucinous adenocarcinoma.
— signet ring cell carcinoma.
— metastatic carcinoma, e.g. direct spread: stomach, pancreas, terminal common bile duct.

Pancreas
(a)Exocrine

— ductal adenocarcinoma (80–90%):
>   tubulo-acinar pattern of malignant ductal epithelium in a desmoplastic stroma.
>   perineural invasion.
>   dysplasia of the adjacent duct epithelium (20–30%).
>   multifocality 15–40%.
>   male preponderance.

— ductal adenocarcinoma variants:
>   mucinous 1–3%.
>   adenosquamous.
>   microglandular/signet ring.
>   oncocytic.
>   clear cell.

— pleomorphic carcinoma (7%):
>   spindle/giant multinucleated cells ± osteoclast-like cells.
>   pure osteoclast-like tumours have a better prognosis than other pleomorphic carcinomas.

— intraductal papillary or mucinous tumours:
>   benign/borderline or malignant according to the degree of dysplasia ± invasion (10–20%).
>   80% are in the head of pancreas and multifocal within the duct system.

— serous macro/microcystic tumours:
>   elderly.
>   mostly benign (microcystic serous adenoma), occasionally malignant.
>   glycogen-rich, clear cuboidal epithelium lining fluid-filled microcysts.

— mucinous cystic tumours:
  > benign/borderline/malignant spectrum of appearance and behaviour tending to malignancy.
  >
  > prognosis relates to the degree of invasion into pancreatic and extrapancreatic tissues.
  >
  > indolent growth with spread to abdominal cavity.
  >
  > middle-aged women, uni-/multilocular.

— solid-cystic-papillary tumour (syn. solid-pseudopapillary tumour):
  > adolescent girls/young women.
  >
  > low malignant potential, usually benign.
  >
  > pseudopapillae covered by several layers of uniform, endocrine-like epithelial cells.
  >
  > necrosis and mucinous cystic change.

— acinar cell carcinoma:
  > 1–2%: uniform cells with cytoplasmic granules resembling normal pancreas.
  >
  > enzyme antibody positive, e.g. lipase, amylase, trypsin.
  >
  > nodal and liver metastases can be present in 50% of cases at diagnosis.

— mixed differentiation carcinoma

— small cell carcinoma:
  > presents at late stage, poor prognosis.

— pancreaticoblastoma:
  > malignant.
  >
  > children.
  >
  > favourable prognosis if resected before metastases; also chemo-/radioresponsive.
  >
  > epithelial (acini, squamous nests) and mesenchymal (spindle cell) components.

(b) Endocrine (islet cell tumours)

— forming a minority of pancreatic neoplasms usually occurring in adults. Small, circumscribed, solid/gyriform/glandular cell patterns with hyaline (± amyloid) stroma.

1. Functional hormonal syndrome (60–85%)
   gastrinoma: pancreatic head, duodenum, gastric antrum, Zollinger-Ellison syndrome
   insulinoma: body and tail
   vipoma: body and tail
   glucagonoma: body and tail

2. Non-functional
   somatostatinoma: also in the duodenum with psammoma bodies and must be distinguished from well-differentiated adenocarcinoma
   PPoma

neurotensinoma
calcitoninoma
small cell carcinoma: ± ectopic ACTH secretion, hypercalcaemia.

Cellular density, atypia and mitoses give some guide as to malignant potential but they are not reliable. Better indicators are:

— tumour type: insulinoma, 85–90% benign; gastrinoma, 60–85% malignant.
— size (> 3 cm), site (e.g. duodenal) and invasion of vessels.
— unequivocal evidence of malignancy is gross invasion of adjacent organs, metastases to regional nodes, liver and other distant sites. Tumour growth is indolent and even patients with metastases can survive several years. Some respond to chemotherapy, e.g. streptozotocin.

Association with multiple endocrine neoplasia (MEN) syndrome: the pancreas is involved in 80–100% of type 1 MEN syndrome, gastrinoma being the commonest (50%).

Mixed exocrine/endocrine carcinoma

— < 1%; bivalent amphicrine cells or adjacent foci of mixed differentiation (the endocrine component being at least one third of the tumour).

Metastatic carcinoma

— direct spread: stomach, colorectum, biliary tract, abdominal mesothelioma/lymphoma.
— distant spread: pleomorphic carcinoma of the pancreas has to be distinguished from metastatic malignant melanoma, sarcoma, choriocarcinoma and large cell lung carcinoma; small cell lung carcinoma and renal carcinoma.

It can be difficult to distinguish adenocarcinoma of the pancreas and adenocarcinoma of the terminal common bile duct from adenocarcinoma of the ampulla of Vater as they share similar histological features: careful examination of the exact anatomical location is required and circumstantial evidence for a point of origin, e.g. an adenomatous lesion in the ampullary mucosa or dysplasia in the pancreatic/bile duct epithelium. Sometimes the only conclusion can be adenocarcinoma of the pancreatico-ampullary-biliary region.

3. Differentiation

Well/moderate/poor.
Pancreatic ductal adenocarcinoma can be graded according to the degree of gland formation in the tumour area

grade 1 (well differentiated)	> 95%
grade 2 (moderately differentiated)	50–95%
grade 3 (poorly differentiated)	5–49%
grade 4 (undifferentiated)	< 5%

Intraduct papillary lesions are:

low-grade   mild nuclear atypia
                 no mitoses
intermediate   moderate nuclear atypia
                 < 5 mitoses/10 high-power fields
high-grade   severe cellular atypia
                 mitoses > 5/10 high-power fields

Endocrine tumours are not graded because of poor correlation with biological behaviour.

4. Extent of local tumour spread

Border: pushing/infiltrative.
Lymphocytic reaction: prominent/sparse.

Ampulla

pTis   carcinoma in-situ
pT1   tumour limited to the ampulla or sphincter of Oddi
pT2   tumour invades duodenal wall
pT3   tumour invades 2 cm or less into pancreas
pT4   tumour invades more than 2 cm into pancreas and/or other adjacent organs.

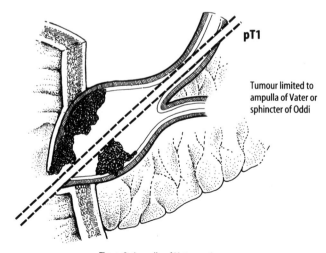

pT1

Tumour limited to ampulla of Vater or sphincter of Oddi

Figure 8. Ampulla of Vater carcinoma.

Pancreas

pTis carcinoma in-situ
pT1   tumour limited to the pancreas, ≤ 2 cm maximum dimension
pT2   tumour limited to the pancreas, > 2 cm dimension

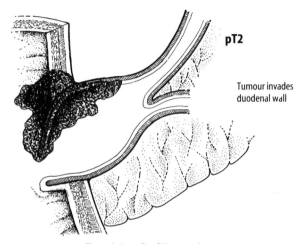

pT2

Tumour invades
duodenal wall

Figure 9. Ampulla of Vater carcinoma.

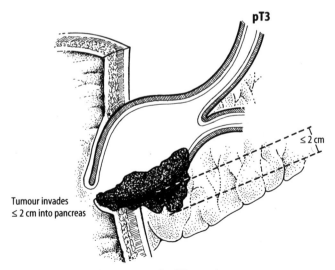

pT3

≤ 2 cm

Tumour invades
≤ 2 cm into pancreas

Figure 10. Ampulla of Vater carcinoma.

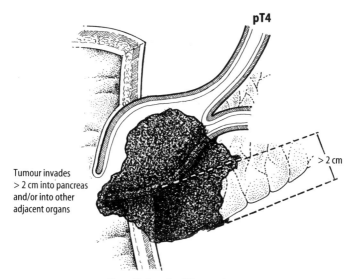

Figure 11. Ampulla of Vater carcinoma.

Tumour invades
> 2 cm into pancreas
and/or into other
adjacent organs

pT4

> 2 cm

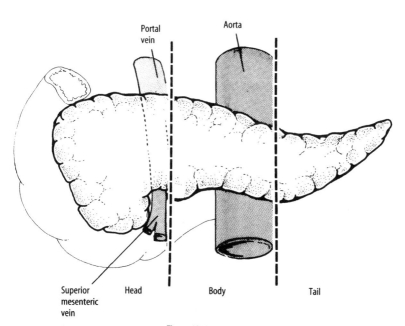

Figure 12. Pancreas.

Portal
vein

Aorta

Superior
mesenteric
vein

Head

Body

Tail

Ampulla of Vater and Head of Pancreas Carcinoma

31

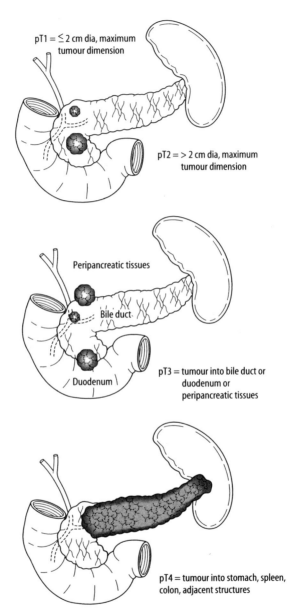

pT1 = ≤ 2 cm dia, maximum tumour dimension

pT2 = > 2 cm dia, maximum tumour dimension

Peripancreatic tissues

Bile duct

Duodenum

pT3 = tumour into bile duct or duodenum or peripancreatic tissues

pT4 = tumour into stomach, spleen, colon, adjacent structures

Figure 13. Head of pancreas carcinoma.

pT3   tumour extends directly into any of: duodenum, bile duct, peripancreatic tissues[1]

pT4   tumour extends directly into any of: stomach, spleen, colon, adjacent large vessels.[2]

5. Lymphovascular invasion

Present/absent.
Intra-/extratumoural.

Perineural space involvement is common in pancreatic carcinoma and lymphovascular invasion is present in up to 50% of cases with spread to local regional nodes at the time of diagnosis. Sites of distant metastases are liver, peritoneum, lung, adrenal, bone, skin and CNS. Regional node involvement is also present in 35–50% of ampullary carcinomas.

6. Lymph nodes

Site/number/size/number involved/limit node/extracapsular spread.
Regional nodes: peripancreatic, pancreaticoduodenal, pyloric and proximal mesenteric.

pN0   no regional lymph node metastasis
pN1   metastasis in regional lymph node(s).

7. Excision margins

Distances (mm) to the gastric, duodenal and pancreatic margins of excision including pancreatic and common bile ducts.

8. Other pathology

Cholestatic jaundice – carcinoma head of pancreas and ampulla.

Ampulla
— duodenal adenoma(s), familial adenomatous polyposis coli (ampullary carcinoma is one of the commonest causes of death in FAPC).

Pancreas
— disseminated intravascular coagulation, thrombophlebitis migrans (25% of cases, particularly with mucin-secreting tumours).

---

[1]Includes retroperitoneum, mesentery and mesocolon, omenta and peritoneum
[2]Includes portal vein, coeliac artery, superior mesenteric and common hepatic arteries and veins.

- gastrointestinal neuroendocrine syndromes, e.g. Zollinger-Ellison syndrome (diarrhoea, gastric hyperacidity with gastric/duodenal/jejunal ulcers), Werner-Morrison syndrome, WDHA syndrome (watery diarrhoea, hypokalaemia, alkalosis).
- chronic pancreatitis shows acinar atrophy, distortion and regenerative changes with stromal fibrosis and residual islet tissue and can mimic pancreatic carcinoma. Similar changes are also seen adjacent to pancreatic carcinoma due to duct obstruction indicating that interpretation and sampling can be problematic. Ductules in chronic pancreatitis tend to retain their lobular architecture, lack significant malignant cytological change and show no invasion of nerve sheaths or peripancreatic fat. Jaundice of short duration in a patient older than 60 years is suspicious of malignancy.

Markers

- neuroendocrine: chromogranin, PGP 9.5, NSE, synaptophysin, ± argyrophil/argentaffin.
- hormonal: specific peptides – insulin, glucagon, gastrin, pancreatic polypeptide, VIP, ACTH, somatostatin.
- exocrine carcinoma: cytokeratins (including CK7), CEA, CA19-9 – expressed in > 80% of ductal lesions.

Prognosis

Prognosis in pancreatic ductal carcinoma is poor with most patients dead within several months. It relates to tumour site (body and tail are worse than head, as it may present early with obstructive jaundice), size (> 4.5 cm is adverse), histological grade and stage. Overall 5 year survival is 2%, even disease confined to the pancreas only reaching 15%. Pancreatic endocrine tumours may present with their associated metabolic or gastrointestinal syndrome and have an indolent time course being of low to intermediate-grade malignancy. Ampullary carcinoma is more favourable than pancreatic or bile duct carcinoma with a 5 year survival of 25–50%. This can improve to 80–85% if the tumour is at an early stage and confined to the sphincter of Oddi (pT1).

9. Other malignancy

Leukaemia
Lymphoma
- usually spread from paraaortic/peripancreatic nodal lymphoma.
- extramedullary plasmacytoma.

Sarcoma
- rare
- leiomyosarcoma, liposarcoma, fibrosarcoma, osteosarcoma.
- exclude secondary from gut or retroperitoneum.

Small Intestinal Carcinoma[1]

1. Gross description

Specimen

— endoscopic/Crosby capsule/laparoscopic or open biopsy/resection.
— weight (g) and size/length (cm), number of fragments.

Tumour

Site

— duodenum (particularly periampullary) 70%.
— jejunum/ileum 30%.
— mucous membrane/muscularis/extra-mural.
— serosal/mesenteric/nodal/single/multifocal.
— mesenteric/anti-mesenteric border.
— Meckel's diverticulum.

Size

— length × width × depth (cm) or maximum dimension (cm).

Appearance

— polypoid/sessile/ulcerated/fleshy/pigmented/yellow/stricture/intussusception ± secondary ischaemic necrosis of the tumour tip/intussusceptum or receiving segment (intussuscipiens).

---

[1]Also refer to Chapter 3.

Duodenal carcinomas tend to be papillary or polypoid, distal carcinoma ulcerated and annular with constriction of the bowel wall (napkin ring-like).

Edge
— circumscribed/irregular.

2. Histological type

Adenocarcinoma
— enteric pattern, well or moderately differentiated: usual type
— anaplastic (poorly differentiated) forms also occur.
— mucinous carcinoma.
— signet ring cell carcinoma.
— adenosquamous carcinoma.

Diagnosis of primary small intestinal adenocarcinoma is by exclusion of spread from more common sites, e.g. colorectum and stomach. Similar to the large intestine there is some evidence for a dysplasia (adenoma)–carcinoma sequence in the adjacent mucosa. Prognosis is poor due to late presentation and advanced stage.

Carcinoid tumour
— NSE/chromogranin ± cytokeratin positive.
— Typically insular pattern, dense fibrous stroma, vascular thickening.
— 20% have carcinoid syndrome implying liver metastases.
— low-grade malignancy: any functioning well differentiated tumour; any tumour with angioinvasion; non-functioning tumour ≥ 2 cm or with invasion beyond the submucosa.
— high-grade malignancy: tumour with a high mitotic rate, cellular atypia or necrosis; poorly differentiated tumours/small cell carcinomas.

Carcinoid tumour has an overall 5 year survival rate of 50–65%. It is better for small lesions (metastatic rate: < 1 cm (2%), 1–2 cm (50%), > 2 cm (80%.)) confined to the wall (85%) than those invading the serosa or beyond (5%). Metastases are to regional nodes and liver (multiple, solid/cystic): also bone, skin and thyroid.

Others
— rare: adenosquamous, sarcomatoid carcinoma; aggressive.

Metastatic carcinoma
— direct spread: colorectum, ovary, stomach, pancreas.
— distant spread: lung, breast and choriocarcinoma.

The bulk of disease is extramural but tumour can invade muscularis and mucous membrane causing obstruction or perforation and mimicking a primary lesion.

Adjacent mucosal dysplasia is a useful pointer and adenoma is present in 24% of primary lesions. Small bowel is a common site of metastatic malignancy with formation of multiple nodules, plaques and strictures causing obstruction.

Metastatic melanoma
— pigmented/multifocal.
— amelanotic/oligomelanotic.
— melanoma requires confirmation with S100, HMB-45, melan-A.

3. Differentiation

Well/moderate/poor – carcinoma.
Low-grade/high-grade – lymphoma, sarcoma.

4. Extent of local tumour spread

Border: pushing/infiltrative.
Lymphocytic reaction: prominent/sparse.

pTis   carcinoma in-situ
pT1   tumour invades lamina propria or submucosa
pT2   tumour invades muscularis propria
pT3   tumour invades through muscularis propria into subserosa or into non-peritonealised perimuscular tissue (mesentery or retroperitoneum) with extension ≤ 2 cm
pT4   tumour perforates visceral peritoneum or directly invades other organs/structures (including loops of small intestine, mesentery, retroperitoneum > 2 cm and abdominal wall via serosa; also for duodenum – invasion of pancreas).

5. Lymphovascular invasion

Present/absent.
Intra-/extratumoural.
Vessel wall fibrosis/stenosis in carcinoid tumour.
Metastatic carcinoma often shows quite extensive lymphovascular invasion in the various layers of the bowel wall.

6. Lymph nodes

Site/number/size/number involved/limit node/extracapsular spread.
Regional nodes: duodenum – pancreaticoduodenal, pyloric, hepatic, superior mesenteric; ileum/jejunum – mesenteric; terminal ileum – ileocolic, posterior caecal.

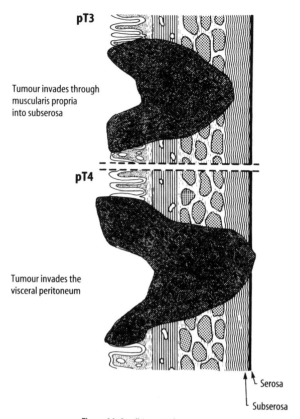

pT3

Tumour invades through
muscularis propria
into subserosa

pT4

Tumour invades the
visceral peritoneum

Serosa

Subserosa

Figure 14. Small intestinal carcinoma.

pN0   no regional lymph node metastasis
pN1   metastasis in regional lymph nodes.

7. Excision margins

Distances (mm) to the nearest longitudinal limit of resection and painted mesenteric margin.

8. Other pathology

There is increased incidence of adenocarcinoma in:

— familial adenomatous polyposis coli, particularly periampullary related to duodenal adenomas: it is a significant cause of mortality in FAPC

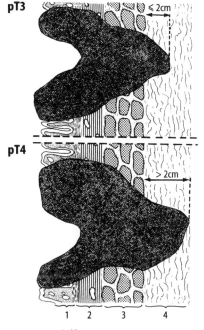

pT3

Tumour invades through muscularis propria and ≤ 2 cm into mesentery or retroperitoneum

pT4

Tumour invades through muscularis propria and > 2 cm into mesentery or retroperitoneum or involves adjacent organs/structures

1. Mucosa
2. Submucosa
3. Muscularis propria
4. Perimuscular tissue
   (mesentery, retroperitoneum)

Figure 15. Small intestinal carcinoma.

— Peutz-Jegher's polyposis (beware epithelial misplacement/pseudo-invasion); rare
— Crohn's disease
— coeliac disease
— ileostomy
— Meckel's diverticulum.

Coeliac disease/ulcerative jejunitis/gluten-induced enteropathy-associated T cell lymphoma (EATCL): change in or lack of responsiveness to a gluten-free diet or presentation as an ulcerative/perforated jejunitis in an older patient can indicate onset of EATCL.

Stricture – carcinoid, metastases.
Intussusception – carcinoid, lymphoma.
Multifocal – carcinoid, lymphoma, malignant melanoma, metastases.
Meckel's diverticulum – carcinoid, adenocarcinoma, leiomyomatous tumours.

Prognosis

Small bowel adenocarcinoma is unusual, being 50 times less common than large bowel carcinoma. Seventy per cent occur in the duodenum, particularly the peri-ampullary region. Presentation is late due to the fluid content of the bowel; many patients already have lymph node metastases and the majority subsequently die from their disease. Five year survival rates are approximately 10–20% with the most important prognostic indicator being depth of spread or stage of disease. Surgical resection is the treatment of choice.

9. Other malignancy

Lymphoma

— MALToma:
>   low/high-grade.
>   B cell (70–90% of bowel lymphoma).
>   centrocyte-like cells with variable numbers of blasts (> 20% = high-grade).
>   lymphoepithelial lesions.
>   monotypic immunoglobulin expression.
>   ± eosinophilia.

— Burkitt's-type/B-lymphoblastic:
>   children (or adults with AIDS).
>   terminal ileum/ileocaecal valve – a high-grade lymphoma.

— multiple lymphomatous polyposis:
>   centrocytic lymphoma or mantle cell lymphoma – small and large bowel disease with numerous polyps.
>   an intermediate-grade lymphoma.

— EATCL: aggressive.

— follicle centre cell (follicular) lymphoma:
>   more usually spread from nodal disease rather than primary.

— immunoproliferative small intestinal disease (IPSID):
>   Mediterranean countries.
>   α chain disease.

— Post-transplant lymphoproliferative disorders:
>   polyclonal/monclonal/disparate morphology and behaviour.
>   some regress on decreasing immunosuppression therapy, e.g. cyclosporin (see Chapter 35).

Prognosis is better for low-grade B cell lymphomas (44–75% 5 year survival) than high-grade B or T cell lymphomas (25–37% 5 year survival). Adverse prognostic indicators are perforation, high-grade histology, multiple tumours and advanced stage.

Gastrointestinal mesenchymal or stromal tumours (GISTs)

— ileum 50%, jejunum 40%, duodenum 10%.

Myogenic: 20% – desmin/smooth muscle actin positive.

Neural: 15% – S100/synaptophysin positive. Also including variants, e.g. GANT – gastrointestinal autonomic nerve tumour (± S100/synaptophysin/NSE/ CD 34, dense core granules and elongate cell processes on electron microscopy – may be associated with von Recklinghausen's disease/MEN syndrome).

Stromal: CD 34 and CD 117 (c-*kit*:tyrosine kinase receptor) positive, with absent or incomplete myogenic/neural differentiation. Putative precursors are the interstitial cells of Cajal, which are gut pacemaker cells located in the deep submucosa and myenteric plexus. Note that there can be marked heterogeneity and focal expression of antigens.

Malignancy relates to: size (> 2–5 cm), cellularity, atypia, cell type (epithelioid is worse than spindle cell), necrosis, margins and mitoses. Prognosis (approximately 50% 5 year survival) is also stage dependent.

DNA ploidy, Ki-67 proliferation indices, loss of CD 34 and CD 117 immunoexpression and morphometry also correlate with these parameters.

Newman et al. 1991.

	Mitoses/30 high-power fields	Lesion type
benign	0–2	spindle cell, no atypia
	0	epithelioid
borderline	2–3	spindle cell, mild atypia
	3–4	spindle cell, no atypia
	1	epithelioid
malignant	> 5	spindle cell, no atypia
	> 3	spindle cell, frank atypia
	> 2	epithelioid.

Emory et al. (1999) note that prognosis in gastrointestinal stromal tumours is dependent on patient age, tumour size (> 5 cm), tumour site and mitotic activity. A robust criterion in stomach tumours is > 5 mitoses/50 high-power fields, but mid- and hindgut lesions are more aggressive (even if mitotic counts are low) than foregut tumours. Behaviour can also be unpredictable, with clinicopathological factors at best being only broadly indicative, and the terminology "gastrointestinal stromal tumours of uncertain malignant potential" is useful. With an established diagnosis of sarcoma histological grading is not a reliable index of metastatic potential and tumour size is a better indicator. Metastases are commonly to peritoneum, liver, pancreas, retroperitoneum and lungs.

Kaposi's sarcoma

— AIDS: 50% of high risk patients have visceral involvement.

Leukaemia

— 14.8–25% of cases.

— granulocytic sarcoma (CD 68/chloroacetate esterase positive).

Colorectal Carcinoma

1. Gross description

Specimen

— biopsy, right or left hemi-/transverse/sigmoid/ subtotal colectomy/anterior or abdominoperineal resection
— weight (g) and size/length (cm), number of fragments.

Tumour

Site

— caecum/ascending colon/hepatic flexure/transverse colon/splenic flexure/descending or sigmoid colon/ multifocal-rectosigmoid (50%) are the commonest sites.
— for rectum: above/at/below the peritoneal reflection; tumours below the reflection have a higher rate of local recurrence. Tumours above/at the reflection anteriorly may involve peritoneum.
— distances (cm) to the dentate line and nearest longitudinal resection limit; these figures can audit the rates of anterior resection versus abdominoperineal resection, with the former being the operation of choice (with total mesorectal excision) for mid- and upper rectal cancers. Low rectal cancers also have higher local recurrence rates.

Size

— length × width × depth (cm) or maximum luminal dimension (cm).

Appearance

— polypoid/annular/ulcerated/mucoid/linitis plastica/stricture/plaque.

Edge

— circumscribed/irregular.

Perforation

— present/absent. Perforation has a higher incidence of local recurrence and poorer prognosis.

2. Histological type

Adenocarcinoma, no specific type (NST)

— 85% of cases.

— diagnostic criteria are: (a) malignant epithelial changes, in (b) a desmoplastic stroma, with (c) invasion beneath the muscularis mucosae.

Mucinous carcinoma

— 10% of cases.

— tumour area >50% mucinous component.

— worse prognosis (5 year survival decreased by 10–15%) compared with an equivalent-stage adenocarcinoma, NST.

Signet ring cell adenocarcinoma

— >50% signet ring cells.

— poor prognosis; rectosigmoid of young people with linitis plastica pattern of annular thickening and stenosis.

— distinguish from secondary carcinoma, e.g. gastric signet ring cell carcinoma in young females, prostate (PSA positive) carcinoma in older males.

Others

— neuroendocrine carcinoma:
　　　　carcinoid/large cell/small cell(right colon, prognosis poor).

— adenocarcinoid:
　　　　composite adenocarcinoma and carcinoid.

— adenosquamous carcinoma:
　　　　caecum.

— squamous cell carcinoma:
　　　　rectal: can be seen in ulcerative colitis/schistosomiasis/amoebiasis; exclude spread from an anal carcinoma or cervical carcinoma. Need intercellular bridges ± keratinisation with no gland/mucin formation.

— undifferentiated carcinoma:
    (a) good prognosis – cf. medullary carcinoma of breast. Circumscribed, expansile margin, solid sheets of tumour cells, intra- and peritumoural lymphocytes (see also HNPCC page 51).
    (b) poor prognosis – pleomorphic and diffusely infiltrative.

— mixed differentiation:
    e.g. adenocarcinoma (NST) with small cell carcinoma.

— metastatic carcinoma:
    transcoelomic spread: stomach, ovary, endometrium, gut, pancreas.
    direct spread: prostate, cervix, kidney.
    distant spread: breast (infiltrating lobular), malignant melanoma, lung.

3. Differentiation

Poor or other.

— 70–80% are moderately differentiated.

— based on the predominant area and not the tumour margins, which can often show poorly differentiated microscopic foci. If there is a substantial component of poor differentiation this should be commented upon. Some authors suggest that a poorly differentiated invasive margin (with budding, microacini and undifferentiated cells) in an otherwise moderately differentiated tumour is predictive of nodal metastases.

4. Extent of local tumour spread

Border: pushing/infiltrative.
Lymphocytic reaction: prominent/sparse.
An expanding growth pattern/margin with a Crohn's-like inflammatory response are good prognostic indicators.
Degree of mesorectal/mesocolic spread from the outer border of the muscularis propria:

< 2 mm	mild
2–5 mm	moderate
> 5 mm	severe.

When the mesenteric or mesorectal circumferential radial margin is involved the degree of tumour spread is an indicator of either advanced disease or alternatively inadequate surgery.

pTis carcinoma in-situ: intraepithelial (within basement membrane) or invasion of lamina propria (intramucosal) with no extension through muscularis mucosae into submucosa
pT1   tumour invades submucosa
pT2   tumour invades muscularis propria

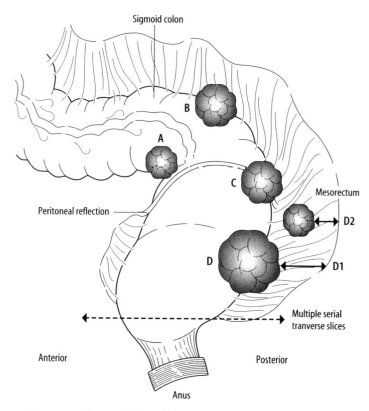

The upper anterior rectum is invested in peritoneum
The anterior mesorectum is thinner (0.75 - 1 cm) than the posterior mesorectum (1.5 - 3 cm)
Cut the resection specimen into multiple serial transverse slices about 5 mm thick
Blocks for histology are:

Above the reflection	A	tumour, rectal wall and serosa
	B	tumour, rectal wall and serosa
		tumour, rectal wall and mesentery
At the reflection	C	tumour, rectal wall and serosa
		tumour, rectal wall and mesorectum
Below the reflection	D	tumour, rectal wall and mesorectum
	D1	distance (mm) of the deepest point of continuous tumour extension to the nearest point of the painted CRM
	D2	distance (mm) of the deepest point of discontinuous tumour extension (or in a lymphatic, node or vessel) to the nearest point of the painted CRM

Figure 16. Rectal carcinoma.

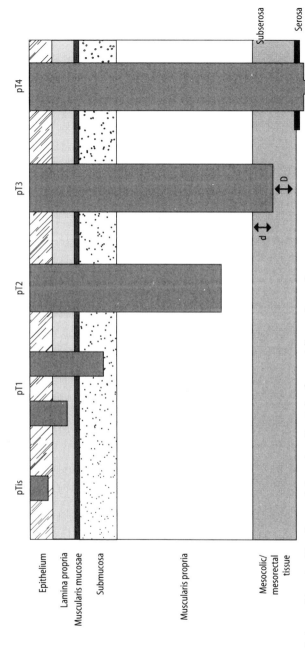

d= tumour distance (mm) from the muscularis propria and is an index of mesorectal/mesocolic spread.
D=tumour distance (mm) to the Circumferential Radial Margin (CRM) of excision of either continuous or discontinuous tumour extension or tumour in a lymphatic, lymph node or vessel. It is an index of adequacy of local excision and degree of spread.

Figure 17. Colorectal carcinoma.

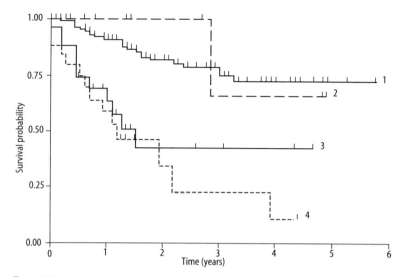

Figure 18. Kaplan-Meier cumulative survival curve for peritoneal involvement (Shepherd NA, Baxter KJ, Love SB. Influence of local peritoneal involvement on pelvic recurrence and prognosis in rectal cancer. J Clin Pathol 1995;48:849–855). *Group 1*, tumour well clear of the closest peritoneal surface; *group 2*, mesothelial inflammatory/hyperplastic reaction with tumour close to but not actually at the peritoneal surface; *group 3*, tumour present at the peritoneal surface with inflammatory reaction/mesothelial hyperplasia/"ulceration"; *group 4*, tumour cells free in peritoneum and adjacent "ulceration".

pT3   tumour invades beyond muscularis propria into subserosa or non-peritonealised pericolic/perirectal tissues
pT4   tumour invades the serosal surface or adjacent organs and/or perforation of visceral peritoneum.

Serosal involvement is tumour either at or ulcerating the serosal surface as this is prognostically worse than tumour in a subserosal inflammatory reaction – about 10% of patients develop peritoneal or ovarian (Krukenberg) deposits.

A minimum of 4 blocks of tumour and bowel wall is necessary to assess the pT stage adequately. The specimen is cut into serial transverse slices 4–5 mm thick, laid out in order and relevant slices selected for blocking.

Multiple carcinomas should be assessed and staged individually.

Direct implantation spread can be seen at anastomoses, peritoneal and abdominal wall wounds.

5. Lymphovascular invasion

Present/absent.
Intra-/extratumoural.
Extramural venous invasion is an adverse prognostic factor: 35% 5 year survival.

6. Lymph nodes

Lymph nodes and liver are the commonest sites of metastases. Also peritoneum, lung, and ovaries and bladder, where the metastases can mimic primary carcinoma of those organs. Immunophenotypical profiles may aid distinction, e.g. ovarian cancer is cytokeratin 7 positive/20 negative and weak for CEA whereas gut cancer is strongly CEA positive and cytokeratin 7 negative/20 positive.

Site/number/size/number involved/limit node/extracapsular spread.
Regional nodes: pericolic, perirectal, those located along the ileocolic, colic, inferior mesenteric, superior rectal and internal iliac arteries.

pN0	no regional lymph node metastasis
pN1	1–3 involved regional lymph nodes
pN2	4 or more involved regional lymph nodes
Dukes' C1	nodes involved but apical node negative
Dukes' C2	suture tie limit apical node positive.

All regional lymph nodes should be sampled for histology:
— a minimum target of 8 will identify the vast majority of Dukes' C lesions (Leeds Group).
— remember to assess the small lymph nodes seen on histology adjacent to the tumour margin. The significance of nodal micrometastases is uncertain.
— comment if an involved lymph node lies adjacent to (≤ 1 mm) the mesorectal CRM (circumferential radial margin) or mesocolic margin as this equates to involvement of that margin.
— a tumour nodule > 3 mm in diameter in the perirectal/pericolic fat without evidence of residual lymph node is classified as a replaced nodal metastasis. If ≤3 mm diameter classify as discontinuous extension, i.e. pT3.
— more than one vascular pedicle suture tie may mean more than one apical node needs to be identified as such.

7. Excision margins

Doughnuts/anastomotic rings/staple gun transections – involved/not involved.
Distances to the: nearest longitudinal resection limit (cm); mesorectal CRM (circumferential radial margin, mm); mesocolic resection margin (mm).
Longitudinal spread beyond the gross edge of a colorectal carcinoma is unusual (<5% of cases) and anterior resection of rectal carcinoma is generally considered satisfactory if a macroscopic clearance of 2–3 cm beyond the lesion edge is feasible.
Block the nearest longitudinal surgical margin if ≤ 3 cm from the tumour edge, or if > 3 cm but with any of: an unusually infiltrative tumour margin, extensive lymphovascular or mesorectal invasion or morphology such as signet ring cell, small cell, undifferentiated carcinoma.
CRM involvement = direct or discontinuous tumour spread, or tumour within a lymphatic, node or vessel ≤ 1 mm from the painted margin. Distances to this

margin are best assessed using transverse serial slices of the resection specimen. Note that non-peritonealised CRMs exist not only in the mesorectum but also where the superior mesorectum joins the inferior aspect of the sigmoid mesentery, and in relation to the posterolateral aspects of the ascending colon.

The prognostic significance of mesocolic margin involvement has not been fully clarified but is clearly an index of spread of disease or adequacy of surgery.

8. Other pathology

Predisposing conditions

Inflammatory: ulcerative colitis/Crohn's disease (1% of colorectal carcinomas), schistosomiasis, juvenile polyposis syndrome (10% risk). Carcinoma in ulcerative colitis occurs in patients with quiescent disease of pancolic distribution and long duration (> 10–20 years). It may be associated with preceding or concurrent mucosal dysplasia above, adjacent to or distant from the tumour. A rectosigmoid biopsy positive for mucosal dysplasia is a good indicator of the presence of carcinoma somewhere in the colorectum. Carcinomas may be multiple, right-sided and in up to one-third of cases difficult to define on endoscopic and gross examination. This is due to aberrant growth patterns with tumour arising in polypoid, villous or flat mucosal dysplasia in a background of mucosa already distorted by the effects of chronic inflammation, e.g. inflammatory polyps and strictures. Therefore interval colonoscopic biopsy of flat mucosa and target biopsy of possible DALMs (dysplasia associated lesion or mass) is employed to detect dysplasia as a marker of potential carcinoma which may be occult and submucosal in location. Prognosis is variable as some lesions present late masked by the symptoms of ulcerative colitis and others are found early at regular (annual/biennial after 8–10 years disease duration) surveillance colonoscopy.

Neoplastic: adenoma(s), familial adenomatous polyposis coli (and the related Gardner's syndrome), previous or synchronous carcinoma(s), HNPCC (see below), hyperplastic polyposis (rare).

The dysplasia – carcinoma sequence indicates that development of adenocarcinoma increases with the size of adenoma, its degree of villous architecture and grade of dysplasia, multiplicity of lesions and age of the patient. A maximum diameter > 2 cm and villous morphology confer approximate cancer risks of 50% and 40% respectively. These risk factors in a rectal adenoma are also good indicators in individual patients for full colonoscopic survey and follow-up to detect right-sided colonic neoplasms.

In the UK severe or high-grade dysplasia is applied to epithelial proliferation of any degree of complexity that is mucosa based, i.e. above the muscularis mucosae. Adenocarcinoma is reserved for those lesions that show invasion below the muscularis mucosae. Terms such as carcinoma in-situ tend to be avoided due to the relative lack of mucosal lymphatics, the rarity of nodal metastases with such lesions and the fear of overtreatment with unnecessary radical resection. However, it is not always possible to demonstrate invasion through the muscularis mucosae on biopsy and malignant epithelial changes with a desmoplastic stromal response are sufficient for a designation of adenocarcinoma.

Sampling error must always be borne in mind in that a dysplastic fragment may not show the adjacent invasive component. Undoubtedly there are also malignant polyps for which terminology such as carcinoma in-situ or intramucosal carcinoma is appropriate. In these circumstances there should be active discussion with the surgeon, emphasising that the process is "mucosa-confined" and comments made on the adequacy of local excision. It should also be checked that the specimen is a complete polypectomy and not simply a diagnostic biopsy from the edge of a larger lesion.

Malignant adenomas

Polyps: therapeutic polypectomy if the adenocarcinoma is:
    (a) well or moderately differentiated,
    (b) clear of the stalk base,
    (c) without lymphovascular invasion.

    resection if the adenocarcinoma is:
    (a) poorly differentiated (22%)*,
    (b) at the stalk base (11%)*,
    (c) shows lymphovascular invasion (18%)*.
    *The risk of lymph node metastases being present.

Resection is more likely if the patient is young and medically fit to obviate the risk of nodal metastases which can occasionally occur with pT1 lesions (4%).

Sessile adenomas with invasion: resection is indicated as this represents invasion of actual mural submucosa (Haggitt level 4) rather than just stalk submucosa (Haggitt levels 1, 2 and 3). Local transanal resection is considered for the very elderly and medically unfit. Indications for more radical surgery are: incomplete tumour excision, muscularis propria invasion, vascular invasion or the presence of a poorly differentiated invasive component.

Flat adenomas: uncommon with a different genetic basis from usual adenomas, difficult to identify endoscopically on gross examination without magnification and dye spray techniques; defined as up to twice the height of the adjacent mucosa – proportionately ($\times 10$ risk) higher grades of dysplasia and frequency of carcinoma. Depressed variants harbour carcinoma in up to 25% of cases, over-express p53 and the DNA aneuploidy rate is increased.

Hereditary non-polyposis colorectal cancer (HNPCC, syn. hereditary mismatch repair deficiency syndrome; hMSH2 and hMLH1 are the two most frequently mutated genes): autosomal dominant with 90% penetrance this forms 2% of colorectal cancer cases requiring three affected family members across two generations with at least one<50 years of age at presentation. Numbers of adenomas are low but they progress quicker, forming carcinomas tending to be right-sided and multiple. Although mucinous or poorly/undifferentiated (medullary-like) in character they are of better prognosis (66% versus 44% 5 year survival). They have expanding or circumscribed margins, intra- and peri-tumoural lymphocytes and are less likely to show distant spread. There is often

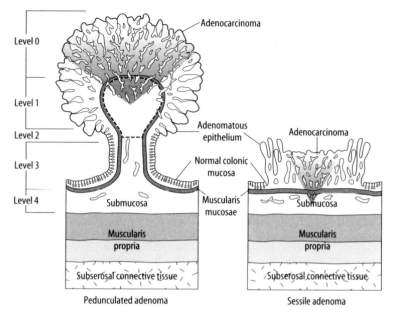

Figure 19. Malignant colorectal polyp. Levels of invasion in a pedunculated adenoma (*left*) and a sessile adenoma (*right*). The *stippled areas* represent zones of carcinoma. Note that any invasion below the muscularis mucosae in a sessile lesion represents level 4 invasion, i.e. invasion into the submucosa of the bowel wall. In contrast, invasive carcinoma in a pedunculated adenoma (*left*) must traverse a considerable distance before it reaches the submucosa of the underlying bowel wall. The *dotted line* in the head of the pedunculated adenoma represents the zone of level 1 invasion. (Haggit RC, et al. Prognostic factors in colorectal carcinomas arising in adenomas: implications for lesions removed by endoscopic polypectomy. Gastroenterology 1985;89:328–336.)

Therapeutic polypectomy:
— carcinoma of well or moderate differentiation.
— levels of invasion 1, 2 or 3.
— no lymphovascular invasion.
— no involvement of the stalk resection margin.

Resection indicated:
— sessile lesion with invasion (level 4).
— pedunculated lesion with level 4 invasion.
— carcinoma poorly differentiated.
— lymphovascular invasion.
— involvement of the stalk resection margin.

a family history of cancer in other viscera, e.g. stomach, small intestine, endometrium, breast, ovary, renal pelvis, and the risk of colonic cancer in a first degree relative of an affected individual is about 50%.

Familial adenomatous polyposis coli: sporadic or familial and autosomal dominant with a high degree of penetrance (chromosome 5q21). A minimum of 100 colorectal polyps is required for a morphological diagnosis and these can vary from unicryptal dysplasia to macroscopic lesions. Usually thousands of polyps are present and, if left untreated, one or more cancers occur on average 20 years earlier than usual colorectal carcinomas. FAPC is also associated with adenomas and periampullary carcinoma in the duodenum (a significant cause of mortality), gastric fundic gland cyst polyps and desmoid tumours (fibromatosis).

Rates for synchronous and metachronous carcinomas range from 5-15%.

Associated conditions

— obstruction leading either to direct tumour perforation (pT4), proximal dilatation, ischaemia and perforation (especially in the caecum) and obstructive enterocolitis. The latter can mimic inflammatory bowel disease with continuous and skip lesions of transmural inflammation either adjacent to or distant from the distal carcinoma.

Markers

— cytokeratin 20 positive/7 negative, CEA, CA19-9, sialomucin/sulphomucin, large intestinal mucus antigen (LIMA)/MUC-2, tumour associated glycoprotein (TAG-72: antibody B72.3) positive. Serum CA125 and CA19-9 may also be elevated. Sixty per cent of cases are p53 positive but this does not appear to be an independent prognostic variable. Microsatellite instability— hMSH2/hMLH1 antibodies.

Adjuvant therapy

— adjuvant radio-/chemotherapy induced tumour regression ± colitis. Adjuvant therapy is used for Dukes' C carcinomas and "bad" Bs, i.e. Dukes' B carcinomas with: perforation, involved serosa, involved deep margin or extramural venous spread. International trials are examining whether treatment should be chemotherapy or radiotherapy in isolation or combination and also pre- or postoperative. Long course (6 weeks) preoperative adjuvant therapy can induce in a significant number of cases (30–50%) marked changes of tumour regression: cell vacuolation, degeneration, apoptosis, necrosis, inflammation, and fibrosis leaving only microscopic residual tumour foci. Its role in reducing tumour bulk at the involved deep margin is uncertain but it does seem to improve resectability. Downstaging of lymph node disease remains controversial although nodes diminish in size and number making harvesting difficult. Response to adjuvant therapy may also depend partly on tumour genotype as to whether the cancer is positive or negative for microsatellite instability or DNA mismatch repair gene deficient or other factors such as tumour tissue levels of thymidylate synthase. Thus tumour characteristics allied to more sophisticated preoperative staging (e.g. endoluminal ultrasound combined with fine needle aspiration cytology of mesorectal nodes) may allow selection of those patients who will benefit most from adjuvant therapy.

Stage

TNM: see above.

| Dukes' | A | tumour limited to the wall, nodes negative |
| | B | tumour beyond the muscularis propria, nodes negative |

	C1	nodes positive, apical node negative
	C2	apical node positive.

Astler Coller modification:

A	tumour confined to the mucosa
B1	tumour limited by muscularis propria, node negative
B2	tumour through muscularis propria, node negative
C1	tumour limited by muscularis propria, node positive
C2	tumour through muscularis propria, node positive.

Jass classification: more often used in a research setting it assesses the extent of local tumour spread, lymph node involvement, quality of the invasive margin and density of lymphocytic infiltrate at that margin to derive a score which allocates the lesion to one of four prognostic groups, giving more refined discrimination than the usual Dukes' staging.

For routine practice Dukes' and pTNM are recommended.

Resection

R0	tumour completely excised locally
R1	microscopic involvement of margin by tumour (to within 1 mm)
R2	macroscopic tumour left behind or gross involvement of margin.

Prognosis

Adverse prognosis

— tumour perforation (pT4) and obstruction.
— mucinous tumour (> 50% tumour area).
— poor differentiation.
— splenic flexure lesion.
— male sex.
— young and old age due to delay in presentation and greater numbers of mucinous and signet ring tumours.

Prognosis relates mainly to tumour stage, differentiation and adequacy of local excision with overall 5 year survival 35–40%.

Stage	Dukes'	5 year survival	Incidence
	A	95%	15%
	B	75%	35%
	C	35%	25%
	D	25%	25%

Differentiation	well	75%	
	poor	30%	
Local excision	CRM positive	20% with 85% risk of local recurrence
	CRM negative	75% with 10% risk of local recurrence.

Not infrequently there is poor correlation between surgical and histological assessment of margin clearance. A positive resection margin (usually the CRM) has strong (×12 risk) prognostic significance for local recurrence and death (×3 risk). It is one of the most important causes of morbidity in rectal cancer. Low rectal cancers also have higher recurrence rates than mid- or upper rectal tumours. For every 100 patients with colorectal cancer it is estimated that 50 will be cured, 10 will die from pelvic recurrence, 5 from lymphatic spread and 35 from haematogenous spread. Sites of spread are regional nodes, liver (75%), lung (15%), bone and brain (5% each). Patients with bone marrow micrometastases are reported by some to have shorter disease-free survival, but the clinical significance of the immunohistochemical and molecular detection of minimal residual disease in lymph nodes and marrow samples which are tumour negative on routine examination awaits results from large international trials.

9. Other malignancy

Gastrointestinal mesenchymal or stromal tumours

— GISTs (Tworek et al. 1999a,b).

The majority are desmin or smooth muscle actin positive with variable S100/CD 34 expression.

Colon

— benign appearing lesions are rare.
— usually aggressive with metastases and death related to: mitoses > 6/50 high-power fields, infiltrative growth pattern into the muscularis propria, mucosal invasion, cellularity, coagulative necrosis.

Anorectal

— lesions arising from the muscularis mucosae (i.e. submucosal leiomyomatous polyp) are usually treatable by local excision or polypectomy.
— lesions arising from the muscularis mucosae are considered malignant if: cellular, > 5 cm diameter, infiltrative into the muscularis propria. However, if originating in the muscularis propria even bland lesions (sparse cellularity, 0–1 mitoses/50 high-power fields) need long term follow-up as there is a tendency for local recurrence and even potential metastases.

Carcinoid tumour

— (a) chronic ulcerative colitis → enteroendocrine cell hyperplasia → microcarcinoids; (b) carcinoid polyp ≤ 1 cm diameter. (a) and (b) are benign and managed by endoscopic surveillance and biopsy. (c) ulcerated tumour: malignancy relates to; size ≥ 2 cm diameter, invasion beyond submucosa, angioinvasion — necessitates resection.
— lesions 1–2 cm diameter are also potentially malignant and require wide local excision.

Chromogranin, PGP 9.5, synaptophysin positive. NB: rectal carcinoid can be falsely positive for prostatic acid phosphatase but is negative for prostatic specific antigen.

Neuroendocrine differentiation can be present in up to 50% of usual type colorectal adenocarcinomas and is not prognostically significant.

Lymphoma

— predisposing conditions are ulcerative colitis and AIDS (which can also result in Kaposi's sarcoma).
— solitary or multifocal.
— of probable mucosa associated lymphoid tissue (MALT) origin (60–70%) with a heterogeneous, polymorphous cell population: low-grade,<20% blasts; high-grade, > 20% blasts.
— B (> 90%) or T cell ± high content of eosinophils.
— prognosis relates to the grade and stage of disease.

Others: centrocytic or mantle cell lymphoma (multiple lymphomatous polyposis), which is of intermediate-grade; rarely follicle centre (follicular) lymphoma spreading from systemic nodal disease; Burkitt's type/B-lymphoblastic in children or adults (with AIDS) in the terminal ileum/ileocaecal valve – a high-grade lymphoma.

Leukaemia

— 50% of children with acute leukaemia who die in relapse.
— chronic lymphocytic leukaemia.
— granulocytic sarcoma (CD 68/chloroacetate esterase positive).
— single/multiple deposits.

Malignant melanoma

— primary or secondary; metastases are commoner.

Kaposi's sarcoma

— AIDS/inflammatory bowel disease
— 50% show visceral involvement, 8% in the hindgut.

Teratoma

— rare; primary in caecum, sigmoid and rectum but exclude spread from ovary or sacrococcygeal area. Choriocarcinoma must be distinguished from adenocarcinoma with trophoblastic differentiation.

6 Vermiform Appendix Tumours

1. Gross description

Specimen

- appendicectomy/right hemicolectomy.
- length and diameter (cm).
- mucocoele/perforation/diverticulum/appendicitis.

Tumour

Site
- tip/base/diverticulum/body.

Size
- length × width × depth (cm) or maximum dimension (cm).

Appearance
- polypoid/sessile/plaque/ulcerated/infiltrative/mucoid/yellow.

Edge
- circumscribed/irregular.

2. Histological type

Carcinoid (endocrine cell) tumours
- 0.5–1.5% of appendicectomies.
- 85% of appendiceal tumours.
- Usually a coincidental finding although it may contribute to appendicitis when at the appendix base (10%).

— NSE, chromogranin, PGP 9.5 positive ± argentaffin/argyrophil (often argentaffin positive only but can be argyrophil positive only, or mixed).

Usual type: 70%, appendiceal tip; solid nests/cords/ribbons/acini of cells; often invasion of muscularis, serosa and lymphatics; benign with appendicectomy the treatment of choice.

Very occasional cases spread to peritoneum, regional nodes and liver and these are usually > 2 cm diameter: size appears to be the main factor predictive of behaviour. Radical surgery should be considered in these circumstances. Invasion of mesoappendix and the appendiceal base are also adverse indicators.

Adenocarcinoid (mucinous/goblet cell carcinoid) type: clusters, strands or glandular collections of mucus-secreting epithelial cells often with a signet ring or goblet cell morphology; a lesser population of endocrine cells is present demonstrated by immunohistochemistry; potential for extra-appendiceal spread (20% of cases), involvement of regional nodes and liver; propensity for transcoelomic spread to involve ovaries and direct spread through the appendix base and into the caecum.

Right hemicolectomy should be considered if there is extensive spread, involvement of the appendix base or tumour pleomorphism and mitoses. The term mixed carcinoid/adenocarcinoma is sometimes used if there is an infiltrating component of colorectal type tumour tissue.

Distinguish from: (1) secondary colorectal carcinoma involving the appendix either directly (e.g. from caecal pouch) or via the peritoneum (signet ring cell carcinoma of rectosigmoid area) and (2) primary colonic-type mucinous adenocarcinoma of appendix which is aggressive in behaviour and requires radical surgery. A pre-existing mucosal adenoma (usually) and the presence of a significant component of endocrine cells in a carcinoid lesion are helpful in this respect.

Adenoma

— 1% of appendicectomies, the majority are benign.
— localised (polypoidal) or diffuse.
— tubular/tubulovillous/villous with variable grades of dysplasia.
— mucinous cystadenoma when associated with mucocoele which may also rupture and result in a localised pseudomyxoma in the mesoappendiceal fat.
— in up to 20% of cases there are adenomas or adenocarcinomas elsewhere in the colorectum.

Adenocarcinoma

— 0.3% of appendicectomies.
— requires invasion through the muscularis mucosae by malignant glands (sometimes but often not with a desmoplastic reaction) and/or the presence of epithelium in extra-appendiceal mucus (cytokeratins and CEA can be useful in demonstrating this).
— identified as primary by a mucosal adenomatous lesion.
— histologically of usual colorectal type, often well differentiated mucinous in character.

— rarely signet ring cell carcinoma – distinguish from adenocarcinoid (chromogranin positive) and metastatic gastric/breast carcinoma (infiltrating lobular type). In this respect it is necessary to know of previous operations to the stomach and breast and these sites may have to be investigated. Breast carcinoma may also be ER/PR positive and cytokeratin 7 positive/20 negative whereas gut cancers are CEA positive and cytokeratin 20 positive/7 negative. The intracytoplasmic vacuoles of lobular carcinoma are PAS-AB positive.

— treatment is right hemicolectomy and regional lymphadenectomy. Prognosis reflects the histological grade of tumour and Dukes' classification, with an overall 5 year survival rate of 60–65% with hemicolectomy but only 20% for appendicectomy alone.

Metastatic carcinoma

— peritoneal spread: colorectum, ovary, stomach.
— distant spread: bronchus, breast.

3. Differentiation

Well/moderate/poor.
Epithelial/enteroendocrine/mixed (the behaviour and prognosis is determined by that of the individual components).

4. Extent of local tumour spread

Border: pushing/infiltrative.
Lymphocytic reaction: prominent/sparse.
Limited to the appendix, into mesoappendix, appendiceal base and caecum.
As in colorectal carcinoma prognosis relates to Dukes' stage:

A   tumour confined to the appendix wall, nodes negative
B   tumour through the appendix wall, nodes negative
C   tumour in regional lymph nodes irrespective of the depth of wall invasion.

In the 5th edition TNM classification appendix is an anatomical subsite of colorectum.

pTis carcinoma in-situ: intraepithelial (within basement membrane) or invasion of the lamina propria (intramucosal) with no extension through muscularis mucosae into submucosa
pT1   tumour invades submucosa
pT2   tumour invades muscularis propria
pT3   tumour invades beyond muscularis propria into subserosa or mesoappendix
pT4   tumour invades the serosal surface or adjacent organs and/or perforation of visceral peritoneum.

5. Lymphovascular invasion

Present/absent.
Intra-/extratumoural.
Serosa/mesoappendix.

Lymphovascular invasion in adenocarcinoma is more significant than in a usual carcinoid tumour where it is quite common with no adverse prognostic effect.

6. Lymph nodes

Site/number/size/number involved/limit node/extracapsular spread.
Regional nodes: ileocolic.
Dukes' C: metastasis in regional lymph nodes.

pN0   no regional lymph node metastasis
pN1   1–3 involved regional lymph nodes
pN2   4 or more involved regional lymph nodes.

7. Excision margins

Distances (mm) to the proximal limit of excision and serosa.

8. Other pathology

Carcinoid syndrome rarely occurs due to the scarcity of appendiceal carcinoid tumours metastatic to the liver.

Mucocoele
Mucocoeles of obstructed or non-obstructed types both result in marked distension of the lumen by abundant mucus. Obstructed mucocoele is effectively a retention cyst lined by variably attenuated, atrophic muscosa. Non-obstructed mucocoeles are due to an abnormality of the underlying mucosa caused either by a hyperplastic (metaplastic) polyp, adenoma or cystadenocarcinoma.

Pseudomyxoma peritonei
Mucocoeles can be associated with rupture or perforation secondary to appendicitis resulting in pseudomyxoma peritonei which is either localised or diffuse. Obstructed mucocoeles and those due to hyperplastic (metaplastic) polyp and adenoma remain localised whereas diffuse pseudomyxoma is due to spillage of either borderline or unequivocally malignant epithelium associated with an appendiceal adenocarcinoma or tumour of uncertain malignant potential. Prognosis relates to the presence of neoplastic epithelial cells within the extra-appendiceal mucus and the presence of mucus away from the vicinity of the appendix elsewhere in the peritoneal cavity. Diffuse pseudomyxoma may be

helped by debulking procedures but is largely refractory to treatment, slowly but relentlessly progressive and causes death by bowel obstruction. In this condition there is also a strong association with intestinal type mucinous tumours of the ovary of borderline malignancy and debate continues as to whether this is merely a synchronous or metachronous association between the ovarian and appendiceal lesions or whether the former represents a metastatic deposit from the latter. Ovarian tumours of mucinous type can show a wide spectrum of intestinal differentiation and it may be that a significant number of these represent metastases from appendiceal, colonic or gastric sites. In addition the appendiceal lesion may not be grossly evident and it is recommended that appendicectomy be carried out, particularly if the ovarian tumours are bilateral and extraovarian disease is present.

Synchronous/metachronous colorectal lesions

The presence of hyperplastic (metaplastic), adenomatous or cystadenocarcinomatous epithelium in the appendix is a marker of concurrent or subsequent epithelial neoplasms elsewhere in the colorectum.

Appendicitis can form an inflammatory appendix mass in the right iliac fossa that mimics colorectal cancer clinically and radiologically. Appendiceal tumours may also present in this fashion.

9. Other malignancy

Malignant lymphoma

— primary (rare) or secondary to systemic/nodal disease.
— Burkitt's lymphoma: ileocaecal angle; childhood; aggressive high-grade disease.

Kaposi's sarcoma

— AIDS.

Anal Canal Carcinoma

1. Gross description

Specimen

— biopsy/resection (local or abdominoperineal).
— weight (g) and size/length (cm), number of fragments.

Tumour

Site

— mucous membrane/muscularis/extra-mural.
— low rectal/anal canal/perianal margin or skin.
— anatomy:

1. upper zone: colorectal mucosa
   _____ dentate line _____
2. transitional/cloacal zone: stratified cuboidal epithelium with surface umbrella cells + anal glands in submucosa
   _____ pectinate line _____
3. lower zone: stratified squamous epithelium continuous with appendage bearing perianal skin.

Size

— length × width × depth (cm) or maximum dimension (cm).

Appearance

— polypoid/sessile/ulcerated/stricture/pigmented/fleshy/mucoid.

Edge

— circumscribed/irregular.

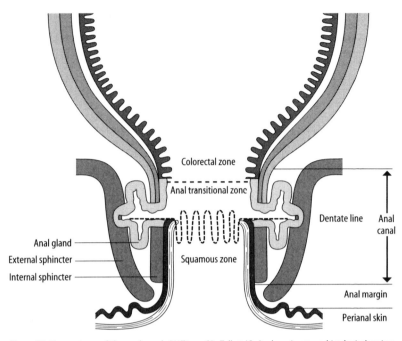

Figure 20. The anatomy of the anal canal. (Williams GR, Talbot IC. Anal carcinoma: a histological review. Histopathology 1994;25:507–516.)

2. Histological type

Anal margin/perianal skin

As for non-melanocytic skin carcinoma (Chapter 20), in particular well-differentiated keratinising squamous cell carcinoma and variants including verrucous carcinoma: also basal cell carcinoma, Bowen's disease, Paget's disease.

Anal canal

Carcinoma of the anal canal is regarded as being a squamous cell carcinoma showing variable degrees of squamous (in > 90% of cases), basaloid (in 65% of cases) and ductular (in 26% of cases) differentiation. Distal canal and anal margin cancers tend to show more overt squamous differentiation (well differentiated).

Squamous cell carcinoma

— keratinising/non-keratinising large cell.

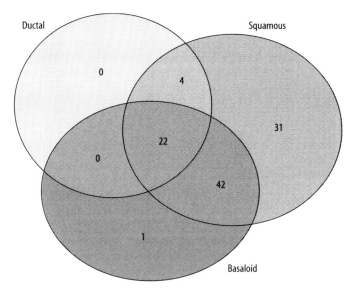

Figure 21. Anal canal carcinoma: overlap in histological subtypes. (Williams GR, Talbot IC. Anal carcinoma: a histological review. Histopathology 1994;25:507–516.)

Basaloid carcinoma

— (syn. cloacogenic/non-keratinising small cell squamous carcinoma).

— palisading nests of basophilic cells with surrounding retraction artefact, central eosinophilic necrosis ± ductular differentiation.

— comprises 50% of anal carcinomas.

— mixed basaloid/squamous types.

— increased incidence in Crohn's disease, smoking, immunosuppression and sexually transmitted disease.

— association with HPV 16/18 and anal intraepithelial neoplasia (AIN).

Others

Mucinous (colloid) adenocarcinoma: in anal fistula which may be associated with Crohn's disease or hindgut duplication.

Anal gland adenocarcinoma: rare; in contrast to anorectal adenocarcinoma lacks O-acetylsialomucin (PAS negative post PB-KOH saponification); late diagnosis, poor prognosis.

Extra-mammary Paget's disease: in 20% an underlying adnexal adenocarcinoma is found.

Neuroendocrine carcinoma: carcinoid/small cell/large cell; carcinoid<2 cm is treated by local excision, if ≥ 2 cm consider more radical surgery.

Spindle cell carcinoma: rare.

Malignant melanoma: primary mucosal origin with adjacent junctional atypia that can be destroyed by surface ulceration; 15% of anal malignancy – aggressive with early spread and death in months (liver, lung metastases).

Metastatic carcinoma: direct spread – low rectal adenocarcinoma (adenocarcinoma of rectal type arising from the colorectal mucosa of the upper anal zone cannot be distinguished from usual rectal carcinoma and is grouped with it); prostatic carcinoma (PSA/PSAP positive); cervical carcinoma.

3. Differentiation

Well/moderate/poor – carcinoma.
Low-grade/high-grade – sarcoma.

4. Extent of local tumour spread

Border: pushing/infiltrative.
Lymphocytic reaction: prominent/sparse.
Depth of spread: submucosa; muscularis of rectum or anal sphincters; extrarectal and extra-anal tissue including ischiorectal fossae and pelvic structures.

At diagnosis the majority have spread through sphincteric muscle into adjacent soft tissue.

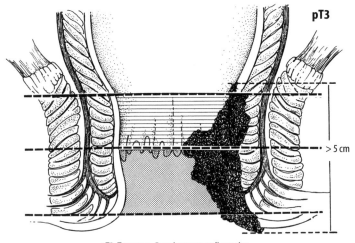

pT3 Tumour > 5 cm in greatest dimension

Figure 22. Anal canal carcinoma.

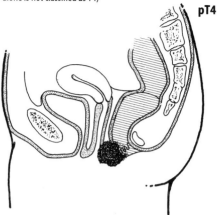

pT4 Tumour of any size invades adjacent organ(s), e.g. vagina, urethra, bladder (involvement of the sphincter muscle(s) alone is not classified as T4)

pT4

Figure 23. Anal canal carcinoma.

pTis carcinoma in-situ
pT1   tumour ≤ 2 cm in greatest dimension
pT2   2 cm<tumour ≤ 5 cm in greatest dimension
pT3   tumour > 5 cm in greatest dimension
pT4   tumour of any size invading adjacent organ(s), e.g. vagina, urethra, bladder.

5. Lymphovascular invasion

Present/absent.
Intra-/extratumoural.
Perineural spread.

Distant metastases at the time of diagnosis are present in 5–10% of cases. Haematogenous spread is to liver, lung and skin.

6. Lymph nodes

Site/number/size/number involved/limit node/extracapsular spread.

Regional nodes: perirectal, internal iliac, inguinal; anal margin tumours go initially to inguinal nodes → iliac nodes; anal canal tumours go initially to haemorrhoidal nodes → perirectal and inguinal nodes.

pN0   no regional lymph node metastasis
pN1   metastasis in perirectal lymph node(s)

pN2   metastasis in unilateral internal iliac and/or inguinal lymph node(s)
pN3   metastasis in perirectal and inguinal lymph nodes and/or bilateral internal iliac and/or inguinal lymph nodes.

Lymph node involvement is present in 10–50% of cases at presentation.

7. Excision margins

Distances (mm) to the nearest longitudinal (rectal or perianal) resection limit and deep circumferential radial margin.

8. Other pathology

Carcinoma of the anal canal (F:M 3:2) is commoner (3:1) than carcinoma of the anal margin (M:F 4:1).

Human papilloma virus infection is a common aetiological agent associated with a spectrum of anal viral lesions, preneoplasia (AIN) and carcinoma. Infection with HIV and other sexually transmitted viruses also contributes.

Condyloma accuminatum, giant condyloma of Buschke-Löwenstein, and Bowen's disease of anal skin are associated with perianal margin/skin squamous carcinoma and its variants. Some authors equate giant condyloma to verrucous carcinoma (indolent growth, exophytic, deep bulbous processes with bland cytology, more aggressive after radiotherapy). Bowenoid papulosis has no significant malignant potential.

Concurrent cervical intraepithelial neoplasia (CIN) and anal intraepithelial neoplasia (AIN) grades I, II, III are associated with anal canal carcinoma, with AIN being present in up to 55% of cases. A premalignant phase or model of progression in AIN is not as well established as in CIN although cancer risk appears to be greatest for high-grade (III) AIN.

The majority of anal canal carcinomas arise in the vicinity of the dentate line from the transitional/cloacal zone and spread preferentially upwards in the submucosal plane thereby presenting as ulcerating tumour of the lower rectum. Due to the differential options of primary adjuvant therapy versus primary resection anal canal carcinoma must be distinguished by biopsy from both rectal adenocarcinoma superiorly and basal cell carcinoma or squamous cell carcinoma of the perianal margin/skin inferiorly.

Anal Paget's disease must be distinguished from Bowen's disease and pagetoid spread of malignant melanoma. Mucin stains and immunohistochemistry are necessary (mucicarmine, PAS ± diastase, cytokeratins, melanoma markers: pigment, S100, HMB-45, melan-A). It may be associated with concurrent or subsequent low rectal adenocarcinoma with the Paget's cells showing intestinal-type gland formation and cytokeratin 20 positivity. Alternatively it is a primary cutaneous lesion lacking intestinal glandular differentiation and cytokeratin 20 positivity (but cytokeratin 7 positive) which may progress to submucosal invasion. The majority remain as intraepithelial malignancy. A further differential diagnosis is pagetoid spread from a primary anorectal signet ring cell carcinoma. Immunohistochemistry is also important in the differential diagnosis of anal basaloid carcinoma (cytokeratins, EMA, CEA positive), malignant melanoma, lymphoma (CD 45 positive), spindle cell carcinoma (cytokeratin positive) and leiomyosarcoma (desmin, smooth muscle actin positive). Distinction between anal canal basaloid carcinoma and basal cell carcinoma of the anal margin is by the anatomical location as well as histological characteristics.

Radiotherapy necrosis.

Leukoplakia with or without AIN is occasionally seen and needs biopsy to establish the presence of dysplasia.

Prognosis

Carcinoma of anal margin/perianal skin is treated primarily by surgery ± adjuvant therapy. Anal canal squamous carcinoma responds well to primary radio-/chemotherapy and abdominoperineal resection is reserved for extensive/recurrent/non-responsive tumours or other lesions such as malignant melanoma and leiomyosarcoma. Perianal carcinoma: 5 year survival 85%; anal canal carcinoma: 5 year survival 65–80%. Adverse prognostic indicators are advanced stage or depth of spread, tumour in inguinal nodes (10–50%) and post-treatment recurrence in the pelvic and perianal regions, e.g. pT1 carcinoma has a 5 year survival of 91%, pT3 16%. Histological grade is not a strong indicator but may be helpful in poorly differentiated squamous cell carcinoma of large cell type. Ductal differentiation in basaloid carcinoma is an adverse factor. Recurrence in men is pelvic and perineal, in women pelvic and vaginal.

9. Other malignancy

Lymphoma/leukaemia
— secondary to systemic/nodal disease.
— AIDS.

Leiomyosarcoma
— low-grade/high-grade based on cellularity, atypia, necrosis, infiltrative margins and mitoses.

Presacral tumours
— teratoma, peripheral neuroectodermal tumours (including Ewing's sarcoma), myeloma, metastatic carcinoma.

Rhabdomyosarcoma
— childhood, embryonal.

Gall Bladder Carcinoma

1. Gross description

Specimen

— laparoscopic/open cholecystectomy.
— size (cm) and weight (g).
— open/intact.
— contents: bile/calculi (number, size, shape, colour).
— lymph nodes: site/size/number.

Tumour

Site
— fundus/body/cystic duct.

Size
— length x width x depth (cm) or maximum dimension (cm).

Appearance
— grossly apparent/inapparent.
— diffuse (65%)/polypoid (30%)/papillary/ulcerated.

Edge
— circumscribed/irregular.

2. Histological type

Adenocarcinoma
— tubular/acinar/papillary: usual type, > 90% of cases.

— intestinal/mucinous/signet ring cell/clear cell: unusual. Distinguish from metastatic stomach or bowel cancer by adjacent mucosal dysplasia.

Adenosquamous carcinoma

Squamous carcinoma

Small cell carcinoma
— and other neuroendocrine lesions, e.g. carcinoid/large cell neuroendocrine carcinoma including composite tumours (carcinoid/adenocarcinoma).
— small cell carcinoma is aggressive and may be a component of usual adenocarcinoma.

Spindle cell carcinoma and carcinosarcoma
— biphasic carcinoma/sarcoma-like components ± specific mesenchymal differentiation; these probably represent carcinomas with variable stromal metaplasia.
— elderly patients, poor prognosis.

Pleomorphic large cell carcinoma

Malignant melanoma
— secondary (15% of disseminated melanoma at autopsy) or rarely primary (nodular, adjacent mucosal junctional change).

Metastatic carcinoma
— direct spread: stomach, colon, pancreas.
— distant spread: breast, lung, kidney.

3. Differentiation

Well/moderate/poor.
— usually well to moderately differentiated arising from a sequence of mucosal intestinal metaplasia and dysplasia.

4. Extent of local tumour spread

Border: pushing/infiltrative.
Lymphocytic reaction: prominent/sparse.
Characteristic perineural spread (25% of cases).

pTis   carcinoma in-situ
pT1   tumour limited to gall bladder wall
       a. lamina propria
       b. muscularis

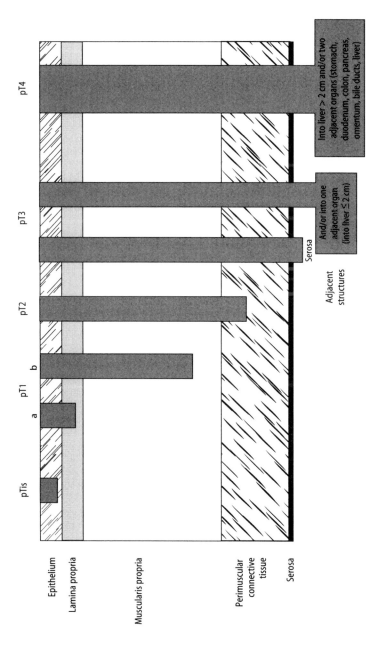

Figure 24. Gall bladder carcinoma.

pT2   tumour invades perimuscular connective tissue
pT3   tumour perforates serosa and/or directly invades one adjacent organ.
       Extension into liver ≤ 2 cm.

pT4   Tumour extends more than 2 cm into liver and/or into two or more adjacent
       organs (stomach, duodenum, colon, pancreas, omentum, extrahepatic bile
       ducts, any involvement of liver) (Figs. 25, 26)

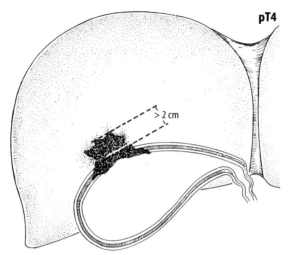

Figure 25. Gall bladder carcinoma.

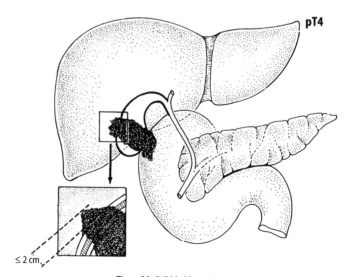

Figure 26. Gall bladder carcinoma.

pT4   tumour extends > 2 cm into liver and/or into two or more adjacent organs (usually stomach, duodenum, colon, pancreas, omentum, extrahepatic bile ducts, liver).

Note that adenocarcinoma may extend into Rokitansky-Aschoff sinuses and this must be distinguished from deeply invasive tumour which shows a lack of low-power lobular organisation, deficient basement membrane and stromal desmoplasia.

5. Lymphovascular invasion

Present/absent.
Intra-/extratumoural.

6. Lymph nodes

Site/number/size/number involved/limit node/extracapsular spread.
Regional nodes: cystic duct node, pericholedochal, hilar, peripancreatic, periduodenal, periportal, coeliac and superior mesenteric.

The regional lymph nodes are the cystic duct node and the pericholedochal, hilar, peripancreatic (head only), periduodenal, periportal, coeliac and superior mesenteric nodes

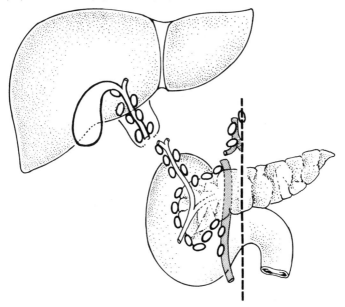

Figure 27. Gall bladder: regional lymph nodes.

pN0   no regional lymph node metastasis
pN1   metastasis in cystic duct, pericholedochal and/or hilar nodes
pN2   metastasis in peripancreatic (head only), periduodenal, periportal, coeliac
       and/or superior mesenteric lymph nodes.

7. Excision margins

Distances (mm) to the proximal limit of the cystic duct and serosa.
Mucosal dysplasia in adjacent gall bladder mucosa, the cystic duct and its limit.

8. Other pathology

Gall bladder carcinoma is cytokeratin and CEA positive.
Adenoma – rare – familial adenomatous polyposis coli (FAPC). As in colorectum
the risk of malignancy increases with size, villousity and degree of dysplasia.

Prognosis

Calculi, chronic inflammatory bowel disease and primary sclerosing cholangitis
are all risk factors, with calculi present in 80–90% of cases in female patients
(F:M 3:1) particularly responsible. Most gall bladder carcinomas are clinically
inapparent and found incidentally as diffuse thickening of the wall at cholecystectomy for gall stones. Prognosis is better if lesions are of papillary type, low
histological grade and confined to the mucous membrane, when resection is
potentially curative (90% 5 year survival). A significant number of carcinomas
are grossly inapparent and a microscopic finding only. However, curative resection is unusual and up to 50% present with regional node metastases and 75%
have involvement of the gall bladder bed liver. In these patients 5 year survival
rates are 5–10%.

9. Other malignancy

Lymphoma/leukaemia
—   MALToma or secondary to systemic nodal disease.

Sarcoma (rare)
—   embryonal rhabdomyosarcoma (children), leiomyosarcoma, angiosarcoma.

Extrahepatic Bile Duct Carcinoma

1. Gross description

Specimen

— cytological brushings and washings/biopsy/resection.
— weight (g) and size/length (cm), number of fragments.

Tumour

Site

— hilum (Klatskin tumour), proximal third (50%: equally between the common hepatic, cystic and upper common bile ducts), intermediate third (25%), distal third including ampulla (10%), multifocal/diffuse (15%).

Size

— length × width × depth (cm) or maximum dimension (cm).
— small and localised (a majority), the entire common bile duct or multifocal throughout the extrahepatic biliary system.

Appearance

— papillary/polypoid: distal third.
— ulcerated/sclerotic/stenotic: proximal two-thirds.

The majority are nodular or sclerosing with deep penetration of the wall, a small minority have a cystic component.

Edge

— circumscribed/irregular.

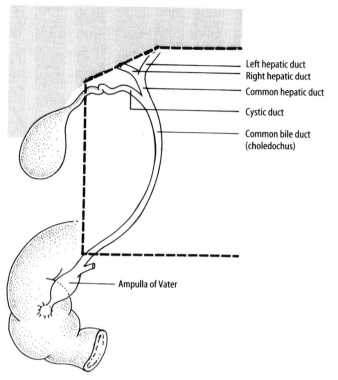

Figure 28. Extrahepatic bile ducts.

2. Histological type

Adenocarcinoma

— intestinal: usual type/well to moderate differentiation ± mucin secretion in a fibrous stroma.

— papillary: well differentiated/distal third

— sclerosing: hilar (Klatskin) tumour. Well to moderately differentiated tubular adenocarcinoma: rarely mucinous or signet ring. Fibrous nodule, short or long segmental stenosis, or papillary. Indolent growth with potentially prolonged survival. Arises in a field of dysplasia and resection limits should be checked for this.

— anaplastic.

— cystadenocarcinoma: a small number are the malignant counterpart of bile duct cystadenoma with variable benign, borderline and focal malignant change. Middle-aged females, resectable, good prognosis.

Adenosquamous carcinoma

Squamous cell carcinoma

Small cell carcinoma
— and other neuroendocrine lesions, e.g. carcinoid tumour.

Carcinosarcoma/spindle cell carcinoma
— cytokeratin positive spindle cells and varying degrees of stromal metaplasia with mesenchymal differentiation.

Malignant melanoma
— metastatic or primary (rare).

Metastatic carcinoma
— colorectum, breast (infiltrating lobular), kidney.

3. Differentiation

Well/moderate/poor.

4. Extent of local tumour spread

Border: pushing/infiltrative.
Lymphocytic reaction: prominent/sparse.

Perineural spread is a characteristic and may be present beyond the resection line causing surgical failure.

pTis   carcinoma in-situ
pT1   tumour invades:
     a. subepithelial connective tissue
     b. fibromuscular layer
pT2   tumour invades perifibromuscular connective tissue
pT3   tumour invades adjacent structures: liver, pancreas, duodenum, gall bladder, colon, stomach.

5. Lymphovascular invasion

Present/absent.
Intra-/extratumoural.

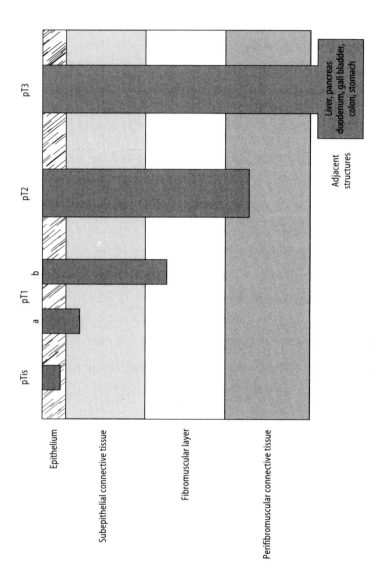

Figure 29. Extrahepatic bile duct carcinoma.

Epithelium	
Subepithelial connective tissue	
Fibromuscular layer	
Perifibromuscular connective tissue	

pTis pT1 a b pT2 pT3

Liver, pancreas, duodenum, gall bladder, colon, stomach

Adjacent structures

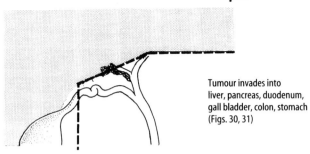

pT3

Tumour invades into
liver, pancreas, duodenum,
gall bladder, colon, stomach
(Figs. 30, 31)

Figure 30. Extrahepatic bile duct carcinoma.

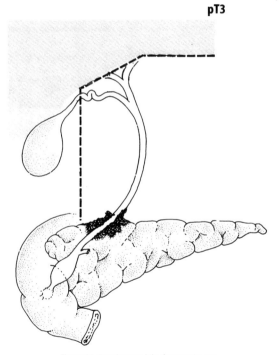

pT3

Figure 31. Extrahepatic bile duct carcinoma.

6. Lymph nodes

Site/number/size/number involved/limit node/extracapsular spread.
Regional nodes: cystic duct, pericholedochal, hilar, peripancreatic (head), periduodenal, periportal, coeliac, superior mesenteric.

pN0 no regional lymph node metastasis
pN1 metastasis in cystic duct, pericholedochal and/or hilar (i.e. in the hepato-
     duodenal ligament) nodes
pN2 metastasis in peripancreatic (head), periduodenal, periportal, coeliac,
     superior mesenteric, posterior pancreatico-duodenal nodes.

Nodal metastases are usually present at the time of diagnosis with subsequent spread to local structures (liver, pancreas, gall bladder, duodenum), lungs and peritoneal cavity.

7. Excision margins

Distances (mm) to the nearest longitudinal and circumferential resection margins of carcinoma and mucosal dysplasia.

8. Other pathology

Ninety per cent of patients (> 60 years, F:M 1:1) present with jaundice and diagnosis is by cholangiography (retrograde endoscopic or percutaneous tran-shepatic) supplemented by fine needle aspiration/brushings/washings cytology and/or biopsy.

Markers (e.g. cytokeratins, CEA) may be helpful in identifying poorly differ-entiated single cell infiltration on biopsy: other markers of bile duct carcinoma are cytokeratins 7 and 19, EMA and CA19-9. There is also overexpression of p53 in contradistinction to normal duct structures.

Frozen section diagnosis of bile duct carcinoma can be difficult due to the presence of ductulo-glandular structures in normal bile duct submucosa and the distortion that can occur in inflammatory strictures.

Dysplasia of adjacent bile duct mucosa must be noted at the resection limits.

Chronic inflammatory bowel disease (ulcerative colitis), primary sclerosing cholangitis, gall stones and choledochal cysts all show an increased incidence. Radiologically it can be difficult to distinguish between primary sclerosing cholangitis and a stenotic carcinoma.

Prognosis

Prognosis is worse for carcinoma of the upper third and hilum which is diffuse and/or multifocal. Distal lesions which are polypoid or nodular are potentially resectable with better prognosis. Despite being a sclerotic, diffuse tumour hilar Klatskin lesions have a well-differentiated morphology and indolent time course. Prognosis of bile duct carcinoma is poor with most patients dead within 2–3 years. It relates to tumour location, stage, histological type and grade. Overall survival is 10% with 25% for lesions of the distal third. This can improve to 50–80% 5 year survival if the tumour is ampullary and of early stage (pT1: limited to the sphincter of Oddi). Treatment for proximal lesions (not as high as the hilar plate) is resection (± hepatic lobectomy) with hepatojejunostomy;

a Whipple's procedure is indicated for distal lesions. Palliative treatment can involve biliary drainage, stenting or radiotherapy.

9. Other malignancy

Lymphoma/leukaemia
— secondary to systemic/nodal disease.

Sarcoma
— embryonal (botryoid) rhabdomyosarcoma in children with direct invasion of abdominal structures, metastases to bone and lungs and poor prognosis. Desmin positive small cells, subepithelial cellular cambium layer, deeper myxoid zone.
— leiomyosarcoma, angiosarcoma.

10

Liver
Carcinoma

1. Gross description

Specimen

— fine needle aspirate/core biopsy/wedge excision/
   partial hepatectomy/R/L lobectomy.
— size (cm) and weight (g).

Tumour

Site

— subcapsular/parenchymal/ductocentric/vascu-
   locentric/lobe/multifocal (particularly when
   cirrhosis is present).

Size

— length × width × depth (cm) or maximum dimension (cm).

Appearance

— hepatocellular carcinoma: solitary/diffuse/multi-
   focal (particularly in cirrhosis)/bile stained/
   venous spread/pedunculated/encapsulated/back-
   ground cirrhosis/haemochromatosis.
— cholangiocarcinoma: papillary/nodular/stenotic/
   scirrhous/multifocal.
— metastatic carcinoma: single/multiple/necrotic/
   umbilicated/mucoid/subcapsular.

Edge

— circumscribed/irregular.

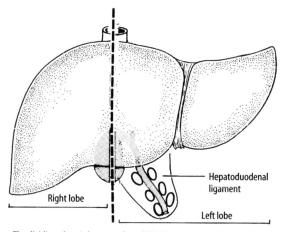

Right lobe

Left lobe

Hepatoduodenal
ligament

The dividing plane is between the gall bladder bed and inferior vena cava

Figure 32. Liver.

2. Histological type

Hepatocellular carcinoma

— trabecular, plate-like or sinusoidal.

— pseudoglandular (acinar).

— solid/scirrhous.

— hepatoid cells (± bizarre or clear cells), bile cytoplasmic staining and canalicular plugging, eosinophilic intranuclear pseudoinclusions, sinusoidal vascular pattern.

— rarely spindle cell or osteoclast-like.

— variants with good prognosis: fibrolamellar carcinoma (90%<25 years old); pedunculated carcinoma; minute, small or encapsulated carcinoma.

Cholangiocarcinoma (intrahepatic)

— scirrhous, solitary or multinodular.

— ductulo-acinar pattern of heterogeneous cuboidal to columnar mucin-secreting cells in a fibrous stroma.

— few survive longer than 2–3 years due to late presentation and limited resectability.

— rarely: signet ring cell; adenosquamous; osteoclast-like; spindle cell (sarcomatoid).

Mixed liver cell/bile duct carcinoma

— rare.

Hepatoblastoma

— 50–60% of childhood liver cancers, 90%<5 years of age.
— usually a large solitary mass. Epithelial component of two cell types (fetal/embryonal hepatocytes or small cell anaplastic) and mesenchyme (25% of cases: osteoid or undifferentiated spindle cells). Treatment is surgery and chemotherapy with a 15–35% long-term survival. Age<1 year, large size and a significant small cell component are adverse factors.

Metastatic carcinoma

— direct spread: stomach, large intestine, pancreas, gall bladder and biliary tree
— distant spread: stomach, colorectum, lung, breast, malignant melanoma, kidney, teratoma.

The tumour distribution may reflect its origin, e.g.:

— colorectum: multiple, large nodules with umbilication, ± mucin, ± calcification.
— gall bladder: bulk of disease centred on the gall bladder bed.
— lung: medium sized nodules.
— breast, stomach: medium-sized nodules or diffuse cirrhotic-like pattern.

NB: carcinoma rarely metastasises to a cirrhotic liver, i.e. the tumour is more likely to be primary.

Resection of some hepatic metastases is done to good effect, e.g. carcinoid tumour, colorectal carcinoma.

3. Differentiation/grade

Well/moderate/poor.

4. Extent of local tumour spread

Border: pushing/infiltrative.
Lymphocytic reaction: prominent/sparse.

The TNM classification applies to hepatocellular carcinoma and intrahepatic cholangiocarcinoma.

pT1   solitary, ≤ 2 cm, no vascular invasion
pT2   solitary, ≤ 2 cm, with vascular invasion
      multiple, one lobe, ≤ 2 cm, no vascular invasion
      solitary, > 2 cm, no vascular invasion
pT3   solitary, > 2 cm, with vascular invasion
      multiple, one lobe, ≤ 2 cm, with vascular invasion
      multiple, one lobe, > 2 cm ± vascular invasion

pT3 Solitary tumour more than 2 cm in greatest dimension with vascular invasion (Fig. 33);
or multiple tumours limited to one lobe, none more than 2 cm in greatest dimension
with vascular invasion (Fig. 34);
or multiple tumours limited to one lobe, any more than 2 cm in greatest dimension
with or without vascular invasion (Figs. 35, 36)

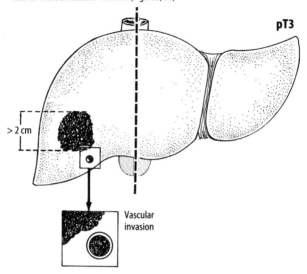

Figure 33. Liver carcinoma.

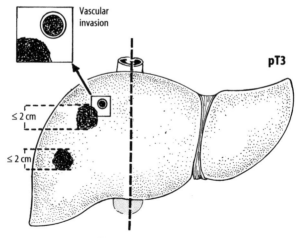

Figure 34. Liver carcinoma.

pT4 multiple, more than one lobe
     invasion of major branch of portal or hepatic veins
     invasion of adjacent organs other than gall bladder, perforation of visceral
     peritoneum.

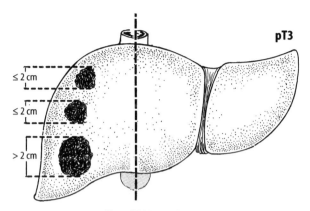

Figure 35. Liver carcinoma.

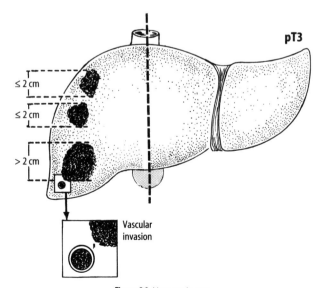

Figure 36. Liver carcinoma.

pT4   Multiple tumours in more than one lobe (fig. 37)
        or tumour(s) involve(s) a major branch of the portal or hepatic vein(s) (Fig. 38);
        or tumour(s) with direct invasion of adjacent organs other than gall bladder;
        or tumour(s) with perforation of visceral peritoneum (Fig. 39)

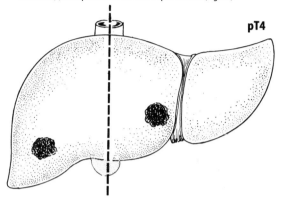

Figure 37. Liver carcinoma.

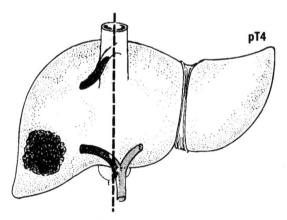

Figure 38. Liver carcinoma.

5. Lymphovascular invasion

Present/absent.
Intra-/ extratumoural.

Note the particular propensity for hepatocellular carcinoma to involve portal tract veins, major branches of portal and hepatic veins and inferior vena cava, ultimately with metastases to lung, adrenal gland and bone. Cholangiocarcinoma

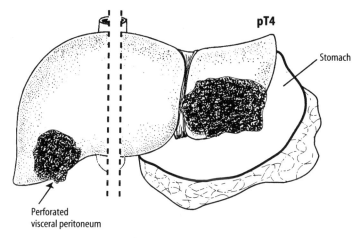

Figure 39. Liver carcinoma.

typically shows perineural invasion with spread to regional lymph nodes, lungs and peritoneum.

6. Lymph nodes

Site/number/size/number involved/limit node/extracapsular spread.

Regional nodes: hilar (hepatoduodenal ligament).

pN0   no regional lymph node metastasis
pN1   metastasis in regional lymph node(s).

7. Excision margins

Distances (mm) to the serosa and limits of excision of parenchyma, bile ducts and veins.

Mucosal dysplasia at the bile duct excision limit.

8. Other pathology

Budd Chiari syndrome secondary to venous invasion

Hepatocellular carcinoma
Risk factors: hepatitis B, C; cirrhosis (present in 60–80% of cases in the West) secondary to viral hepatitis, alcohol, congenital bile duct atresia, alpha-1-antitrypsin

deficiency, haemochromatosis, etc.; small /large cell liver cell dysplasia – there is a strong association between large cell dysplasia and hepatitis B surface antigen; small cell dysplasia (enlarged nucleus, decreased volume of cytoplasm) is regarded as being a more important risk factor for development of carcinoma; adenomatous hyperplastic nodules or macroregenerative nodules in a background of cirrhosis – 2–3 cm, ± fibrous rim, ± cytoarchitectural atypia (plates 3 cells thick, irregular edges, loss of reticulin, ± dysplasia).

Staining: tumour positive for AFP (25%: high specificity but low sensitivity) and polyclonal CEA in bile canaliculi; also EMA, CAM 5.2 (but not AE1), ER/PR. PAS positive cytoplasmic glycogen, intracellular PAS positive globular inclusions, loss of pericellular reticulin.

Cholangiocarcinoma
Risk factors: primary sclerosing cholangitis/ulcerative colitis/liver fluke/biliary tree anomaly. Treatment is surgical (partial/total hepatic resection ± liver transplantation) but prognosis is poor with overall mean survival ≤ 2 years.

Staining: cytokeratins (7,19), EMA, CEA, CA19-9, mucin positive. Also CAM 5.2 (low molecular weight cytokeratin, as for hepatocellular carcinoma) and AE1 (high molecular weight cytokeratin, negative in hepatocellular carcinoma).

Differential diagnosis of hepatic mass lesions

Focal nodular hyperplasia: young to middle-aged women, usually solitary and asymptomatic; radiological and gross central scar with proliferating bile ducts, plates 2 or 3 cells thick, cirrhosis-like nodule with adjacent normal parenchyma.

Hepatocellular adenoma: middle-aged women with acute abdominal presentation, history of oral contraception; no portal tracts or central veins, liver cell plates > 2 cells thick, retention of reticulin pattern and sinusoidal Kupffer cells (CD 68 positive).

Hepatocellular carcinoma: evidence of risk factors, e.g. cirrhosis; plates > 2 cells thick, loss of reticulin pattern and Kupffer cells, look for vascular invasion; serum AFP markedly elevated in 40–75% of cases: CT/MRI scan shows the location of the lesion, its extent of invasion and multicentricity.

Poorly differentiated metastatic carcinoma: specific histological appearance (e.g. small cell carcinoma lung), immunogenicity (e.g. PSA positive) or histochemical feature (e.g. mucin positive – this cannot distinguish secondary adenocarcinoma from primary cholangiocarcinoma).

Sometimes the distinction between adenoma and well-differentiated hepatocellular carcinoma is not possible and the subsequent clinical course establishes the diagnosis. Fine needle aspiration cytology of hepatic mass lesions is useful for simple cysts, abscesses and some metastatic cancers (e.g. small cell lung carcinoma). Secondary adenocarcinoma cannot always be distinguished from cholangiocarcinoma and previous history is important eg resection for colorectal carcinoma. Fine needle aspiration is reasonably robust for moderately differentiated hepatocellular carcinoma but may need to be supplemented by core/open biopsy in poorly differentiated carcinomas (to exclude metastatic cancers) and well-differentiated lesions (to exclude adenoma, focal nodular hyperplasia, cirrhosis). Useful diagnostic features for hepatocellular carcinoma are: hepatoid cells (polygonal with central nucleus), nuclear/nucleolar enlargement, a trabecular pattern, nuclear pseudoinclusions, bile secretion and an absence of bile duct epithelial and inflammatory cells. Immunostaining may also be helpful.

Prognosis

Treatment of hepatocellular carcinoma depends on surgical resection ± liver transplantation. Chemotherapy is used for recurrent or inoperable tumours. Prognosis relates to tumour size (> 5 cm), cell type or differentiation, encapsulation, multifocality, high serum AFP levels, vascular invasion and the presence or absence of a background cirrhosis (an adverse indicator). Five year survival is at most 10–15% and more usually about 3%. The majority die within several months of presentation with liver failure, haemorrhage and infection. Small tumours (< 3–5 cm) and variants such as fibrolamellar and pedunculated carcinoma are potentially curable.

Fibrolamellar carcinoma
— large eosinophilic cells in a fibrous stroma, potentially resectable.
— 50% cure rate.
— serum AFP not raised, no cirrhosis. May also have areas of usual liver cell carcinoma and cholangiocarcinoma.

Pedunculated carcinoma
— inferoanterior aspect right lobe, up to 1 kg weight.

Minute, small encapsulated carcinoma
— 2–5 cm, encapsulated by fibrous tissue.
— 90-100% 5 year survival if no angio-invasion.

9. Other malignancy

Lymphoma/leukaemia
— secondary involvement by Hodgkin's/non-Hodgkin's lymphoma or leukaemia: lymphoma, mainly portal; leukaemia, mainly sinusoidal; mixed patterns of distribution.
— primary lymphoma is rare but of more favourable prognosis – solitary/ multiple masses or diffuse and high-grade large B cell in type.

Angiosarcoma
— cirrhosis, PVC, thorotrast exposure, commonest sarcoma of liver.

— exclude peliosis (well-differentiated angiosarcoma) and primary and secondary carcinoma (poorly differentiated angiosarcoma).

Epithelioid haemangioendothelioma

— fibrous masses with cords and tube-like structures of epithelioid cells, cytoplasmic vacuoles, CD31 positive.
— of low to intermediate grade malignancy: also seen in skin, lung and bone.

Kaposi's sarcoma

— AIDS.

Embryonal sarcoma

— 15% 5 year survival in patients of 6–10 years of age.
— spindle/stellate/pleomorphic/rounded cells.

Embryonal rhabdomyosarcoma

— < 5 years of age, poor prognosis, desmin positive small cells.
— arises from major bile ducts near the porta hepatis.

Leiomyosarcoma, fibrosarcoma

— rare.
— exclude sarcomatoid liver carcinoma and more commonly secondary sarcoma, e.g. gastrointestinal stromal tumour.

Carcinoid tumour

— usually represents metastases from gastrointestinal tract.

Mimics of malignancy

— abscess, sclerosed haemangioma, inflammatory myofibroblastic or pseudotumour (spindle cells in a storiform pattern, plasma cells).

Head and Neck Cancer

- Lip and Oral Cavity Carcinoma

- Oropharyngeal Carcinoma (with comments on nasopharynx and hypopharynx)

- Paranasal Sinus Carcinoma

- Laryngeal Carcinoma

- Salivary Gland Tumours

- Thyroid Gland Tumours

General Comments

See: Royal College of Pathologists. Minimum dataset for head and neck carcinoma histopathology reports. London. November 1998.

Basic rules are applied to carcinomas arising at various sites in the upper aerodigestive tract (lip, oral cavity, pharynx, paranasal sinuses and larynx), 95% of which are squamous cell carcinoma.

The surgeon should mark clinically relevant resection margins in the primary specimen and lymph node territories in neck dissections.

Prognosis

Prognosis relates to carcinoma:

Type
— e.g. keratinising squamous carcinoma versus undifferentiated nasopharyngeal carcinoma; this also influences treatment modality, e.g. surgery in the former, chemo-/radiotherapy in the latter.

Grade
— the majority are moderately differentiated but identify well and poorly differentiated lesions.

Size
— maximum diameter.

Depth
— maximum depth of invasion below the luminal aspect of the surface measured from the level of the adjacent mucosa.

Invasive edge
— a cohesive versus non-cohesive pattern of infiltration; the latter equates to single cells, small groups or multiple thin (< 15 cells across) strands of cells at the deep aspect of the tumour.

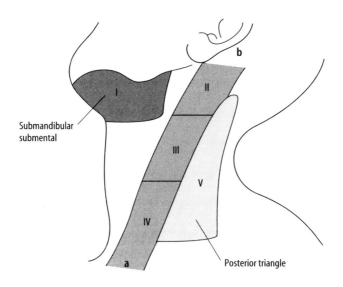

a (Origin) and b (Insertion) of sternocleidomastoid muscle

Figure 40. Lymph node groups in block dissection of the neck.

Margins of excision

> 5 mm	clear
1–5 mm	close to; also high risk of recurrence if the invasive edge is non-cohesive or shows vascular invasion
< 1 mm	involved.

Note also the presence of severe dysplasia at the resection edge.

Lymphovascular and perineural spread
— strong indicators of local recurrence.

Bone invasion
— distinguish erosion of the cortex from infiltration of the medulla.

Lymph node status
— number identified and number involved at each anatomical level of the neck dissection.   `
— an important prognostic factor is involvement of the lower cervical nodes, that is level IV (lower jugular chain deep to the lower one-third of sternocleidomastoid muscle) and level V (posterior triangle of neck behind the posterior border of sternocleidomastoid).

- maximum dimension of the largest nodal deposit.
- extracapsular spread.
- the significance of micrometastases is uncertain but should be counted as involved.

Lip and Oral Cavity Carcinoma

1. Gross description

Specimen

— fine needle aspirate/diagnostic or (wedge) excision biopsy/resection, e.g. glossectomy/neck dissection.
— size (cm) and weight (g).

Tumour

Site

— lip: external upper.
            external lower.
            commissures.

— oral cavity:
        buccal mucosa – lips/cheek/retromolar areas/bucco-alveolar sulci.
        upper alveolus and gingiva (upper gum).
        lower alveolus and gingiva (lower gum).
        hard palate.
        tongue – dorsal surface and lateral borders; (anterior two-thirds); inferior (ventral) surface.
        floor of mouth.

The commonest sites are, in order of decreasing frequency, lip (90% lower), lateral borders of tongue, anterior floor of mouth and the soft palate complex (soft palate, anterior pillar of fauces and retromolar areas).

Multifocal lesions are not uncommon, both synchronous and metachronous.

Size

— length × width × depth (cm) or maximum dimension (cm).

Appearance

— verrucous/warty/nodular/sessile/plaque/ulcerated.

Edge

— circumscribed/irregular.

2. Histological type

Squamous cell carcinoma

— 90% of cases.
— large cell/small cell.
— keratinising/non-keratinising.
— verrucous: elderly, tobacco usage, exophytic and keratotic with a pushing deep margin of cytologically bland bulbous processes. Locally invasive but may become aggressive after radiotherapy.
— spindle cell: pleomorphic, cytokeratin positive, distinguish from sarcoma. A more obvious in-situ or invasive squamous component may be seen and nodal metastases can show a spectrum of epithelial and spindle cell changes. Prognosis relates to the depth of invasion.
— basaloid: poor prognosis, nests of basaloid cells with necrosis.
— adenoid squamous: poor prognosis, acantholytic pattern.
— adenosquamous: poor prognosis, mixed differentiation.

Salivary gland tumours

— there is a higher frequency in the oral cavity (particularly palate) of carcinoma of minor salivary gland origin, e.g. polymorphous low-grade adenocarcinoma (cytological uniformity with architectural diversity), adenoid cystic carcinoma, mucoepidermoid carcinoma.

Small cell carcinoma

— aggressive: pure or with a squamous component.

Malignant melanoma

— Japanese/Africans, palate and gingiva, ± adjacent junctional activity; prognosis poor with nodal and distant metastases common.
— lip: desmoplastic melanoma. Show S100 positivity to distinguish from fibrous tissue; ± neurotropism.

Metastatic carcinoma

— lung, breast, kidney, gut, malignant melanoma.

3. Differentiation

Well/moderate/poor.

— usually moderately differentiated whereas carcinomas at the base of the tongue can be poorly differentiated/undifferentiated and immunohistochemistry for cytokeratins is needed to distinguish from malignant lymphoma.

4. Extent of local tumour spread

Border: pushing/infiltrative.
Lymphocytic reaction: prominent/sparse.

pTis carcinoma in-situ
pT1   tumour ≤ 2 cm in greatest dimension
pT2   tumour > 2 cm but ≤ 4 cm in greatest dimension
pT3   tumour > 4 cm in greatest dimension
pT4   Lip: tumour invades adjacent structures, e.g. through cortical bone, inferior alveolar nerve, floor of mouth, skin of face
      Oral cavity: tumour invades adjacent structures, e.g. through cortical bone, into deep (extrinsic) muscle of tongue, maxillary sinus, skin.

Cancers of the lip and lateral borders of the tongue may remain localised for considerable periods of time prior to invasion of local adjacent structures.

5. Lymphovascular invasion

Present/absent.
Intra-/extratumoural.
Perineural spread: predictor of local recurrence.

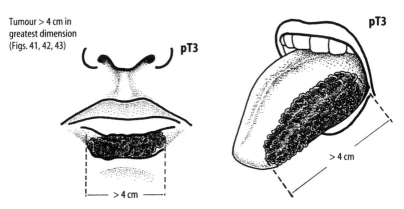

Tumour > 4 cm in greatest dimension (Figs. 41, 42, 43)

pT3

pT3

> 4 cm

> 4 cm

Figures 41, 42. Lip and oral cavity carcinoma.

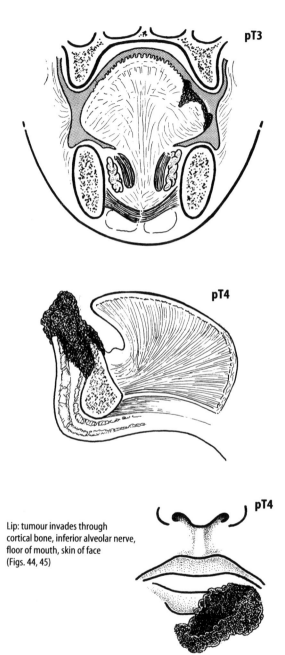

pT3

pT4

Lip: tumour invades through
cortical bone, inferior alveolar nerve,
floor of mouth, skin of face
(Figs. 44, 45)

pT4

Figures 43, 44, 45. Lip and oral cavity carcinoma.

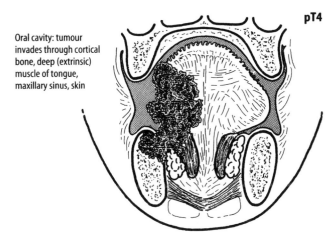

Oral cavity: tumour invades through cortical bone, deep (extrinsic) muscle of tongue, maxillary sinus, skin

Figure 46. Lip and oral cavity carcinoma.

6. Lymph nodes

Metastases are mainly lymphatic with the more anterior the tumour the lower the position of the cervical nodes involved. Nodal metastases may also undergo cystic degeneration with central straw-coloured fluid and viable cells at the tumour margin only. Residual paucicellular masses of keratin with a foreign body reaction may result from radiation therapy. These features should be borne in mind on fine needle aspiration of cervical nodes and a careful search made for malignant cells, which may be very well differentiated. A common differential diagnosis is branchial cyst.

Site/number/size/number involved/limit node/extracapsular spread.
Regional nodes: cervical.

pN0   no regional lymph node metastasis
pN1   metastasis in a single ipsilateral node ≤ 3 cm
pN2   metastasis in:
      a. ipsilateral single node > 3 cm to 6 cm
      b. ipsilateral multiple nodes ≤ 6 cm
      c. bilateral, contralateral nodes ≤ 6 cm
pN3   metastasis in a lymph node > 6 cm.

7. Excision margins

Distances (mm) to the nearest painted excision margins.

8. Other pathology: predisposing factors

Clinical

leukoplakia	thin, smooth	
	thick, fissured	cancer risk rises
	granular, verruciform	
	erythroleukoplakia 25–33% risk	
erythroplakia	50% cancer risk.	

Histological: dysplasia

— mild/moderate/severe. Most clinical examples of leukoplakia do not show histological dysplasia although if present it indicates a greater predisposition to carcinoma. Note that carcinoma can also arise from lesions with no dysplasia.

Others

— smokeless tobacco keratosis.
— chronic hyperplastic candidosis; this may also mimic squamous carcinoma histologically and treatment of infection is advised prior to any designation of malignancy.
— human papilloma virus (HPV 16,18): aetiological factor contributing to verrucous and squamous carcinoma.
— smoking, alcohol, post-transplant immunosuppression.

Squamous carcinoma is positive for a range of cytokeratins (excluding CK 20); this is of use in the distinction of spindle cell carcinoma from sarcoma.

Prognosis

Prognosis relates to tumour site, stage and histological grade.

lip	90% 5 year survival
anterior tongue	60% 5 year survival
posterior tongue, floor of mouth	40% 5 year survival.

Treatment is by surgery and/or radiotherapy supplemented by chemotherapy depending on the site and stage of disease.

9. Other malignancy

Lymphoma

— Waldeyer's ring is the commonest site of oropharyngeal non-Hodgkin's lymphoma but it can arise in gingiva, buccal mucosa and palate. Most are B cell and diffuse although others, e.g. T cell NHL and anaplastic large cell lymphoma do occur. Some are MALT derived whereas others are of nodal type, e.g. centrocytic (mantle cell). Prognosis relates to histological type and grade and stage of disease. There is an increasing incidence with AIDS.

Leukaemia

— direct infiltration or ulceration with opportunistic infection, e.g. herpes simplex virus, cytomegalovirus. Gingival involvement is seen in 4% of acute myeloid leukaemia. Rarely granulocytic sarcoma (CD 68/chloroacetate esterase positive) is the first presentation of disease.

Plasmacytoma

Odontogenic/osseous cancers by direct spread

Sarcoma

— Kaposi's sarcoma: AIDS, palate.
— leiomyosarcoma: cheek.
— rhabdomyosarcoma: embryonal – children.
— synovial sarcoma: young adults, cheek, tongue, palate.

Oropharyngeal Carcinoma
(with comments on nasopharynx and hypopharynx)

1. Gross description

Specimen

— fine needle aspirate/biopsy/tonsillectomy/adenoidectomy/pharyngectomy/pharyngooesophagectomy/neck dissection.
— weight (g) and size (cm), number of fragments.

Tumour

Site
Oropharynx: lies between the soft palate and tip of the epiglottis.

Boundaries:

1. anterior wall	posterior third tongue, vallecula
2. lateral wall	tonsil, tonsillar fossa and pillars
3. posterior wall	
4. superior wall	inferior surface soft palate, uvula.

Nasopharynx: superiorly from the skull base and delineated inferiorly by the superior surface of the soft palate.

Hypopharynx: delineated anteriorly by the larynx and aryepiglottic folds, laterally the piriform sinus and superiorly the oropharynx at the level of the hyoid bone. It lies below the tip of the epiglottis down to the start of the oesophagus at the postcricoid area.

Size
— length × width × depth (cm) or maximum dimension (cm).

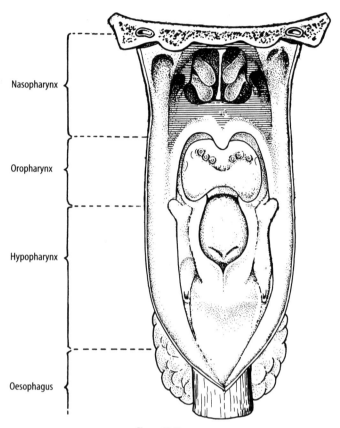

Figure 47. Pharynx

Appearance
— polypoid/sessile/ulcerated/fleshy.

Edge
— circumscribed/irregular.

2. Histological type

Squamous cell carcinoma
— 70% of cases predominantly well-differentiated keratinising.
— keratinising/non-keratinising.
— large cell/small cell.

— verrucous: exophytic, hyperkeratotic, pushing deep margin of cytologically bland bulbous processes; local invasion and may become aggressive post radiotherapy.
— spindle cell/adenoid squamous/squamous/adenosquamous; rare, all of worse prognosis.

Basaloid squamous cell carcinoma
— aggressive; nests of basaloid cells with necrosis.

Transitional type carcinoma
— 10%.
— features intermediate between squamous and transitional cell carcinoma.

Undifferentiated carcinoma
— 15%
— absence of squamous or glandular differentiation.
— particularly nasopharynx.

Adenocarcinoma salivary type, e.g.
— adenoid cystic carcinoma.
— acinic cell tumour.
— mucoepidermoid carcinoma.

Malignant melanoma
— primary or secondary, poor prognosis.

Neuroendocrine carcinoma
— carcinoid/atypical carcinoid/small cell carcinoma.

Metastatic carcinoma
— renal cell carcinoma, breast, lung, gut.

3. Differentiation

Well/moderate/poor.
— mainly well-differentiated keratinising but varies according to tumour site, e.g. nasopharyngeal carcinoma is of undifferentiated type. Carcinoma of the tonsil and base of the tongue also tend to be poorly differentiated.

4. Extent of local tumour spread

Border: pushing/infiltrative.
Lymphocytic reaction: prominent/sparse.

Oro-(hypopharynx)

pT1   tumour ≤2 cm in greatest dimension (hypopharynx – and limited to one subsite)

pT2   2 cm<tumour ≤4 cm in greatest dimension (hypopharynx – and more than one subsite)

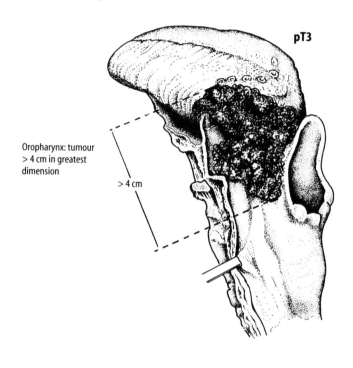

Oropharynx: tumour > 4 cm in greatest dimension

> 4 cm

pT3

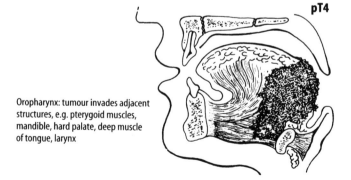

Oropharynx: tumour invades adjacent structures, e.g. pterygoid muscles, mandible, hard palate, deep muscle of tongue, larynx

pT4

Figures 48, 49. Oropharyngeal carcinoma.

pT3 tumour > 4 cm in greatest dimension (hypopharynx – or with fixation of hemilarynx)

pT4 tumour invades adjacent structures, e.g. pterygoid muscles, mandible, hard palate, deep muscle of tongue, larynx (hypopharynx – thyroid/cricoid cartilage, carotid artery, soft tissues of neck, pre-vertebral fascia/muscles, thyroid and/or oesophagus).

Nasopharynx

pT1 tumour confined to nasopharynx

pT2 tumour into oropharynx and/or nasal fossa

pT3 tumour into bone and/or nasal sinuses

pT4 intracranial extension and/or into cranial nerves, hypopharynx, orbit.

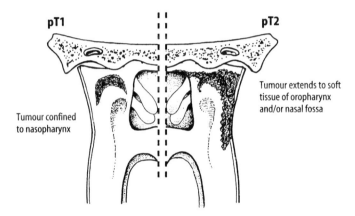

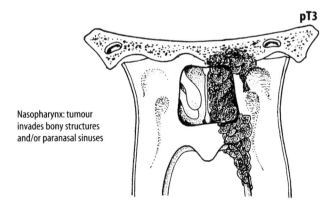

Figures 50, 51. Nasopharyngeal carcinoma.

5. Lymphovascular invasion

Present/absent.
Intra-/extratumoural.

6. Lymph nodes

Site/number/size/number involved/limit node/extracapsular spread.
Regional nodes: cervical

Oro- and hypopharynx
pN0   no regional lymph node metastasis
pN1   metastasis in a single ipsilateral node ≤ 3 cm in greatest dimension
pN2   a. metastasis in a single ipsilateral node > 3 cm but ≤ 6 cm in greatest dimension
        b. metastasis in multiple ipsilateral nodes ≤ 6 cm in greatest dimension
        c. metastasis in bilateral or contralateral nodes ≤ 6 cm in greatest dimension
pN3   metastasis in node > 6 cm in greatest dimension.

Nasopharynx
pN1   unilateral nodal metastasis ≤ 6 cm, above supraclavicular fossa
pN2   bilateral nodal metastasis ≤ 6 cm, above supraclavicular fossa
pN3   metastasis in nodes > 6 cm or in supraclavicular fossa.

Presentation in up to 10% of cases is with upper cervical lymph node metastases mimicking malignant lymphoma. Cervical metastases of nasopharyngeal carcinoma may also show a necrotising granulomatous nodal reaction. Carcinomas of the base of the tongue and oropharynx tend to metastasise to the retropharyngeal nodes and rarely (6%) the posterior triangle of neck.

7. Excision margins

Distances (mm) to the nearest longitudinal and circumferential excision margins.

8. Other pathology

Concurrent carcinoma bronchus, oropharyngolaryngeal ring: 10–15%.
    Primary treatment of oropharyngeal and hypopharyngeal carcinoma is surgical ± adjuvant radio-/chemotherapy, with the majority of lesions being well-differentiated keratinising squamous cell carcinoma. In contrast primary treatment of nasopharyngeal carcinoma is radio-/chemotherapy. The majority of nasopharyngeal carcinomas are of undifferentiated type comprising a syncytial arrangement of enlarged tumour cells with a prominent nucleolus and an accompanying lymphoid stroma. The tumour (undifferentiated and

non-keratinising variants) is strongly associated with Epstein-Barr virus infection, which can be shown by in-situ hybridisation techniques. Markers are helpful in distinguishing carcinoma (cytokeratins, EMA) from high-grade lymphoma (CLA–CD 45) and malignant melanoma (S100, HMB-45, melan-A). Nasopharyngeal carcinoma has a biphasic age presentation (15–25 years, 60–90 years) with the keratinising squamous cell variant occurring in the older age group. Nasopharynx has separate pT and pN staging in the TNM system. Hypopharynx may also be submitted with a laryngectomy specimen due to spread from a laryngeal carcinoma.

Prognosis

Prognosis of oropharyngeal carcinoma relates to tumour site, stage and histological grade, with 20–40% 5 year survival rates for the posterior tongue, tonsil and palate. Undifferentiated carcinoma has a very poor prognosis. However, the radiosensitivity of nasopharyngeal carcinoma results in complete remission in 80% of cases and 10 year survival rates of 40%. The keratinising squamous cell variant in the older age group is of worse prognosis as are cancers with lower cervical rather than upper cervical lymph node metastases.

9. Other malignancy

Leukaemia

Lymphoma
— large B cell non-Hodgkin's lymphoma.
— centrocytic (mantle cell) lymphoma: intermediate-grade.
— MALToma with recurrence in other MALT sites, e.g. stomach, Waldeyer's ring.
— angiocentric T cell lymphoma: aggressive.

Plasmacytoma/myeloma
κ, λ light chain restriction. Look for evidence of systemic disease, e.g. serum immune paresis, Bence-Jones proteinuria, radiological lytic bone lesions.

Sarcoma
— children: embryonal rhabdomyosarcoma (subepithelial cellular cambium layer; deeper myxoid zone; desmin positive, ± myoglobin, ± sarcomeric actin).
— young adults: synovial sarcoma; pharynx, palate.
— Kaposi's sarcoma: AIDS.

Nasopharyngeal chordoma (locally destructive), olfactory neuroblastoma, primitive neuroectodermal tumour.

Paranasal Sinus Carcinoma

1. Gross description

Specimen

— fine needle aspirate/biopsy/resection, e.g. maxillectomy, craniofacial resection/neck dissection.
— weight (g) and size (cm), number of fragments.

Tumour

Site
— maxillary sinus, ethmoid sinus, sphenoid/frontal sinuses.
— mucosal/osseous/extrinsic.

Size
— length × width × depth (cm) or maximum dimension (cm).

Appearance
— exophytic/papillary/mucoid/sclerotic/chondroid/osseous.

Edge
— circumscribed/irregular.

2. Histological type

Squamous cell carcinoma
— 75% of cases.
— keratinising/non-keratinising.

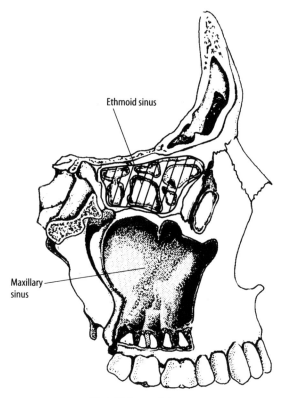

Figure 52. Paranasal sinuses.

— large cell/small cell.
— usually moderately differentiated ± keratinisation.

Transitional carcinoma

— possible origin in transitional (inverted) papilloma which is a benign but locally recurrent sinonasal tumour: a papillary exophytic neoplasm with features intermediate between transitional and squamous epithelia. Complicated by carcinoma in 3% of cases which is either focal (good prognosis) or diffusely infiltrative (25% survival rate).

Anaplastic carcinoma

— undifferentiated nasopharyngeal type.
— pleomorphic/spindle cell/small cell (neuroendocrine) types – necrosis/mitoses/vascular invasion.

Adenocarcinoma

— polypoid/well-differentiated intestinal pattern/woodworker's tumour (wood-dust exposure)/middle turbinate or ethmoid sinus/locally aggressive and recurrent.
— mucoepidermoid carcinoma.
— acinic cell tumour.
— adenoid cystic carcinoma.
— adenocarcinoma of no specific type.

Malignant melanoma

— rare (commoner in nasal cavity), 2% of malignant paranasal tumours, antrum, ethmoid, frontal sinuses.
— ± adjacent mucosal junctional activity.
— poor prognosis (most dead within 5 years).

Metastatic carcinoma

— renal, lung, breast, gut, malignant melanoma.

3. Differentiation

Well/moderate/poor.

The majority are moderately differentiated but this varies according to tumour site and type, e.g. undifferentiated nasopharyngeal carcinoma.

4. Extent of local tumour spread

Border: pushing/infiltrative.
Lymphocytic reaction: prominent/sparse.

pTis   carcinoma in-situ.

Maxillary sinus
pT1   tumour limited to the antral mucosa
pT2   tumour causes erosion or destruction of bone, except posterior antral wall
pT3   tumour invades any of: posterior wall maxillary sinus, subcutaneous tissues, skin of cheek, floor/medial wall orbit, infratemporal fossa, pterygoid plates, ethmoid sinus(es)
pT4   tumour invades orbital contents or any of: cribriform plate, base of skull, nasopharynx, sphenoid, frontal sinus.

Ethmoid sinus
pT1   tumour confined to ethmoid ± bone erosion
pT2   tumour extends into nasal cavity
pT3   tumour extends to anterior orbit and/or maxillary sinus

pT4   tumour invades intracranial cavity, orbital apex, sphenoid, frontal sinus, skin of nose.

Presentation is not infrequently late with bone destruction already present.

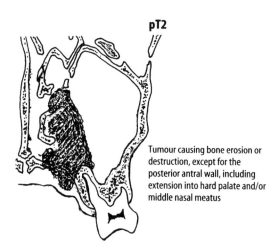

pT2

Tumour causing bone erosion or destruction, except for the posterior antral wall, including extension into hard palate and/or middle nasal meatus

Tumour invades any of the following: bone of posterior wall of maxillary sinus, subcutaneous tissues, skin of cheek, floor or medial wall of orbit, infratemporal fossa, pterygoid plates, ethmoid sinuses (Figs. 54, 55)

pT3

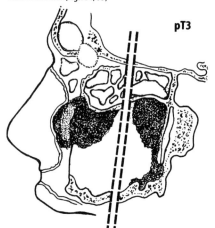

pT3

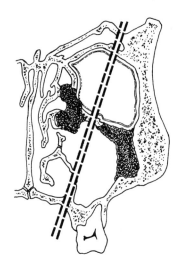

Figures 53–55. Maxillary sinus carcinoma.

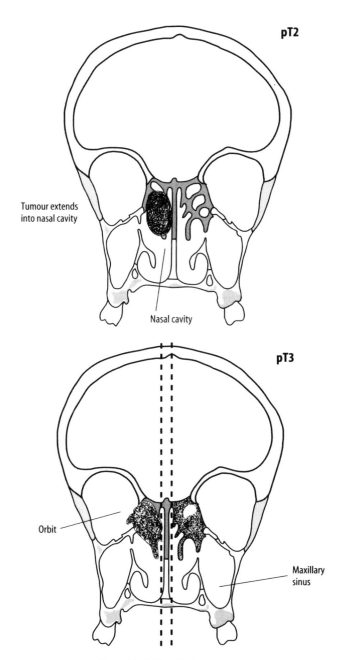

pT2

Tumour extends into nasal cavity

Nasal cavity

pT3

Orbit

Maxillary sinus

Figures 56, 57. Ethmoid sinus carcinoma.

5. Lymphovascular invasion

Present/absent.
Intra-/extratumoural.

6. Lymph nodes

Site/number/size/number involved/limit node/extracapsular spread.
Regional nodes: cervical.

pN0 no regional lymph node metastasis
pN1 metastasis in a single ipsilateral node ≤ 3 cm in greatest dimension
pN2 a. metastasis in a single ipsilateral node > 3 cm but ≤ 6 cm in greatest
      dimension
      b. metastasis in multiple ipsilateral nodes ≤ 6 cm in greatest dimension
      c. metastasis in bilateral or contralateral nodes ≤ 6 cm in greatest
      dimension
pN3 metastasis in a node > 6 cm in greatest dimension.

7. Excision margins

Distance (mm) to the nearest painted excision margin.

8. Other pathology

Malignant tumours are more common than benign in the paranasal sinuses with
the reverse being the case in the nasal cavity. Equivalent nasal cavity tumours
have a better prognosis. Markers are of use in differentiating carcinoma from
malignant melanoma and lymphoma. Fifty-five per cent of sinonasal malignancies occur in the maxillary sinus, 35% in the nasal cavity and 9% in the ethmoid
sinus. The majority of lesions (75%) are squamous cell carcinoma and its variants with adenocarcinoma representing only 5–10% of cases. About 10% of
patients present with nodal metastases.

Prognosis

Prognosis is strongly related to tumour stage. Treatment is by a combination of
surgery and radiotherapy with 5 year survival about 60%. Undifferentiated carcinoma has a very poor prognosis and histologically squamous and glandular
differentiation are precluded by definition. Undifferentiated carcinoma of
nasopharyngeal type is radiosensitive with remission in 80% and 10 year survival
in 40%.

9. Other malignancy

Lymphoma

— large B cell lymphoma; CD 20 positive.

— angiocentric T cell lymphoma (sinonasal NK (natural killer)/T cell lymphoma):

    destructive nasal/midline tumour.
    large areas of zonal necrosis.
    vasculocentric/destructive.
    polymorphic tumour cells (CD 56 positive/CD 3 ±) which may be hard to recognise amongst the inflammatory infiltrate.
    EBV associated.
    poor prognosis.

Plasmacytoma/myeloma

— development of myeloma may take a number of years.

— κ, λ light chain restriction and clinical evidence of myeloma, e.g. elevated ESR, serum immune paresis, Bence-Jones proteinuria, radiological lytic bone lesions.

Rhabdomyosarcoma (embryonal – children), angiosarcoma, fibrosarcoma, malignant fibrous histiocytoma, chondrosarcoma, osteosarcoma.

Olfactory neuroblastoma, primitive neuroectodermal tumour

— small, round blue cell tumour aggregates (± rosettes) in a vascular stroma with calcification. Tumours confined to the nasal cavity have a reasonable prognosis while those in the nasal cavity and paranasal sinuses an intermediate outlook. Extra-nasal/paranasal and visceral lesions are of poor prognosis. Treatment is by a combination of surgery and radiotherapy. Overall 5 year survival is 50–60% with a tendency for late recurrences. Variably S100 and GFAP positive immunohistochemistry aids in distinction from the differential diagnoses of malignant melanoma, lymphoma, plasmacytoma and embryonal/alveolar rhabdomyosarcoma.

Pituitary carcinoma

Chordoma

— locally destructive low-grade malignancy derived from notochordal remnants – characteristic vacuolated physaliphorous cells.

Malignant meningioma

Ewing's sarcoma, malignant teratoma

Laryngeal Carcinoma

1. Gross description

Specimen

— biopsy/hemi-/partial or total laryngectomy/neck dissection.
— size (cm) and weight (g).

Tumour

Site

supraglottic   30%
glottic   60%   } transglottic   5%
infraglottic   5%

Supraglottis: from the tip of the epiglottis to the true cords including the aryepiglottic folds, false vocal cords and ventricles.

Glottis: true cords and anterior commissure.

Subglottis: from the lower border of the true cords to the first tracheal cartilage.

Anterior/posterior/lateral(right, left)/commissural/ventricles/false cords.
Anterior glottis is the commonest site.

Size

— length × width × depth (cm) or maximum dimension (cm).

Appearance

— polypoid/verrucous/plaque/ulcerated/multifocal.

Edge

— circumscribed/irregular.

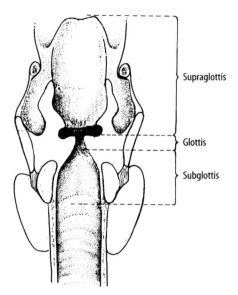

Figure 58. Larynx.

2. Histological type

Squamous cell carcinoma
— 90% of cases.
— large cell/small cell.
— keratinising/non-keratinising.

Verrucous squamous carcinoma
— exophytic, hyperkeratotic, pushing deep margin of cytologically bland bulbous processes arising in the glottis. Locally invasive, rarely metastatic, radiation may result in anaplastic change.

Papillary squamous carcinoma
— exophytic fronds, covered by in-situ type epithelium with focal invasion at the base.

Spindle cell carcinoma
— glottic, elderly, ± history of irradiation for previous carcinoma. A minor squamous element is present (in-situ or invasive) with a major variably pleomorphic fibrosarcoma-like component. Diffuse or focal cytokeratin positivity suggests that it is a metaplastic form of carcinoma. Prognosis is better if polypoid and superficial than infiltrative when the outlook is

poor. Distinguish from sarcoma and bizarre post-irradiation granulation tissue.

Basaloid squamous cell carcinoma
— nests of basaloid cells with peripheral palisading and necrosis: aggressive.

Undifferentiated carcinoma

Neuroendocrine carcinomas
— chromogranin/NSE/± CAM 5.2 positive.
— well differentiated – carcinoid tumour.
— moderately differentiated – atypical carcinoid tumour.
— poorly differentiated – small cell/large cell carcinoma.

Atypical carcinoid and large cell neuroendocrine carcinoma are commoner in the larynx than carcinoid tumour and are aggressive lesions with 50% mortality.

Adenocarcinoma
— salivary type, e.g. adenoid cystic, mucoepidermoid carcinomas of mucosal gland origin.
— adenocarcinoma of no specific type.

Metastatic carcinoma
— direct spread: thyroid, oesophagus.
— distant spread: malignant melanoma, kidney, breast, pancreas, colon, ovary, prostate.

3. Differentiation

Well/moderate/poor.

4. Extent of local tumour spread

Border: pushing/infiltrative.
Lymphocytic reaction: prominent/sparse.

Anterior
— mucous membrane, cricothyroid membrane, thyroid cartilage, thyroid gland, strap muscles, jugular vein.

Superior
— base of epiglottis, vestibular folds, pyriform fossa and limits.

Inferior
— trachea and limit.

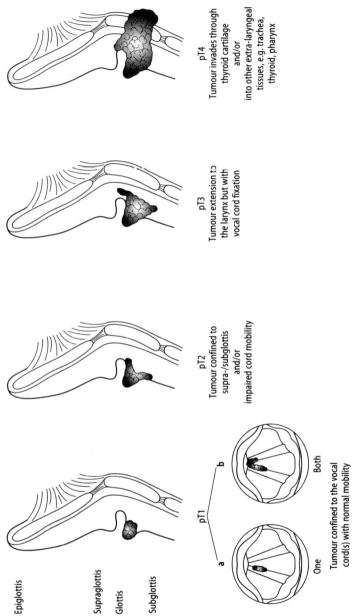

Figure 59. Laryngeal carcinoma: glottic.

Epiglottis

Supraglottis

Glottis

Subglottis

pT1
Tumour confined to the vocal cord(s) with normal mobility

a — One

b — Both

pT2
Tumour confined to supra-/subglottis and/or impaired cord mobility

pT3
Tumour extension to the larynx but with vocal cord fixation

pT4
Tumour invades through thyroid cartilage and/or into other extra-laryngeal tissues, e.g. trachea, thyroid, pharynx

pTis   carcinoma in-situ
pT1*   tumour confined to one subsite*, normal cord mobility
pT2*   tumour invades more than one subsite*, impaired cord mobility
pT3   tumour limited to larynx. Fixation of 1 or 2 cords
pT4   tumour through thyroid cartilage and/or extends beyond larynx to, e.g.
        trachea, soft tissues of neck, thyroid, oesophagus.

*Exact details depend on whether the tumour site is supraglottic, glottic or subglottic.

5. Lymphovascular invasion

Present/absent.
Intra-/extratumoural.

6. Lymph nodes

The incidence of nodal metastases at presentation varies according to the site of the primary tumour from glottic (< 10%) to supra-/infraglottic (30–50%). Well differentiated carcinomas are less likely to metastasise than poorly differentiated cancers.

Site/number/size/number involved/limit node/extracapsular spread.
Regional nodes: cervical.

pN0   no regional lymph nodes involved
pN1   metastasis in single ipsilateral node ≤ 3 cm diameter
pN2   metastasis in:
       a. single ipsilateral node > 3 cm diameter but ≤ 6 cm
       b. ipsilateral multiple nodes ≤ 6 cm
       c. bilateral, contralateral nodes ≤ 6 cm
pN3   metastasis in node > 6 cm diameter.

7. Excision margins

Distances (mm) to the tracheal limit, aryepiglottic fold and pre-laryngeal anterior fascia of infiltrating carcinoma and any mucosal dysplasia or carcinoma in-situ.

8. Other pathology

Laryngeal carcinoma is predominantly (> 95%) in males who smoke and are 50–60 years of age. Smokers and heavy voice users can develop keratosis with hoarseness and thickened white cords on laryngoscopy. A proportion may be associated with dysplasia and progression to carcinoma in-situ and eventually over a period of years squamous carcinoma. These premalignant changes can be treated by local excision, laser or irradiation. Carcinoma in-situ may be leukoplakic, erythroplakic or inapparent and biopsy is necessary.

Radionecrosis

— post-radiotherapy confluent necrosis which may lead to local airway obstruction and necessitate resection.

Concurrent carcinoma bronchus/oropharynx

— 10–15%.

Verrucous squamous cell carcinoma has to be distinguished from benign squamous epithelial papilloma and hyperplasia by its pushing deep margin. It can also co-exist with squamous carcinoma of usual type. Beware granular cell tumour with overlying pseudoepitheliomatous hyperplasia – the granular cells (Schwann cell origin) are S100 protein positive.

Juvenile laryngeal papillomatosis (multiple squamous papillomas of the upper respiratory tract) is a rare cause of squamous cell carcinoma, usually after radiotherapy.

Prognosis

Prognosis relates to tumour site, stage and histological grade. Early (pTis, pT1) glottic and supraglottic carcinoma may be treated by local excision, laser or radiotherapy. Advanced carcinoma, infraglottic and transglottic tumours usually necessitate laryngectomy supplemented by radiotherapy.

Site-related 5 year survival:

glottic	80%
supraglottic	65%
transglottic	50%
subglottic	40%.

Stage-related 5 year survival:

glottic	I	90%
	II	85%
	III	60%
	IV	< 5%.

Most glottic carcinomas are well to moderately differentiated while non-glottic carcinomas are more frequently moderately to poorly differentiated.

9. Other malignancy

Lymphoma/leukaemia

— primary MALToma or secondary to nodal/systemic disease.

— sinonasal (angiocentric) T/NK cell lymphoma.

Plasmacytoma/myeloma

— initially localised but generally becomes part of disseminated myeloma. Look for κ, λ light chain restriction and evidence of systemic disease (elevated ESR, serum immune paresis, Bence-Jones proteinuria, radiological lytic bone lesions).

Sarcoma, particularly low-grade chondrosarcoma and rhabdomyosarcoma (embryonal – childhood), occasionally angiosarcoma, liposarcoma, fibrosarcoma

Malignant melanoma

— primary or secondary (commoner). S100, HMB-45, melan-A positive.

Kaposi's sarcoma

— AIDS.

Salivary Gland Tumours

1. Gross description

Specimen

— parotid/submandibular/minor (oral).
— conservative superficial/radical parotidectomy, submandibulectomy, excision of oral tumour (sublingual glands, or minor salivary glands of mucosal origin), neck dissection.
— size (cm) and weight (g).

Tumour

Site

— salivary gland/nodal.
— bilateral: Warthin's tumour, pleomorphic adenoma, acinic cell tumour.

Size

— length × width × depth (cm) or maximum dimension (cm).

Appearance

— solid/cystic.
— mucoid/chondroid/necrotic/fleshy/scirrhous.

Edge

— circumscribed/irregular.

Gland

— intra-salivary lymph nodes/nerves.

2. Histological type (WHO)

Adenomas
— pleomorphic; 70% of salivary gland tumours, 80% in the parotid.
— myoepithelioma.
— basal cell.
— Warthin's tumour (adenolymphoma).
— oncocytoma.
— canalicular.
— sebaceous.
— ductal papilloma (inverted/intra-ductal/sialadenoma papilliferum).
— cystadenoma (papillary/mucinous).

Carcinomas
— acinic cell.
— mucoepidermoid: low-grade/well differentiated, high-grade/poorly differentiated.
— adenoid cystic: cribriform/tubular/solid.
— polymorphous low-grade.
— epithelial/myoepithelial.
— salivary duct.
— basal cell.
— sebaceous.
— oncocytic.
— papillary cystadenocarcinoma.
— mucinous.
— adenocarcinoma, no special type (NST).
— squamous.
— carcinoma in pleomorphic adenoma (ex-PSA) usually adenocarcinoma, no special type.
— myoepithelial.
— small cell.
— undifferentiated.
— carcinosarcoma.

Lymphoma
— extranodal lymphoma of salivary gland (MALToma).
— lymphoma of salivary gland nodes (nodal lymphoma).

Metastatic carcinoma
— squamous cell carcinoma of head and neck region and upper aerodigestive tract, malignant melanoma, renal cell carcinoma, lung and breast carcinoma, prostate, large bowel carcinomas. The metastasis is to adjacent or intra-

salivary lymph nodes and the enlargement mimics a primary lesion. Note that secondary carcinoma of the submaxillary region is commoner than a primary neoplasm.

3. Differentiation

Well/moderate/poor.

4. Extent of local tumour spread

Border: pushing/infiltrative.
— infiltrative margins are a useful diagnostic feature of malignancy in low-grade lesions, e.g. polymorphous low-grade adenocarcinoma.
Lymphocytic reaction: prominent/sparse.
Perineural space involvement particularly adenoid cystic carcinoma resulting in intractable facial pain.
Skin, subcutis.

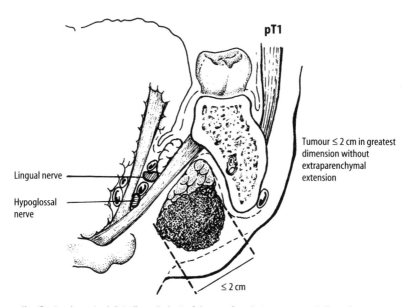

pT1

Lingual nerve

Hypoglossal nerve

Tumour ≤ 2 cm in greatest dimension without extraparenchymal extension

≤ 2 cm

Classification determined clinically on the basis of absence of paralysis or macroscopically on the basis of no extraparenchymal extension. Frontal section through the premolar region

Figure 60. Salivary gland carcinoma.

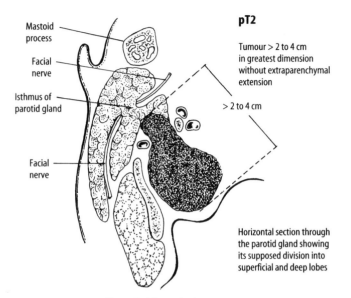

pT2

Tumour > 2 to 4 cm in greatest dimension without extraparenchymal extension

Mastoid process

Facial nerve

Isthmus of parotid gland

> 2 to 4 cm

Facial nerve

Horizontal section through the parotid gland showing its supposed division into superficial and deep lobes

Figure 61. Salivary gland carcinoma.

Tumour having extraparenchymal extension without seventh nerve involvement and/or more than 4 cm but not more than 6 cm in greatest dimension (Figs. 62, 63)

pT3

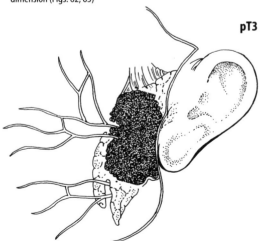

Figure 62. Salivary gland carcinoma.

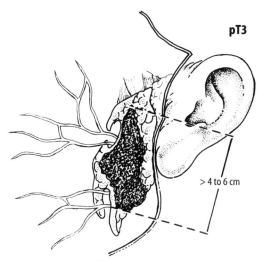

pT3

> 4 to 6 cm

Figure 63. Salivary gland carcinoma.

Tumour invades base of skull, seventh nerve, and/or exceeds 6 cm in greatest dimension (Figs. 64, 65)

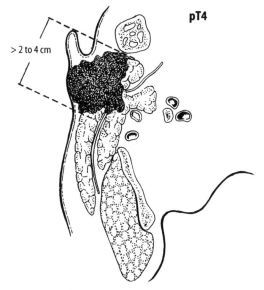

pT4

> 2 to 4 cm

Figure 64. Salivary gland carcinoma.

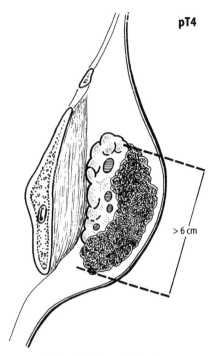

Figure 65. Salivary gland carcinoma.

pT1   tumour ≤2 cm, without extraparenchymal extension*
pT2   tumour > 2 to 4 cm, without extraparenchymal extension*
pT3   tumour with extraparenchymal extension, and/or > 4 to 6 cm
pT4   tumour invades base of skull, seventh nerve, and/or > 6 cm.

*Extraparenchymal extension is clinical or macroscopic evidence of invasion of skin, soft tissues, bone or nerve; microscopic evidence is not sufficient.

The TNM classification applies to major salivary glands: parotid, submandibular and sublingual. Minor salivary gland tumours (i.e. from the mucosa of the upper aerodigestive tract) are classified according to anatomical site, e.g. lip.

5. Lymphovascular invasion

Present/absent.
Intra-/extratumoural.

6. Lymph nodes

Intra-/extraglandular.
Site/number/size/number involved/limit node/extracapsular spread.
Regional nodes: cervical.

pN0   no regional lymph nodes involved
pN1   metastasis in single ipsilateral node ≤3cm
pN2   metastasis in:
      a. single ipsilateral node > 3 cm but ≤ 6 cm
      b. ipsilateral multiple nodes ≤ 6 cm
      c. bilateral or contralateral nodes ≤ 6 cm
pN3   metastasis in lymph node > 6 cm.

Regional nodes are the commonest site of metastasis followed by lungs and bone.

7. Excision margins

Distance (mm) to the nearest painted excision margin.

Pleomorphic adenomas should not be surgically enucleated as the irregular margin can lead to residual tumour and local recurrence.

8. Other pathology

Fine needle aspiration cytology has an important role to play in the primary diagnosis of salivary gland enlargement and is capable of designating benignity and malignancy in a majority of cases. It can indicate non-neoplastic disorders such as simple cysts, abscess and fatty infiltration. The separation of benign from malignant salivary tumours results in more appropriate surgery (superficial conservative versus radical parotidectomy) or the avoidance of it (lymphoma, secondary carcinoma). The experienced cytopathologist can in many cases obtain sufficient material to stipulate the tumour subtype. Some pitfalls are cystic lesions (simple cyst versus cystic salivary tumour, e.g. mucoepidermoid carcinoma, acinic cell tumour or metastatic squamous carcinoma), clear cell lesions (primary epithelial or myoepithelial tumour versus secondary renal, lung or thyroid carcinoma), metastases (primary squamous or mucoepidermoid carcinoma versus secondary squamous carcinoma), the onset of low grade lymphoma in lympho(myo-)epithelial sialadenitis and distinction from extranodal lymphoma and chronic sialadenitis. The technique is obviously reliant on representative sampling of the tumour and there can be a degree of cytological overlap between subtypes, e.g. pleomorphic adenoma, adenoid cystic carcinoma and polymorphous low-grade adenocarcinoma.

Necrotising sialometaplasia of minor salivary glands in the mouth and palate can mimic carcinoma, e.g. mucoepidermoid carcinoma. It presents as an ulcerating lesion in middle-aged men.

There is a higher incidence of carcinoma in minor salivary glands (e.g. polymorphous low-grade adenocarcinoma of the palate or floor of mouth): palate 44%, submaxillary glands 38%, parotid 17% of salivary carcinomas.

Salivary tumours with clear cells tend to be malignant, and must also be distinguished from secondary renal cell carcinoma. A wide range of salivary tumours can show clear cell differentiation: acinic cell, mucoepidermoid, epithelial-myoepithelial, sebaceous, clear cell carcinomas and malignant myoepithelioma. Abdominal investigation may be necessary to distinguish metastatic renal cell carcinoma (vascular stroma, glycogen/fat-rich cells), S100, melan-A and HMB-45 clear cell melanoma, and thyroglobulin clear cell thyroid carcinoma. Primary clear cell carcinoma of low-grade arises in minor salivary glands, has uniform clear cells in a dense hyalinising stroma and is locally infiltrative.

Acinic cell tumours have deceptively bland granular cells with a variably solid, follicular or microcystic pattern but can still infiltrate and metastasise; more aggressive pleomorphic variants occur. Overall recurrence can be seen in 10–30% and death in about 6%. Peak incidence is in the third decade of life but, like mucoepidermoid carcinoma, acinic cell tumours are seen in childhood and teenage years. Gross invasion, cellular pleomorphism and incomplete primary excision are adverse indicators.

Mucoepidermoid carcinoma shows a spectrum of epidermoid and mucous cells in varying proportions (mucin stains may be necessary). Well-differentiated lesions may be largely cystic with only mural tumour. Poorly differentiated (high-grade) lesions are more solid, squamoid and infiltrative. The mucin and keratin can be extruded into the interstitium causing an inflammatory reaction. Tumour grade dictates prognosis.

Adenoid cystic carcinoma forms 5% of salivary gland neoplasms but 20% of the carcinomas with equal distribution between the parotid and minor glands (palate). It shows biphasic cell differentiation (epithelial/myoepithelial: cytokeratin/S100 and smooth muscle actin positive) and biphasic histochemical staining of PAS positive luminal mucus and alcian blue positive matrix. It typically shows indolent perineural spread with late lymph node involvement; it is slow growing but highly malignant and locally recurrent. Prognosis relates to a solid growth pattern, stage and incomplete primary excision, with radical surgery being the treatment of choice.

Polymorphous low-grade adenocarcinoma is characterised by cellular uniformity and architectural diversity (solid/cribriform/single cell/ductal/papillary): palate (second commonest after adenoid cystic carcinoma), local recurrence in 21%, nodal metastases in 6.5% and distant metastases in 1.8%. A somewhat more aggressive tumour is the related low-grade papillary adenocarcinoma.

Epithelial/myoepithelial carcinoma recurs in one-third of cases, comprising ductal cells and outer clear myoepithelial cells in a biphasic pattern. Death can occur in 7% and nuclear atypia in > 20% of cells is an adverse prognostic factor. Occasionally one element dedifferentiates resulting in carcinomatous or sarcomatous overgrowth.

Myoepithelial carcinoma is a spindle cell lesion with mitotic activity, nuclear atypia, necrosis and invasion.

Ductal carcinoma resembles high-grade ductal carcinoma in-situ of the breast. It shows aggressive behaviour with poor prognosis: 70% die within 3 years.

Patients are > 50 years of age and the male to female ratio is 3:1 with parotid being the main site.

Primary squamous cell carcinomas (5–10%) occur mostly in the parotid gland and are aggressive with 5 year survival rates of 40%. Metastases to the parotid gland from other sites must be excluded, commonly upper aerodigestive tract or skin. Some primary lesions represent mucoepidermoid carcinoma or carcinoma within a mixed tumour.

Carcinoma in pleomorphic adenoma (3–4% of cases) is unusual and manifests itself as regrowth or facial pain in an existing lesion present for 15–30 years (9.5% risk after 15 years). In descending order of frequency the malignancy is carcinoma (adenocarcinoma of no specific type, poorly differentiated ductal and undifferentiated), malignant myoepithelioma, carcinosarcoma and metastasising pleomorphic adenoma. Prognosis relates strongly to the degree of extension of the malignancy beyond the capsule of the original benign tumour.

Basal cell carcinoma is the malignant counterpart of basal cell adenoma except that it shows infiltration, perineural and vascular invasion. It occurs in the patient's parotid gland, 50–60 years of age.

Carcinosarcoma, small cell carcinoma and undifferentiated carcinoma (some of which are EBV related similar to nasopharyngeal carcinoma) have poor prognosis.

Most low-grade tumours of mucoepidermoid or acinic cell type can be treated by superficial parotidectomy whereas more radical surgery with sacrifice of the facial nerve is needed for large (> 4 cm), higher-grade or advanced carcinomas. Submaxillary tumours are treated by total removal of the gland.

Prognosis

Prognosis relates to tumour stage, anatomical location and histological type and grade.

— minor salivary gland tumours have a higher incidence of recurrence and metastases than equivalent parotid lesions.

— examples of 5 year survival rates: low-grade mucoepidermoid, 90–95%; high-grade mucoepidermoid, 50–60%; squamous cell carcinoma, 40%.

— histological type:
  better prognosis: low-grade mucoepidermoid/acinic cell tumours
  worse prognosis: high-grade mucoepidermoid/acinic cell tumours; adenoid cystic carcinoma, malignant mixed tumour; salivary duct carcinoma, squamous carcinoma.

9. Other malignancy

Rhabdomyosarcoma
— children. Note that mucoepidermoid and acinic cell tumours can also typically occur in childhood and young adults.

Malignant fibrous histiocytoma, fibrosarcoma, malignant peripheral nerve sheath tumour

— adults

Lymphoma

— 2–5% of salivary gland neoplasms.

— 20% have Sjögren's syndrome or LESA (lymphoepithelial or myoepithelial) sialadenitis.

— one third are diffuse large B cell lymphoma, of nodal or parenchymal origin.

— one third are follicular lymphoma, usually of nodal origin.

— one third are MALToma; LESA has a ×40 increased risk of developing low-grade lymphoma and 15–20% do so over a variable period of 5-20 years. MALToma is characterised by lymphoepithelial lesions surrounded by broad haloes or sheets of centrocyte-like (marginal zone/monocytoid) B cells. Other features include monotypic plasma cells and follicular colonisation. High-grade transformation to large cell lymphoma can occur. PCR demonstration of clonality does not reliably predict those lymphoid lesions that will progress to clinical lymphoma.

Thyroid Gland Tumours

1. Gross description

Specimen

— fine needle aspirate/partial or total thyroidectomy/
  left or right lobectomy/isthmectomy
— size (cm) and weight (g).

Tumour

Site

— left/right lobe, isthmus,multifocal.

Size

— length × width × depth (cm) or maximum dimension (cm).

Appearance

— solid/cystic/calcified/haemorrhagic/pale/tan/
  papillary.

Edge

— circumscribed/irregular.

Gland

— uniform, nodular, atrophic, pale in colour.

2. Histological type (WHO)

Follicular adenoma
— usual type: macrofollicular; microfollicular; embryonal/fetal.
— variants: hyalinising trabecular; oxyphil (Hurthle).

Papillary carcinoma
— usual type: psammomatous.
— variants with worse prognosis:
        diffuse sclerosing.
        tall cell.
        columnar cell.
        trabecular.
        diffuse follicular.
— variants with better prognosis:
        encapsulated.
        papillary microcarcinoma (< 1 cm).
— variants with usual prognosis:
        follicular/solid/oxyphil (Hurthle).

Follicular carcinoma
— widely invasive:
        follicular/trabecular/solid patterns.
        cytological features of malignancy, e.g. atypia/mitoses/necrosis.
— minimally invasive:
        encapsulated – angioinvasive with potential for metastases or capsular invasion with equivocal potential for metastases.
— variants: oxyphil (Hurthle)/clear cell.

Undifferentiated (anaplastic) carcinoma
— old age; 5–10% of cases; rapid growth with involvement of vital neck structures and death in 6 months. Treatment (surgery, radiotherapy) is usually palliative.
— spindle/squamoid/giant cells ± cartilage/osseous metaplasia ± a differentiated component i.e. evidence of origin from a more usual thyroid carcinoma, e.g. papillary carcinoma.

Poorly differentiated carcinoma
— "insular" carcinoma – large solid nests of small round uniform tumour cells (medullary-like); older age; grossly invasive; aggressive behaviour.
— also includes carcinomas with solid, scirrhous and trabecular patterns and/or of tall cell or columnar type either alone or as part of a carcinoma of more usual type.

Small cell carcinoma

Medullary carcinoma

— 5–10% of cases, including mixed medullary/follicular.

Miscellaneous

— signet ring carcinoma, squamous carcinoma, mucoepidermoid carcinoma, carcinoma with thymus-like differentiation.

Metastatic carcinoma

— direct spread: upper aerodigestive tract, metastases in cervical lymph nodes.
— distant spread: malignant melanoma, breast, kidney, lung. Renal cell carcinoma can mimic primary clear cell carcinoma of thyroid; renal carcinoma may be multiple, clear cells with glycogen and fat, a vascular stroma with haemorrhage and thyroglobulin negative.

3. Differentiation

Well/moderate/poor.

4. Extent of local tumour spread

Border: pushing/infiltrative.
Lymphocytic reaction: prominent/sparse.
Perineural space involvement.
Solitary/multifocal, one or two lobes.
Involvement of lesion capsule, extracapsular spread.
Involvement of thyroid capsule, extrathyroid spread.

pT1   tumour ≤ 1 cm in greatest dimension*
pT2   1 cm<tumour ≤ 4 cm in greatest dimension*
pT3   tumour > 4 cm in greatest dimension*
pT4   tumour of any size extending beyond the thyroid capsule.

*Limited to thyroid.

All categories may be subdivided: (a) solitary tumour, (b) multifocal tumour.

5. Lymphovascular invasion

Present/absent.
Intra-/extratumoural.

Papillary carcinoma tends to lymphatic spread, follicular carcinoma to vascular spread.

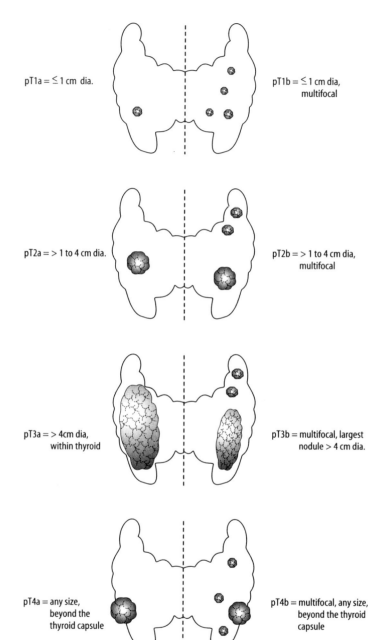

pT1a = ≤ 1 cm dia.

pT1b = ≤ 1 cm dia, multifocal

pT2a = > 1 to 4 cm dia.

pT2b = > 1 to 4 cm dia, multifocal

pT3a = > 4cm dia, within thyroid

pT3b = multifocal, largest nodule > 4 cm dia.

pT4a = any size, beyond the thyroid capsule

pT4b = multifocal, any size, beyond the thyroid capsule

Figure 66. Thyroid carcinoma.

Histopathology Reporting

6. Lymph nodes

Site/number/size/number involved/limit node/extracapsular spread.
Regional nodes: cervical, upper mediastinal

pN0   no regional lymph nodes involved
pN1   metastasis in regional lymph node(s)
    a. ipsilateral cervical
    b. bilateral, midline, or contralateral cervical or mediastinal.

7. Excision margins

Distances (mm) to the nearest painted capsule and surgical excision margins.

8. Other pathology

Thyroid carcinoma is commoner in females (2.5:1) with the most frequent subtypes being papillary carcinoma (60%) and follicular carcinoma (20%). Previous irradiation predisposes to papillary carcinoma. Papillary carcinoma occurs in younger patients (average age 40 years), is multifocal in a significant proportion of cases (20%) and shows a tendency to lymphatic and lymph node spread (40–50%). Despite this, prognosis is excellent with a low disease-related mortality of about 5%. Papillary carcinoma may undergo cystic change with only residual mural tumour – a potential pitfall on fine needle aspiration cytology. Invasion is not necessary for its diagnosis, which is mainly cytological. Diagnostic features are a combination of optically clear (orphan Annie) ground glass, over-lapping nuclei with longitudinal grooves and nuclear pseudoinclusions. Stromal (not intrafollicular) and tumour cell related psammoma bodies are present (50% of cases) and the stroma may be hyalinised, calcified or ossified. Architectural patterns are papillary, follicular or solid. The cells are thyroglobulin, cytokeratin and vimentin positive. Variants with an excellent prognosis are encapsulated carcinoma (totally surrounded by a capsule) and papillary microcarcinoma (< 1 cm diameter: nodal metastases in 30%). Diffuse sclerosing (sclerosing, numerous psammoma bodies, solid foci, squamous metaplasia, heavy lympho-cytic infiltrate), diffuse follicular, tall cell (older patients, papillary, oncocytic cell with height twice the width) and columnar cell (nuclear stratification) and trabecular variants have significantly worse outlooks with a high risk of lymph node and distant metastases and disease-related mortality of up to 25%.

Follicular carcinoma tends to be in older patients than papillary carcinoma (50–60 years), unifocal and spreads via the blood stream to lung and bone. Minimally invasive carcinoma has an excellent prognosis with lymph node metastases in<5% of cases whereas widely invasive tumour has a mortality of 30–35%. Multiple blocks (say 8–10) of the lesion and its capsule are required for the distinction between follicular adenoma and minimally invasive follicular carcinoma; diagnostic criteria are invasion of the capsule and/or its vessels. Cytological appearances of the epithelium are not helpful as adenomas may be markedly atypical, although solid, trabecular and microfollicular growth patterns can be a low-power clue. Carcinoma often has a thick, partly desmoplastic fibrous capsule and its full width must be traversed to qualify as invasion. The invasive tumour front may then form a second fibrotic interface with the parenchyma giving a dumbbell type of distribution. Vascular invasion, which is a more reliable indicator of malignancy, requires vessels to be:

a. within or outside the capsule, i.e. extratumoural,
b. of venous rather than capillary calibre with a definite muscular wall and endothelial lining, and
c. partially or completely plugged by tumour in the lumen with a definite point of attachment to the vessel wall.

Note that capsular invasion needs to be distinguished from rupture following fine needle aspiration cytology which often shows organising haemorrhage and a reparative response. Ultrasound and isotope scan examinations are combined with fine needle aspiration cytology in the investigation of a wide range of thyroid enlargement. Cytology can be diagnostic in:

— inflammatory/autoimmune goitres:
    Hashimoto's thyroiditis (lymphocytes, Askanazy epithelial cells, colloid poor).
    de Quervain's thyroiditis (lymphocytes, giant cells, degenerate follicular cells).
    Riedel's struma (spindle cells, scant aspirate).
    abscess (polymorph rich).
— simple goitre: multinodular colloid/adenomatous (characteristically colloid rich/cell poor).
— simple thyroid cyst: watery colloid and macrophages, scanty follicular cells.
— solitary, solid thyroid nodule: papillary carcinoma and medullary carcinoma (see above and below).
    Adenoma and minimally invasive follicular carcinoma cannot be distinguished on fine needle aspiration cytology. They are designated follicular lesion or neoplasm and are recognised by a variable cell rich/colloid poor pattern usually distinguishing them from simple goitres. Surgical excision is necessary for the histological assessment of capsular and vascular invasion.
— malignant goitre:
    widely invasive follicular carcinoma (cytological features of malignancy).
    malignant lymphoma (dispersed atypical lymphoid cells, lymphoglandular bodies).
    anaplastic carcinoma (spindle/giant cells with atypia).

A higher proportion of Hurthle cell neoplasms are malignant than follicular neoplasms of usual type. Once again capsular and vascular invasion are the hallmarks of malignancy. Hurthle cell carcinomas are aggressive with 5 year mortality rates of 20–40%. Follicular carcinomas are thyroglobulin, cytokeratin and vimentin positive.

Medullary carcinoma (C-cell differentiation) is in the majority of cases (80%) sporadic and unifocal. The hereditary forms occur in younger patients, can be multifocal and bilateral, associated with C-cell hyperplasia, C-cell tumourlets and the multiple endocrine neoplasia (MEN) syndromes types II and III. Its morphology is heterogeneous, but usually comprises polygonal or plump spindle cells with a nested, trabecular or solid pattern. The hyalinised stroma can be calcified and is typically positive for amyloid and the cells are CEA, calcitonin and chromogranin positive. Lymph node metastases are seen in 30–60% of cases but 5 year survival is 80%. High serum calcitonin levels are associated with an adverse prognosis. Family members should be genetically screened to establish the hereditary cases (autosomal dominant) and prophylactic thyroidectomy can be offered to affected children. Treatment is surgical with radio-/chemotherapy of limited use.

Poorly differentiated carcinoma (70% 5 year survival) has a prognosis inter-mediate between that of usual thyroid carcinoma (90–95% 5 year survival) and anaplastic carcinoma. It is more frequently associated with old age, lymph node metastases and extrathyroid extension.

Anaplastic (syn. undifferentiated or sarcomatoid) carcinoma requires immunohistochemistry to distinguish it from high-grade lymphoma, malignant melanoma and angiosarcoma:

carcinoma	low molecular weight cytokeratin positive
lymphoma	CD 45, CD 20 (B) , CD 3 (T)
melanoma	S100, HMB-45, melan-A
angiosarcoma	CD 31, factor VIII positive.

Prognosis

Prognosis is worse in:

— male patients.
— patients > 50–60 years of age.
— large tumours:<1.5 cm, excellent; > 3.5–5 cm, poor.
— multicentric tumours.
— unencapsulated tumours.
— widely invasive tumours with extrathyroid extension.

Low-grade malignancy
— minimally invasive follicular carcinoma.
— papillary carcinoma.

Intermediate-grade malignancy
— widely invasive follicular carcinoma.
— medullary carcinoma.
— poorly differentiated carcinoma.
— lymphoma.

High-grade malignancy
— undifferentiated carcinoma
— angiosarcoma.

Most solitary thyroid neoplasms are treated by lobectomy ± isthmectomy or subtotal thyroidectomy. Total thyroidectomy tends to be reserved for worse prognosis subtypes of papillary carcinoma, widely invasive follicular carcinoma, medullary carcinoma (particulary if familial) and undifferentiated carcinoma (if operable). Other treatment modalities are tumour suppression by administration of thyroxine or radioactive iodine (papillary and follicular carcinoma) and radiotherapy (incompletely excised carcinomas or undifferentiated carcinoma).

9. Other malignancy

Lymphoma
— lymphocytic/Hashimoto's thyroiditis/MALToma.
— low-grade: centrocyte-like cells, lymphoepithelial lesions, follicle loss/ destruction.
— high-grade: blast cells.

The majority of lesions are large cell and there is some evidence for progression from Hashimoto's thyroiditis through low-grade to high-grade MALToma. Clinical onset can be rapid with compression of neck structures.

Overall 5 year survival is 50–80% and spread can occur to other MALT sites, e.g. gut. Advanced age, size (> 10 cm) and stage of disease can worsen 5 year survival rates to 40%.

Primary Hodgkin's disease is extremely rare.

Plasmacytoma
— as part of systemic myeloma: elevated ESR, serum immune paresis, Bence-Jones proteinuria, radiological lytic bone lesions.

Angiosarcoma
— overlaps with undifferentiated carcinoma – a pleomorphic tumour with vasoformative areas in elderly patients. Endothelial markers (CD31, factor VIII) are required for confirmation.

Respiratory and Mediastinal Cancer

Lung Carcinoma

Malignant Mesothelioma

Mediastinal Cancer

Lung
Carcinoma

1. Gross description

Specimen

— exfoliative or aspiration cytology/bronchial biopsy/thoracoscopic biopsy/wedge resection/ sleeve resection/segmentectomy/(bi-)lobectomy/ pneumonectomy (extra-/intrapericardial).

— resection can be either open or thoracoscopic.

— size (cm) and weight (g)/number of fragments.

Tumour

Site

— central (main/segmental bronchus):<2 cm or ≥ 2 cm from carina; RUL/RML/RLL/LUL/LLL.

— peripheral (parenchymal/pleural).

Size

— length × width × depth (cm) or maximum dimension (cm).

Squamous carcinomas can attain a large size and remain localised whereas small cell carcinomas can be small primary lesions but with extensive local and distant spread.

Appearance

— necrosis/haemorrhage/mucoid/cavitation.

— polypoid/nodular/ulcerated/stenotic.

— endobronchial/bronchial/extrabronchial.

Squamous cell carcinoma frequently cavitates, central carcinoid is polypoid or nodular, small cell carcinoma is submucosal and bronchostenotic or shows extrinsic compression.

Edge

— circumscribed/irregular.

Pulmonary changes

— scar: peripheral adenocarcinoma.
— fibrosis/asbestosis.
— partial and hilar or total: abscess/pneumonia; bronchiectasis; atelectasis.

2. Histological type (WHO)

Squamous carcinoma

— 50% of cases; requires nuclear stratification, intercellular bridges, ± keratinisation.
— large cell/small cell.
— keratinising/non-keratinising.
— spindle cell (see carcinosarcoma): cytokeratin positive ± vimentin positive.
— basaloid: poor prognosis, nests of basaloid cells with necrosis.
— papillary: cytological atypia distinguishes it from papilloma.

Small cell carcinoma

— 25% of cases; small round/fusiform nuclei ($\times$ 2–3 lymphocyte size) with granular chromatin, moulding and an inconspicuous nucleolus, DNA crush and vessel artefact, fir tree hyaline stroma, apoptosis and mitoses. The nuclear features are the diagnostic characteristic of small cell carcinoma. Note that there can be a scattered population of large bizarre (polyploid) cells.
— oat.
— intermediate: larger nucleus/more cytoplasm.
— combined: + non-small cell component.

Adenocarcinoma

— 15% (50% in females) of cases; 35% endobronchial, 65% are peripheral, 75% involve the pleura at presentation; higher resectability rates than squamous carcinoma.
— acinar.
— papillary.
— solid with mucus formation ($\geqslant$5 PAS/AB-diastase positive cells in at least two high-power fields).
— bronchioloalveolar: peripheral; single/multiple or pneumonic infiltrate with lepidic spread along alveolar walls and no stromal, vascular or pleural invasion.

Large cell carcinoma

— no evidence of squamous or glandular differentiation although they probably represent poorly differentiated forms of these.

— giant cell, clear cell, lymphoepithelioma-like, basaloid and neuroendocrine variants.

  In primary clear cell carcinoma (rare) exclude clear cell change in squamous or adenocarcinoma, secondary thyroid, salivary or renal cell carcinoma, malignant melanoma and benign clear cell (sugar) tumour of lung (HMB-45 and glycogen positive).

Miscellaneous

— adenosquamous carcinoma, pulmonary blastoma, carcinosarcoma (all with mixed differentiation).

— pulmonary endodermal tumour or adenocarcinoma of foetal type.

— pulmonary blastoma: adults, peripheral, solitary, large; well-differentiated foetal-type tubular glands in a cellular embryonal stroma; poor prognosis.

— carcinosarcoma: pulmonary or polypoid bronchial mass; squamous (or large cell/adeno-) carcinoma with fibrosarcoma-like spindle cells (cytokeratin positive representing carcinoma with stromal metaplasia of varying degrees) ± heterologous mesenchymal differentiation, e.g. cartilage, bone, striated muscle; poor prognosis. Overlaps with pleomorphic (spindle cell) carcinoma.

Note that only about 40% of primary lung carcinomas are of homogeneous histological type and mixed differentiation and patterns are reasonably common, e.g. squamous and small cell components, acinar and papillary adenocarcinoma.

Neuroendocrine tumours

— 5% of primary pulmonary neoplasms.

— NSE, chromogranin, synaptophysin positive.

— argyrophil (Grimelius) positive.

— carcinoid: central/peripheral; nodal metastasis in 5–15%, 70% 10 year survival.

— atypical carcinoid: central/peripheral; spindle cells; cell atypia; necrosis (usually punctate); mitoses 2–10/10 5/10 high power fields; nodal metastasis in 50%.

— large cell neuroendocrine carcinoma: 34% 5 year survival: significant numbers of endocrine cells present rather than just a non-small cell carcinoma with focal endocrine differentiation.

Salivary gland-type adenocarcinoma

— bronchial mucosal gland origin.

— adenoid cystic carcinoma: indolent growth but prognosis is poor with late metastases to nodes and lung parenchyma common.

— mucoepidermoid carcinoma: prognosis is determined by the histological grade.

Metastatic carcinoma

— multiple/bilateral/well defined/rapid growth/nodular or mass lesions: breast, gut, kidney, sarcoma, malignant melanoma, ovary, germ cell tumour.

— lymphangitis carcinomatosis: stomach, breast, pancreas, prostate, lung.

— cavitation in a mass lesion: squamous carcinoma, gut, leiomyosarcoma.

— endobronchial polypoid mass: breast, kidney, gut, sarcoma.

— vasculo-embolic: breast, stomach, liver, choriocarcinoma.

— bronchioloalveolar pattern of spread: gut, pancreas (metastases are more pleomorphic and necrotic than bronchioloalveolar carcinoma); prostate.

In limited biopsy material a positive diagnostic yield is increased by multiple biopsies (5 or 6) examined histologically through at least three levels, the aim being to designate basic neoplastic categories, e.g. primary versus secondary, small cell versus non-small cell carcinoma, neuroendocrine (carcinoid) lesions and lymphoma. This is due to tumour heterogeneity and poor observer agreement at subclassifying moderately to poorly differentiated cancers of non-small cell type. Designation of small cell carcinoma is reasonably robust and it must be distinguished from carcinoid, malignant lymphoma and small cell variant of squamous carcinoma. The presence of carcinoma in-situ and a lack of demonstrable invasion is not unusual in biopsies and must be correlated with the clinical findings. It may be representative of the lesion if derived from a segment of thickened, irregular mucosa. However, in the presence of an obvious bronchoscopic abnormality and radiological mass lesion it usually represents the edge of an invasive carcinoma. Squamous metaplasia may be entirely non-specific, associated with a carcinoma or overlying a lesion such as carcinoid tumour or small cell carcinoma when it can be atypical and suggest a cytological diagnosis of non-small cell carcinoma in brushings material. Sometimes the main biopsy fragments are negative but dyscohesive clusters of cytologically malignant cells lie in mucus separate from the epithelial surface. Close correlation with cytology preparations, e.g. bronchial brushings and washings and transbronchial fine needle aspirates increases diagnostic yield and accuracy with agreement rates of 70–90% for small cell carcinoma, well-differentiated squamous and adenocarcinomas. Cytology is particularly helpful where there is biopsy sampling error, extensive biopsy crush artefact, e.g. small cell carcinoma and extrabronchial or peripheral cancers. Cell yield and preservation can be high when biopsy fragments are negative or uninterpretable. Conversely the tissue pattern and capability for immunohistochemistry in a positive biopsy can be helpful in specific situations, e.g. primary versus secondary adenocarcinoma, small cell carcinoma versus lymphoma. Thoracoscopic biopsy is used for patients suspected of having malignancy but in whom bronchial biopsy and cytology are negative and in suspected bilateral disseminated disease. Other sources of a positive diagnosis are radiologically guided fine needle aspiration of peripheral lung tumours, pleural fluid cytology and fine needle aspiration cytology or biopsy of cervical or supraclavicular lymph nodes. These approaches should be considered when the tumour is difficult to diagnose by conventional means, the patient is unfit for bronchoscopy or there is suspected disseminated disease. Thus a tissue diagnosis is obtained providing staging information, a basis for adjuvant therapy and exclusion of unrelated non-respiratory malignancy, e.g. malignant lymphoma.

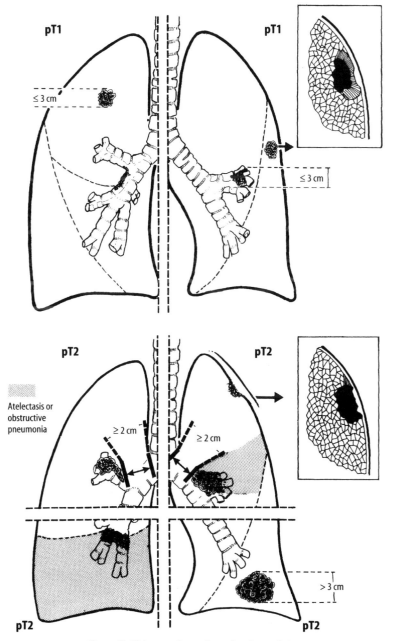

Figures 67, 68. Lung carcinoma. For explanation see below.

3. Differentiation

Well/moderate/poor.
Small cell carcinoma and large cell carcinoma are by definition poorly differentiated.

4. Extent of local tumour spread

Border: pushing/infiltrative.
Lymphocytic reaction: prominent/sparse.
Distance to the proximal bronchial limit (mm).
Distance to the mediastinal limit (mm).
Distance to the pleura (mm).

— visceral pleural invasion is recognised by infiltration of the inner elastin layer in the submesothelial plane. Note that the pleura can be distorted without actual true invasion and use of an elastin stain is helpful.

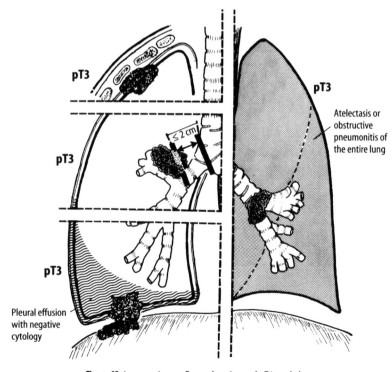

Figure 69. Lung carcinoma. For explanation and pT4 see below.

Distance to the pericardium (mm).
Mucosa, cartilage plates, parenchyma.
Tumour necrosis.

pTx   positive cytology
pTis carcinoma in-situ
pT1   tumour ≤ 3 cm diameter, surrounded by lung/visceral pleura and not inva-
      sive proximal to a lobar bronchus
pT2   tumour > 3 cm diameter or involves main bronchus 2 cm or more distal
      to the carina, or visceral pleura. Partial atelectasis, extending to hilum but
      not the entire lung
pT3   tumour of any size invading chest wall, diaphragm, mediastinal pleura,
      parietal pericardium or tumour of main bronchus<2 cm distal to the
      carina or total atelectasis
pT4   tumour of any size invading the mediastinum, heart, great vessels, trachea,
      oesophagus, vertebral body, carina, or, tumour with malignant pleural effu-
      sion. Separate tumour nodules in the same lobe.

Some 60–75% of lung cancers are incurable at presentation due to extensive local
or distant spread with symptoms developing late in the disease course. Spread
is by direct extension along the bronchus (proximally and distally), direct into
the lung parenchyma and to the mediastinum and pleura when diaphragm and
chest wall may be involved. Distant metastases are commonly seen in the liver,
lung elsewhere (by lymphovascular or aerogenous spread), adrenals, bone, kidney
and CNS (particuarly adenocarcinoma). A majority of small cell carcinomas have
extensive metastatic spread at the time of diagnosis.

5. Lymphovascular invasion

Present/absent.
Intra-/extratumoural.
Common (80%) in lung cancer and along with nodal metastases is an adverse
prognostic indicator.

6. Lymph nodes

Site/number/size/number involved/limit node/extracapsular spread.
Regional nodes: intrathoracic, scalene, supraclavicular

pN0   no regional lymph node metastasis
pN1   metastasis in ipsilateral peribronchial/hilar/intrapulmonary nodes
pN2   metastasis in ipsilateral mediastinal/subcarinal nodes
pN3   metastasis in contralateral mediastinal, contralateral hilar, ipsi-/contralat-
      eral scalene or supraclavicular nodes.

Cervical, scalene or mediastinal lymph node fine needle aspiration or biopsy is
sometimes used to establish a diagnosis of carcinoma in patients suspected of having a malignancy but in whom bronchial biopsy and cytology are negative, when it
represents recurrent disease, or who are medically unfit for invasive procedures.

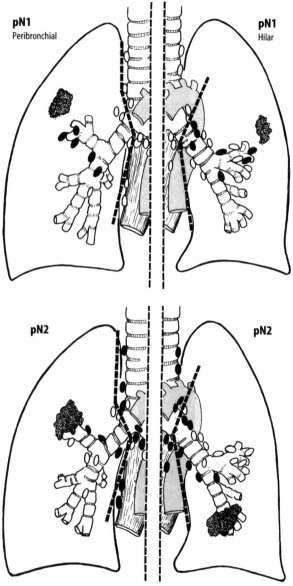

pN1 Metastasis in ipsilateral peribronchial and/or ipsilateral hilar lymph nodes
and/or intrapulmonary nodes including involvement by direct extension
(Fig. 70)

pN1
Peribronchial

pN1
Hilar

pN2

pN2

pN2 Metastasis in ipsilateral mediastinal and/or subcarinal lymph nodes

Figures 70, 71. Lung carcinoma. For explanation see above.

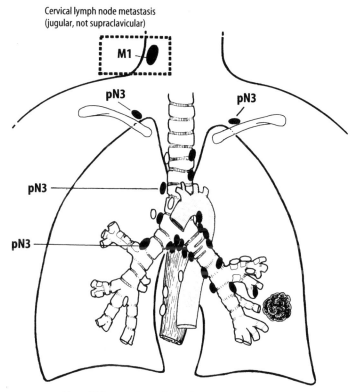

pN3 Metastasis in contralateral mediastinal, contralateral hilar, ipsilateral or contralateral
scalene or supraclavicular lymph node(s) (Fig. 72)

Figure 72. Lung carcinoma. For explanation and pT4 see above.

7. Excision margins

Distances (mm) to the proximal bronchial, vascular and mediastinal limits and
pleura.

The presence of significant dysplasia at the bronchial mucosal limit can be a
marker of potential local recurrence.

8. Other pathology

Atelectasis
Bronchiectasis
Pneumonia
— suppurative   } the extent of change helps determine pT stage.
— lipoid (endogenous)

Lymphangitis carcinomatosa: can be diagnosed on transbronchial biopsy and is characterised by involvement of peribronchial and perivascular lymphatics.

Asbestos bodies/asbestosis/mesothelioma: 5% of lung cancer deaths.

Scar/fibrosis in lung periphery: adenocarcinoma.

Lung cancer is multiple (either synchronous or metachronous) in up to 5% of cases and associated with independent cancers of the head and neck region in 10–20% of cases.

Metastatic carcinoma may be single or multifocal, diffuse or nodular, endo-bronchial, parenchymal, lymphovascular, vasculo-embolic or pleural. Knowledge of the clinical history and direct comparison of morphology with the primary tumour are important. This can be supplemented by specific immune markers, e.g. thyroglobulin, prostate specific antigen, CA 125 (ovary), ER/GCDFP-15 (breast), surfactant antibody (50% of lung adenocarcinomas). Surgical resection of germ cell tumour and carcinomatous (e.g. colorectum) pulmonary metastases is not infrequent, the appearances of which can be greatly altered by adjuvant therapy: tumour necrosis, inflammation, fibrosis and tissue maturation. Similarly chemotherapy of metastatic osteosarcoma can result in pulmonary nodules of mature bone with no residual malignant tissue.

Atypical adenomatous hyperplasia (usually <5mm dia) of adjacent lung parenchyma is regarded as a precursor of malignancy and is seen in 10% of resected lung carcinomas especially peripheral or bronchioloalveolar carcinoma (BAC). BAC is either of bronchial goblet cell, type II pneumocyte or peripheral Clara cell origin and is categorised as non-mucinous (solitary, good prognosis, 60–75% of cases) or mucinous (multifocal, bilateral,worse prognosis). Surfactant antibody positivity is useful for distinguishing from secondary carcinoma, e.g. large bowel. BAC has a slightly better prognosis than other lung cancers.

Extrapulmonary effects: e.g. small cell carcinoma and Cushings syndrome (ACTH), carcinoid syndrome, diabetes insipidus (ADH), gynaecomastia.

Immunophenotype

— small cell carcinoma:
    ± neurone specific enolase, ± chromogranin, ± CAM 5.2 (paranuclear dot reactivity). Immunonegative in 25% of cases.

— squamous cell carcinoma:
    cytokeratin positive.
    ± EMA, vimentin, CEA.

— spindle cell carcinoma:
    cytokeratin positive, vimentin positive.

— adenocarcinoma:
    cytokeratin (7), EMA, CEA positive, ± vimentin, CD 15 positive, surfactant antibody positive (PE 10: 50% of cases).

— bronchioloalveolar carcinoma:
    surfactant antibody (PE 10) positive, cytokeratin positive.

Prognosis

Prognosis in lung cancer (overall 13% 5 year survival) relates to weight loss, performance status, cell type (small cell carcinoma has 2% long-term survival and

90% present with locally advanced or systemic disease), cell differentiation (well differentiated is better than poorly differentiated) and tumour stage (only 10–20% of non-small cell carcinomas are potentially curable by resection). An important therapeutic distinction must be made between small cell carcinoma (adjuvant chemo-/radiotherapy) and non-small cell carcinoma (surgery ± radiotherapy). This can be achieved with a relatively high level of consistency (kappa = 0.86) whereas subtyping of non-small cell carcinoma shows poor inter-observer agreement (kappa = 0.25; Burnett et al., 1994). A general guide to suitability for surgical resection is non-small cell cancer > 2 cm from the carina and without mediastinal lymph node involvement i.e. ≤ pT2 N1. International trials are currently examining the role of neoadjuvant therapy in non-small cell carcinoma more advanced than stage pT2 N1. The significance of occult bone marrow micrometastases detected by immunohistochemistry is uncertain. Prognosis improves if the carcinoma is "early" or "occult" with positive cytology but negative chest radiology: preoperative chemotherapy may also be beneficial.

Operable (localised)	*5 year survival*
squamous/large cell	35%
adenocarcinoma	
well differentiated	75%
poorly differentiated	35%
overall	50%
small cell	10%

Non-operable (extensive)	*5 year survival*
squamous cell	6%
small cell	2%.

10. Other malignancy

Leukaemia

— 50–60% of acute leukaemias.

— 15–40% of chronic leukaemias.

— rarely granulocytic sarcoma; CD 68/chloroacetate esterase positive.

Lymphoma

— primary MALToma or secondary to nodal/systemic disease: designation depends on the constituent cell type and clinicopathological staging of the extent of disease. There may also be a previous history of nodal lymphoma.

MALT lymphoma

— commonest primary lung lymphoma.

— sixth/seventh decade.

— ± Sjögren's syndrome or rheumatoid arthritis.

— central mass with peripheral tracking along septa, bronchovascular bundles and pleura.

— solitary or multifocal ± spread to other MALT sites.

— limited resection ± chemo-/radiotherapy.

— 5 year survival 80–90%, most are low-grade but can transform to high-grade.

— most large B cell (high-grade) pulmonary lymphomas probably originate in low-grade MALToma.

High-grade lesions are easily assessed as malignant but must be distinguished from other tumours, e.g. non-small cell carcinoma, using immunohistochemistry. Low-grade lesions are characterised by a dense monomorphic population of centrocyte-like cells, absence or colonisation of reactive follicles and local invasion. B cell predominance, light chain restriction and immunoglobulin heavy/light chain monoclonal gene rearrangements are confirmatory in distinction from a lymphoid interstitial pneumonitis. Mass lesions previously designated pseudolymphoma are now considered to be low-grade MALTomas.

Primary or secondary Hodgkin's disease

— usually secondary to spread from mediastinal disease.

— parenchymal nodules or endobronchial plaque/nodules.

Angiocentric T cell lymphoma

— on a spectrum with B cell lymphomatoid granulomatosis/angiocentric immunoproliferative lesion and associated with EBV.

— prognosis (poor) is dictated by the histological grade and extrapulmonary lesions are common (kidneys, liver, brain, spleen).

Intravascular lymphoma

— malignant angioendotheliomatosis or angiocentric large B cell lymphoma: skin, CNS and adrenal gland involvement with poor prognosis.

Epithelioid haemangioendothelioma (intravascular bronchioloalveolar tumour)

— a vascular tumour of intermediate-grade malignancy (CD 31 positive) in young adult females; slow progression; association with liver and skin lesions.

Kaposi's sarcoma

— AIDS.

Angiosarcoma

— primary or secondary.

Malignant melanoma

— usually secondary, intraparenchymal or endobronchial.

Sarcomas including synovial sarcoma, leiomyosarcoma, rhabdomyosarcoma (embryonal children, pleomorphic adults)

In any lung sarcoma it is important to exclude the more common possibilities of either a primary elsewhere or a lung carcinoma with sarcoma-like morphology.

Malignant Mesothelioma

1. Gross description

Specimen

— pleural or laparoscopic aspiration cytology or biopsy/ pleurectomy/omentectomy.
— size (cm) and weight (g).

Tumour

Site

— pleural (visceral/parietal)/pericardial/peritoneal.
— pleura (> 90%) is the commonest site.

Size

— length × width × depth (cm) or maximum dimension (cm).

Appearance

— localised (solitary)/diffuse/nodular/plaque/infiltrative/cystic change.

Edge

— circumscribed/irregular.

2. Histological type

Localised (solitary) fibrous tumour

— rare/solitary/visceral pleura, circumscribed/ smooth or bossellated.
— "patternless" fibroblasts and vessels with bland cytology, 90% benign, CD 34 positive.

— now regarded as arising from subserosal fibrous tissue rather than from mesothelium.

Well differentiated multicystic peritoneal mesothelioma
— on the surfaces of the uterus, ovary, bladder, rectum and pouch of Douglas it is potentially locally recurrent and invasive into retroperitoneum, bowel mesentery and wall – differential diagnosis of lymphagitic (lining cells are cytokeratin negative) and peritoneal inclusion cysts and cystic malignant mesothelioma. Fifty per cent recur over many years and can occasionally lead to death. Some have a previous history of surgery, endometriosis or pelvic inflammatory disease.

Well-differentiated papillary peritoneal mesothelioma
— middle aged women. Rare, with most being an incidental finding at hysterec tomy, localised and benign but can be extensive and diffuse nodular serosal/omental disease with ultimately progression and ascites.

Diffuse malignant mesothelioma
— epithelial (50%):   tubulopapillary
                        microglandular
                        solid (epithelioid)
                        small cell 6%
                        pleomorphic (large cell)
                        lymphohistiocytoid1%
                        deciduoid
                        signet ring cell.

— sarcomatoid (20%):   fibroblastic/fibrosarcomatous-like
                        muscle-like
                        fibrous (desmoplastic) 5–10%
                        angiomatoid
                        chondroid/osseous.

— mixed (biphasic) (30%).

Metastatic carcinoma
— lung/breast/stomach/ovary/prostate/kidney carcinomas, malignant melanoma, soft tissue sarcoma and germ cell tumours can all mimic mesothelioma on histology, and even gross distribution of disease. Knowledge of relevant previous history and close clinicopathological correlation is needed.

3. Differentiation

Well/moderate/poor.
— probably best regarded as a minority of well-differentiated lesions (e.g. papillary and multicystic peritoneal variants) and others which are not graded. Sarcomatoid lesions are considered poorly differentiated, epithelial lesions as well to moderately differentiated.

4. Extent of local tumour spread

Border: pushing/infiltrative.
Lymphocytic reaction: prominent/sparse.

The TNM classification applies to pleural mesothelioma only.

pT1   tumour limited to ipsilateral parietal and/or visceral pleura
pT2   tumour invades any of: ipsilateral lung, endothoracic fascia, diaphragm, pericardium
pT3   tumour invades any of: ipsilateral chest wall muscles, ribs, mediastinal organs or tissues
pT4   tumour directly extends to any of: contralateral pleura, contralateral lung, peritoneum, intra-abdominal organs, cervical tissues.

Spread is typically pleural, encasing the lung with extension along fissures and septa and into subpleural lung parenchyma. Nodal spread and distant metastases (up to 30% of cases) occur late in the disease course.

Contiguous spread through the diaphragm with involvement of abdominal organs is not infrequent.

pT1   Tumour limited to ipsilateral parietal and/or visceral pleura (Fig. 73)

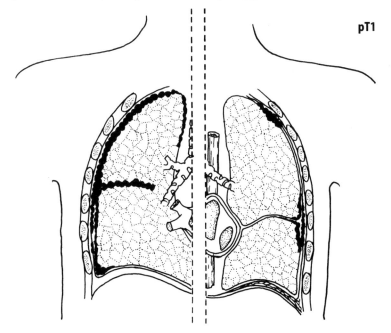

Figure 73. Pleural mesothelioma.

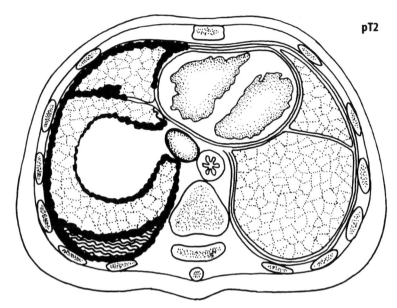

pT2

Tumour invades any of: ipsilateral lung, endothoracic fascia, diaphragm, pericardium (Fig. 74)

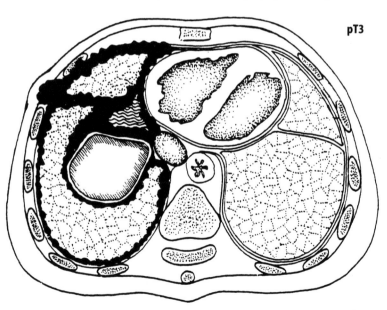

pT3

Tumour invades any of: ipsilateral chest wall muscle, ribs, mediastinal organs or tissues (Fig. 75)

Figures 74, 75. Pleural mesothelioma.

pT4 Tumour directly extends to any of the following:
     contralateral pleura, contralateral lung, peritoneum,
     intra-abdominal organs, cervical tissues (Figs. 76, 77)

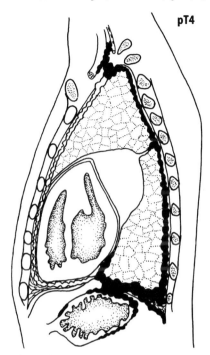

Figure 76. Pleural mesothelioma.

Peritoneal disease is usually secondary to pleural tumour but can also be primary and asbestos related. Pericardial disease usually represents spread from pleural tumour.

Flat or granular pleura adjacent to tumour nodules may show cytological atypia constituting "mesothelioma in-situ" and although unusual in pleural biopsies this can be a useful indicator of potential for progression to invasion.

5. Lymphovascular invasion

Present/absent.
Intra-/extratumoural.

6. Lymph nodes

Site/number/size/number involved/limit node/extracapsular spread.
Regional nodes: intrathoracic, scalene, supraclavicular.

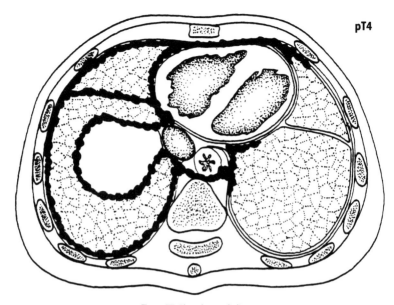

Figure 77. Pleural mesothelioma.

pN0 no regional lymph node metastasis
pN1 metastasis in ipsilateral peribronchial and/or hilar lymph nodes, including involvement by direct extension
pN2 metastasis in ipsilateral mediastinal and/or subcarinal lymph nodes
pN3 metastasis in contralateral mediastinal, contralateral hilar, ipsilateral or contralateral scalene or supraclavicular lymph nodes.

7. Excision margins

Distance (mm) to the nearest painted excision margin of local resection for limited disease.

8. Other pathology

Asbestos exposure, pleural plaques, subpleural fibrosis, asbestosis, bronchogenic carcinoma.

Two to three per cent of people with exposure to significant amounts of asbestos develop malignant mesothelioma. The consequences of asbestos fibre exposure can be both dose-related and idiosyncratic. Some individuals require minimal exposure to develop asbestos-related disease while others with extensive fibre burden do not. Classically there is a long lag period of 20–50 years until illness develops. Exposure can also be second-hand, e.g. washing spouse's contaminated clothing. Fibre burden can only really be assessed by incineration of lung tissue and quantitation by scanning electron microscopy. Identification by light microscopy correlates with a significant fibre load. Exposure is usually occupation related. A typical clinical history of mesothelioma is a unilateral opaque chest radiograph with necessity for multiple, repeated pleural taps. Note that the tumour may infiltrate chest wall through the biopsy needle track.

Markers

A number of malignant tumours metastatic to the pleura can mimic malignant mesothelioma. These include adenocarcinoma of lung, spindle cell carcinoma/carcinosarcoma of lung, renal cell carcinoma, malignant melanoma, lymphoma and leukaemia, ovarian carcinoma, thymoma and sarcoma. There is no one specific marker for mesothelioma and diagnosis often relies on exclusion of metastatic carcinoma and sarcoma by immunohistochemistry, clinical history, examination and radiology. Radiology is very useful in demonstrating the distribution of disease, e.g. diffuse pleural thickening versus an intrapulmonary/hilar mass with pleural thickening (lung carcinoma) or multiple discrete lung nodules with pleural thickening (metastatic carcinoma).

Useful immune marking is positivity with one or more of CEA, BerEP4 and Leu M1 (CD 15) (Table 18.1), indicating adenocarcinoma and excluding mesothelioma (although some cases can be Ber EP4 positive). HBME-1 and thrombomodulin give variable results. Other putatively positive mesothelioma markers such as calretinin, cytokeratin 5/6, N- and E- cadherin await further assessment.

Adenocarcinoma may be PAS-diastase resistant for mucin (60% of cases).

Sarcomatoid mesothelioma may co-express cytokeratin, vimentin and muscle-specific actin. Differential diagnosis is spindle cell lung carcinoma or primary or secondary sarcoma with similar immunophenotypic co-expression eg epithelioid leiomyosarcoma or synovial sarcoma. Desmoplastic mesothelioma (> 50% of the tumour is poorly cellular fibrous tissue) must be distinguished from fibrous pleurisy (inflammatory and reactive looking) and pleural plaque (acellular basket-weave pattern of collagen) neither of which show parenchymal or chest wall infiltration or strongly cytokeratin positive spindle cells within the fibrous tissue.

Solitary fibrous tumour of pleura is cytokeratin negative, CD34 positive.

Table 18.1.

Antibody	Epithelial mesothelioma	Reactive mesothelioma cells	Pulmonary adenocarcinoma
cytokeratin	+	+	+
vimentin	+	±	±
EMA	+	-	+
HBME-1	±	+	-
thrombomodulin	±	-	-
CEA	-	-	+
Leu M1 (CD15)	-	-	+
Ber EP4	-	-	+

Other markers include:
— S100, HMB-45, melan-A (melanoma).
— CD 45, CD 20, CD 3 (B/T cell lymphoma).
— thyroglobulin (thyroid papillary carcinoma).
— CA125 (ovarian serous carcinoma).
— PAS, cytokeratin, EMA, vimentin, abdominal ultrasound/CT scan (renal cell carcinoma).
— PSA, PSAP (prostate carcinoma).
— βHCG, AFP, PLAP (germ cell tumour).
— ER/PR, GCDFP-15 (breast carcinoma).
— CA19-9, CEA, CK 20 (gut carcinoma).

Morphological markers of mesothelial malignancy versus reactive mesothelial hyperplasia are: cytological atypia and cellularity, necrosis and invasion of subpleural connective tissue, i.e. the extent, atypia and invasiveness of the mesothelial cell population in an adequate specimen. In a significant minority of cases diagnosis may not be able to be made at first presentation but the possibility raised from a constellation of atypical features in the pleural fluid cytology and biopsy.

Reactive mesothelial hyperplasia and dense inflammatory fibrosis do not clinically progress as does mesothelioma with repeated clinical presentations and the need for symptomatic relief by paracentesis. Some well-differentiated lesions pursue such a biological course over a span of several years but normally the clinical progression is relatively rapid indicating a malignant diagnosis. Reactive mesothelial hyperplasia may be seen in pulmonary infarction, tuberculous pleuritis, rheumatoid arthritis, systemic lupus erythematosus and overlying primary or secondary neoplasms.

Prognosis

Prognosis of diffuse malignant mesothelioma relates to stage but is generally poor with the majority of patients dying from their disease within 1–3 years. Spindle cell tumours are more aggressive than epithelial variants. Adjuvant chemotherapy combined with resection of limited disease can occasionally result in prolonged remission with 3 year survival rates 15–30%, but only a small minority of patients are suitable. Symptomatic relief may be gained by multiple paracentesis of malignant pleural or peritoneal fluid supplemented by intracavitary chemotherapy; this may act either directly on the tumour cells reducing secretions or produce a loculated, sclerosant effect. Well-differentiated multicystic and papillary peritoneal mesotheliomas are regarded as being of borderline or low malignant potential.

Mediastinal Cancer

1. Gross description

Specimen

— percutaneous or thoracoscopic fine needle aspirate/(core) biopsy/resection.
— number of fragments and their length (mm).
— size (cm) and weight (g).

Tumour

Site

— mediastinal boundaries:

lateral	pleural cavities
anterior	sternum
posterior	spine
superior	thoracic inlet
inferior	diaphragm

— superior: thymoma and thymic cysts.
malignant lymphoma.
nodular goitre thyroid.
ectopic parathyroid lesions.

— anterior: thymoma and thymic cysts.
malignant lymphoma.
germ cell tumours.
metastatic carcinoma.
thyroid/parathyroid lesions.
mesenchymal lesions – lipoma, lymphangioma, haemangioma.

— middle: metastatic carcinoma.
malignant lymphoma.
pericardial/bronchogenic cysts.

— posterior: neural tumours – neurilemmoma, neurofibroma, ganglioneuroma, ganglioneuroblastoma, malignant schwannoma, neuroblastoma, paraganglioma.

gastroenteric cysts.

Size

— length × width × depth (cm) or maximum tumour dimension (cm).

Appearance

— circumscribed/encapsulated/infiltrative/fleshy/pale/pigmented/cystic/necrotic/haemorrhagic, e.g. thymoma can be encapsulated or infiltrative, solid/cystic or multiloculated whereas lymphoma is fleshy and pale ± necrosis and sclerosis. Teratoma can be cystic, solid, necrotic or haemorrhagic, neurilemmoma is encapsulated.

Edge

— circumscribed/irregular.

2. Histological type

Metastatic carcinoma

— the commonest mediastinal malignant tumour (particularly in the middle mediastinum) and can mimic a primary thymic tumour both clinically and radiologically, e.g. small cell carcinoma lung can have a small primary lesion with extensive direct or nodal spread to the mediastinum.
— direct spread: lung, oesophagus, pleura, chest wall, vertebra, trachea.
— distant spread: breast, thyroid, nasopharynx, larynx, kidney, prostate, testicular (or ovarian) germ cell tumour, malignant melanoma.

Identify a residual nodal rim of lymphoid tissue at the tumour edge to indicate metastasis.

Malignant lymphoma

— occurs in decreasing order of frequency in the anterior, superior and middle mediastinum; it is the commonest primary neoplasm of the middle mediastinum. Thymic or nodal based. Specific thymic/mediastinal features are:

Hodgkin's disease: young females, nodular sclerosis in type; fibrotic/lobulated ± thymic epithelial cysts; radiotherapy; prognosis depends on the stage of disease.

Lymphoblastic lymphoma: acute dyspnoea in adolescent males; mediastinal + cervical/supraclavicular and axillary disease; ± Hassall's corpuscles and can therefore mimic thymoma; small to medium-sized lymphoid cells, apoptosis, tdt positive – usually T cell (CD 3) and high Ki-67 index.

Large cell lymphoma: young females presenting with superior vena cava syndrome; sclerosis/fibrosis – banded and pericellular. CD 45, CD 20 positive,

Ki-67 positive in > 70% of cells; spread to pericardium, pleura, lung, sternum and chest wall common.

MALToma: occasionally.

Germ cell tumours

— 20% of mediastinal tumours/cysts.
— thymus based with a primary origin in extragonadal germ cells.
— exclude metastases from a clinical or occult testicular/ovarian germ cell tumour, particularly if there is associated retroperitoneal disease.
— mature cystic teratoma: the commonest germ cell tumour and similar to that in the ovary.
— immature teratoma: rare; immature epithelium, mesenchyme or neural elements.
— embryonal carcinoma, yolk sac tumour, malignant teratoma intermediate, choriocarcinoma (third decade, gynaecomastia) – all require chemotherapy and are less responsive with a higher relapse rate and lower survival than equivalent testicular lesions. Serum HCG and AFP levels are raised in >90% of non-seminomatous germ cell tumours.
— seminoma: PLAP positive, cytokeratin negative; 69% 10 year survival; the seminoma cells can be obscured by granulomatous inflammation, reactive lymphoid follicular hyperplasia or thymic epithelial cysts and immunomarkers are helpful.

Neurogenic tumours

— posterior mediastinum.
— children: derived from the sympathetic nervous system: neuroblastoma, ganglioneuroblastoma, ganglioneuroma.
— adults: derived from the peripheral nervous system: neurilemmoma, neurofibroma ± cystic degeneration. Malignant peripheral nerve sheath tumour: de novo or in von Recklinghausen's disease, ± enteric glands, ± rhabdomyoblasts (Triton tumour). Poor prognosis with pleural and pulmonary spread.

Sarcoma

— rarely primary – liposarcoma, synovial sarcoma.

Thymoma

— anterosuperior mediastinum.
— solid, yellow/grey, lobulated ± cystic change: 80% are encapsulated and easily excised, 20% are infiltrative. It comprises a dual population of cytokeratin positive epithelial cells and T marker (CDs 1, 3, 4, 8) positive lymphocytes of variable maturity. Classification which can reflect invasiveness and prognosis relies on:

1. the character of the epithelial cells and lymphocytes
2. the relative proportion of these cells
3. their cellular atypia, and,

4. the organoid architecture: lobulated corticomedullary differentiation; epithelial lined glands and cysts; Hassall's-like corpuscles; perivascular spaces.

Individual tumours can show some heterogeneity in these features.

Medullary (6%):
  spindle shaped epithelial cells.
  scanty to moderate numbers of mature lymphocytes.
  thick capsule.
  excellent prognosis.

Mixed (composite) (20%):
  elderly patients, thick capsule, excellent prognosis.
  biphasic, lobulated.
  medullary component plus component of round to stellate epithelial cells (vesicular nucleus, inconspicuous nucleolus) with numerous lymphocytes.

Predominantly cortical (organoid) (7%):
  lymphocyte rich, organoid corticomedullary areas (thymus-like).
  less prominent epithelial component and expansile edge with local invasion common.

Cortical (42%):
  young patients.
  large round/polygonal epithelial cells with vesicular nucleus.
  lesser component of intervening immature lymphocytes.
  lobulated, fibrous septa, locally invasive.

Well-differentiated thymic carcinoma (17%):
  predominantly epithelial (small cells with mild nuclear atypia).
  few lymphocytes.
  lobulated, sclerotic, invasive.

Thymic carcinoma (8%):
  clear-cut cytological features of malignancy.
  exclude metastasis from lung or elsewhere.
  90% are either squamous cell carcinoma (+ keratinisation) or non-keratinising; lymphoepithelioma-like carcinoma (similar to that of nasopharyngeal carcinoma).

Others:
  spindle cell carcinoma (carcinosarcoma).
  clear cell carcinoma.
  basaloid carcinoma.
  mucoepidermoid carcinoma.
  papillary carcinoma.
  small cell carcinoma.
  undifferentiated large cell carcinoma.
  carcinoid (classic/spindle cell/pigmented/with amyloid/atypical).

3. Differentiation/grade

Metastatic carcinoma

— well/moderate/poor.

Malignant lymphoma
— low-grade: MAL Toma.
— high-grade: diffuse large cell lymphoma; lymphoblastic lymphoma.

Germ cell tumours
— seminoma.
— non-seminomatous: mature/immature; malignant, e.g. embryonal carcinoma, yolk sac tumour, MTI, choriocarcinoma.

Neurogenic tumours
— small round blue cell: neuroblastoma component.
— low-grade/high-grade: sarcoma.
— thymoma: see above.

4. Extent of local tumour spread

Border: pushing/infiltrative.
Lymphocytic reaction: prominent/sparse.

For all tumours:

— confined to the mediastinal nodes.
— confined to the thymus.
— into the mediastinal connective tissues.
— into other organs, e.g. pleura, lung, pericardium, main vessels.

Thymoma
I   encapsulated
II   minimally invasive: capsule traversed and into the mediastinal connective tissue
III   widely invasive: into pleura, lung, pericardium, main vessels
IV   metastatic: into intra-/extrathoracic lymph nodes and/or haematogenous metastases, e.g. cervical nodes, lung, liver, bone and ovary (they can occur after a lag period of months to years after diagnosis).

5. Lymphovascular invasion

Present/absent.
Intra-/extratumoural.

6. Lymph nodes

Site/number/size/number involved/limit node/extracapsular spread.
Regional nodes: intrathoracic, scalene, supraclavicular nodes

Thymoma

pN0   no regional lymph nodes involved

pN1   metastasis to anterior mediastinal lymph nodes

pN2   metastasis to intrathoracic lymph nodes other than the anterior mediastinal lymph nodes

pN3   metastasis to extrathoracic lymph nodes.

7. Excision margins

Distances (mm) to the nearest painted margins of excision.

8. Other pathology

Mediastinal neoplasms can present in a number of ways:

1.   during staging or follow up (chest radiograph, CT or MRI scan) of a patient with a known cancer elsewhere, e.g. lung carcinoma, colorectal carcinoma, non-Hodgkin's lymphoma/Hodgkin's disease, or testicular/ovarian germ cell tumour,

2.   as an incidental finding on chest radiograph in a patient who may or may not have ill-defined symptoms, e.g. dyspnoea,

3.   as a finding in the investigation of a patient with other presenting features, e.g. pneumonia or pleural effusion,

4.   as superior vena cava syndrome due to malignant infiltration or compression of local structures, e.g. lung carcinoma (primary or secondary), malignant lymphoma,

5.   as a paraneoplastic syndrome, e.g. ACTH or inappropriate ADH secretion.

Therefore, knowledge of a relevant past medical history is fundamental in determining the nature of the underlying abnormality. Tissue diagnosis can be obtained by percutaneous/thoracoscopic/transbronchial fine needle aspirate or needle core biopsy with material provided not only for routine morphology but, importantly, ancillary techniques such as immunohistochemistry to aid distinction between diagnoses such as metastatic carcinoma, lymphoblastic or large cell lymphoma and thymoma. However, in some cases, due to the limitations of these sampling techniques, invasive mediastinal incisional biopsy may be required. Prior to this it should be determined whether a more convenient source of tissue diagnosis is available, e.g. palpable supraclavicular or cervical lymphadenopathy or pleural fluid cytology.

Tumour site within the mediastinum is an important clue to tumour type, e.g. middle mediastinal disease is most likely to be metastatic carcinoma or malignant lymphoma whereas anterosuperior mediastinal lesions are more likely to be thymus-based cancers, e.g. thymoma, germ-cell tumours and lymphoma.

Markers

Thirty to forty-five per cent of thymoma patients have myasthenia gravis; other paraneoplastic syndromes relate to the mediastinal cancer type, e.g. small cell lung carcinoma with ACTH or inappropriate ADH secretion.

Thymic carcinoid tumour is associated with carcinoid tumour at other sites, e.g. bronchus, ileum and type I multiple endocrine neoplasia (MEN I) syndrome.

Immunohistochemistry
— metastatic carcinoma: cytokeratins, CEA, EMA, BerEP4, CD 15 (Leu M1), ± vimentin.
— Hodgkin's disease: CD 15, CD 30.
— non-Hodgkin's lymphoma: CD 45, CD 20, CD 3, CD 30, κ/λ light chain restriction, molecular gene rearrangements.
— lymphoblastic lymphoma: tdt, CD 10, CD 99 (O 13).
— seminoma: PLAP (cytokeratin negative).
— embryonal carcinoma/yolk sac tumour: cytokeratins, HCG, AFP, (± PLAP – in embryonal carcinoma).
— thymoma: cytokeratins, EMA, CEA, S100 positive interdigitating reticulum cells; variably mature T lymphocytes CDs 1, 3, 4, 8.

Cystic change
— multilocular thymic cysts: multilocular; adherent to mediastinal structures due to inflammation and fibrosis mimicking an invasive thymic tumour; cubocolumnar or squamous epithelial lining.
— 50% of thymic nodular sclerosing Hodgkin's disease.
— thymic seminoma.

Prognosis

Prognosis obviously relates to the nature of the underlying pathological abnormality and to whether it represents primary or secondary disease. Cancer subtype also determines the choice of therapy, e.g. surgery, chemotherapy or radiotherapy. Note that prebiopsy or presurgical radiotherapy and chemotherapy can induce tumour apoptosis, necrosis and hyalinisation which can lead to difficulties in accurate classification of disease.

In thymoma several rules apply:

1. tumours with predominantly bland spindle/oval cells are usually encapsulated and of excellent prognosis,

2. tumours with predominantly round/polygonal epithelial cells have a course related to the relative predominance of epithelial cells over lymphocytes and any cellular atypia that is present, and

3. the encapsulation of the tumour, or its lack of encapsulation and any signs of invasion at surgery along with completeness of excision are, irrespective of the histological subtype, the best markers of future clinical behaviour.

Medullary and mixed thymoma tend to present at stages I or II, predominantly cortical or cortical more often stage III or IV. However, prognosis is usually 90–100% 5 year survival, patients with myasthenia gravis doing worse than those without. Treatment is surgical supplemented by radiotherapy if there is local recurrence (2–10% of cases, more usually the predominantly cortical and cortical types). Distant metastases may need chemotherapy. Well differentiated thymic carcinoma has an 80% 5 year survival. Thymic carcinoma may require a combination of surgery, radiotherapy and chemotherapy for bulky local disease or distant spread. Disease course relates to tumour type being either aggressive (death in 6 months to 2 years in non-keratinising carcinoma, sarcomatoid/clear cell/undifferentiated carcinomas), intermediate (squamous cell carcinoma, carcinoid tumour) or indolent (mucoepidermoid/basaloid carcinomas).

Skin Cancer

- Non-Melanocytic Skin Carcinoma

- Malignant Melanoma

Non-Melanocytic Skin Carcinoma

1. Gross description

Specimen

— smear cytology/curettage/punch biopsy/excision biopsy/Mohs' surgery.
— size: length × width × depth (cm).

Tumour

Site

— anatomical site: limbs/trunk/head/neck/perineum/ epidermal/dermal/subcutaneous.

Size

— length × width × depth (mm) or maximum dimension (mm).

Appearance

— verrucous/warty/nodular/exophytic/sessile/ulcerated/invaginated/cystic/haemorrhagic/necrotic.

Edge

— circumscribed/irregular.

2. Histological type

Squamous cell carcinoma

— large cell/small cell.
— keratinising/non-keratinising.
— 80% are well differentiated and keratinising.

— variants: clear cell – elderly, scalp.
 signet ring cell.
 basaloid.
 spindle cell.
 pseudoglandular (adenoid) and pseudoangiosarcomatous.
 verrucous – sole of foot and anal margin, locally invasive: exophytic with deep margin of cytologically bland bulbous processes.

Basal cell carcinoma

— superficial multifocal.
— micronodular.
— infiltrative.
— nodulo-cystic.
— keratotic (with squamous metaplasia).
— morphoeic.
— adenoid.
— metatypical/basosquamous – configuration of a basal cell carcinoma but with more nuclear atypia, a fibroblastic response and foci of malignant squamous differentiation. It is somewhat intermediate between basal and squamous carcinomas of usual type.

Adnexal carcinoma

— hair follicle differentiation.
— sebaceous differentiation: epithelioma/carcinoma
— ductal differentiation: apocrine; eccrine.

Paget's disease

— extramammary sites are vulva, perineum, scrotum, axillae: see Chapters 7 and 27.

Neuroendocrine carcinoma: Merkel cell

— head/neck, extremities, elderly.
— chromogranin/NSE/cytokeratin 20 positive, paranuclear dot CAM 5.2 positive.
— ± overlying basal or squamous carcinoma (in-situ or invasive).
— clinically exclude secondary small cell carcinoma of lung (CK 20 negative).
— poor prognosis, local recurrence and nodal metastases are common; treatment is primary excision with wide margins.

Dermal tumours

— fibrohistiocytic, neural, muscular, vascular, adipose.

Leukaemia

— 5–10% of leukaemia cases: sometimes as a first manifestation of disease but more often secondary to widespread systemic or recurrent disease.

Lymphoma: primary
— disease confined to skin for at least 6 months after complete staging.
— T cell 65 %: B cell 25%.
  T cell, indolent behaviour:
      mycosis fungoides ± follicular mucinosis.
      Pagetoid reticulosis.
      anaplastic large cell, CD 30 positive.
      lymphomatoid papulosis.
  T cell, aggressive behaviour;
      Sézary syndrome.
      anaplastic large cell, CD 30 negative.
      pleomorphic medium/large cell.
      subcutaneous panniculitis-like lymphoma.
  B cell, indolent behaviour:
      follicle centre lymphoma.
      mantle zone lymphoma.
      marginal zone lymphoma (good prognosis – a minority have *Borrelia burgdorferi* organism as a chronic antigenic stimulus).
  B cell, intermediate behaviour:
      large cell lymphoma of the lower legs in elderly women
      5 year survival 58%.
  B cell, aggressive behaviour:
      large cell lymphoma in other clinical settings
      lymphoblastic lymphoma in children and adults – tdt positive.

Lymphoma: secondary
— secondary to nodal/systemic disease.

For staging of lymphoma refer to Chapter 35.

Metastatic carcinoma
— kidney, breast, gut, lung, oral cavity, ovary, malignant melanoma.
— single/multiple nodule(s) commonly on the trunk and head and neck regions, sometimes in the vicinity of the primary lesion.
— some metastases can be epidermotropic and simulate a primary lesion.
— secondary small cell carcinoma of lung or gut carcinoid can mimic Merkel cell tumour.

3. Differentiation

Well/moderate/poor.

4. Extent of local tumour spread

Border: pushing/infiltrative.
Lymphocytic reaction: prominent/sparse.

pTis   carcinoma in-situ
pT1   tumour ≤ 2 cm in greatest dimension
pT2   tumour > 2 cm but ≤ 5 cm in greatest dimension
pT3   tumour > 5 cm in greatest dimension
pT4   tumour invades deep extradermal structures (cartilage, skeletal muscle, bone).

5. Lymphovascular invasion

Present/absent.
Intra-/extratumoural.

6. Lymph nodes

Site/number/size/number involved/limit node/extracapsular spread.
Regional nodes: those appropriate to the site of the primary tumour

pN0   no regional lymph node metastases
pN1   metastasis in regional lymph node(s).

7. Excision margins

Distances (mm) to the nearest painted excision margins, either of quadrant blocks if specimen size allows or serial slices (toast racked).

Adequate treatment is based on successful complete primary excision or, if there is initial margin involvement, on secondary re-excision.

8. Other pathology

Basal cell carcinoma (comprising basaloid cells with peripheral palisading, mitoses and a point of attachment to the epidermis) is the commonest skin cancer in Caucasians. It is non-metastatic but locally infiltrative, the infiltrative, micronodular and superficial multifocal variants being more likely to recur. The metatypical/basosquamous (with malignant squamous component) type is also more aggressive. Distant metastases are exceedingly rare. Squamous cell carcinoma is more prone to lymph node metastases particularly if > 2 cm diameter or > 2 mm in thickness, poorly differentiated or with perineural spread. Morphologically it shows nuclear stratification, intercellular bridges ± keratinisation. Variants such as clear cell, spindle cell and pseudoglandular (acantholytic) typically occur on the head and neck of the elderly and tend to recur locally with a reasonable prognosis. General prognostic indicators for squamous carcinoma are stage, level of dermal invasion and tumour thickness. Recurrent tumours tend to be ≥ 4 mm thick with involvement of the deep dermis and fatal tumours at least 1 cm thick with extension into subcutaneous fat.

Predisposing lesions to cutaneous carcinoma are:
— actinic keratosis/solar elastosis; sun exposure.
— PUVA treatment for psoriasis.
— varicose ulcers, lichen planus, hidradenitis suppurativa.
— immunosuppression post transplant, HIV.
— Bowen's disease – indolent progression to carcinoma.
— condyloma acuminatum, Bowenoid papulosis, HPV infection – perineum/ perianal margin squamous carcinoma.
— epidermodysplasia verruciformis, xeroderma pigmentosum.
— naevus sebaceous of Jadassohn.
— naevoid basal cell carcinoma syndrome.

Double pathology may be encountered, e.g. basal or squamous cell carcinoma overlying Merkel cell tumour, basal cell carcinoma and syringocystadenoma papilliferum in naevus sebaceous of Jadassohn, basal cell carcinoma and dermatofibroma.

Mohs' surgery is often used for resection of recurrent basal cell carcinoma of the face; it involves submission of circumferential margins and multiple painted serial blocks examined by frozen section as a guide to completeness of excision.

Pseudoepitheliomatous (pseudocarcinomatous) hyperplasia may be seen in association with: chronic venous stasis, ulceration, chronic inflammation, e.g. pyoderma gangrenosum, and overlying neoplasms, e.g. granular cell tumour.

Distinction between carcinoma in-situ and invasive squamous carcinoma can be difficult and some of these lesions should be designated "best regarded as squamous carcinoma"; treatment (primary surgical excision ± radiotherapy) is the same for both.

Sebaceous carcinoma may be periocular and aggressive or extraocular and non-aggressive; it forms a spectrum of behaviour with sebaceous epithelioma (local recurrence). For information on sweat gland carcinoma refer to Hollowood (1999).

Skin carcinoma varies greatly in its immunophenotypic expression –

Immunophenotypic expression

Squamous cell carcinoma: high molecular weight cytokeratins, EMA, CEA positive; Ber EP 4 negative.

Basal cell carcinoma: low molecular weight cytokeratins, Ber EP 4 positive; EMA, CEA negative.

Adnexal carcinomas: usually EMA and CEA positive, and differential molecular weight cytokeratin expression according to their differentiation; generally CAM 5.2 (low molecular weight) and AE1 (intermediate molecular weight) positive.

Some centres use smear cytology with immediate reporting to distinguish basal cell from non-basal cell cutaneous carcinoma to facilitate a one-stop assessment and institution of treatment.

9. Other malignancy

Sarcoma

Dermal and subcutaneous soft tissue tumours may have classical clinical features, e.g. angiosarcoma of the scalp in the elderly and Kaposi's sarcoma in AIDS. However, they are classified according to their cell of origin; malignancy is assessed by cellularity, cellular atypia, mitotic activity and infiltrative margins. Immunocytochemistry is often very useful in determining histogenesis, e.g. desmin, actin (muscular), S100 (neural, melanocytic (also HMB-45, melan-A), chondroid, adipose), CD 31, factor VIII (vascular), CD 68 (histiocytic) and CD 34 (dermatofibrosarcoma). Examples are: cutaneous leiomyosarcoma, dermatofibrosarcoma protuberans, angiosarcoma, epithelioid haemangioendothelioma, malignant nerve sheath tumour, liposarcoma and extraskeletal myxoid chondrosarcoma (usually extending from deep soft tissues).

Kaposi's sarcoma is found in the elderly (solitary) or young (AIDS, multiple). The early patch/plaque phase is subtle, characterised by linear "vascular" slit-like spaces in the dermal collagen orientated parallel to the epidermis; later there is a sieve-like pattern with extravasation of red blood cells and spindle cell proliferation.

Immunocytochemistry is also important in the differential diagnosis of cutaneous spindle cell lesions, viz. spindle cell carcinoma versus malignant melanoma, leiomyosarcoma, metastatic sarcoma and atypical fibroxanthoma. Other morphological clues are dysplasia of the surface squamous epithelium (carcinoma), junctional activity and melanin pigmentation (melanoma), Touton-like giant cells (AFX) and eosinophilic fusiform spindle cells (leiomyosarcoma). Clinical history is important to exclude a metastasis.

A further indication for immunohistochemistry is in the distinction between Merkel cell tumour (CD 20/NSE/neurofilament/EMA), lymphoma (CD 45 (lymphoblastic – tdt/CD 99)), PNETs (CD99 ± NSE/neurofilament) and small cell malignant melanoma (S100/HMB-45/melan-A).

Lymphoma

Immunocytochemistry (for cell lineage and light chain restriction) and molecular studies (T cell receptor gene and immunoglobulin heavy chain gene rearrangements) are also of use in cutaneous lymphoma. T cell lymphomas show epidermotropism while B cell lymphomas often have a dermal grenz zone and a "bottom-heavy" infiltrate extending into the subcutis. Low-grade T cell lymphomas have a horizontal band-like dermal growth pattern while high-grade lesions and B cell lymphomas are sharply demarcated with a nodular, vertical and three-dimensional growth. Molecular studies are particularly helpful in inflammatory conditions simulating cutaneous lymphoma, e.g. lymphocytoma cutis and lymphomatoid reactions to drugs and insect bites. Designation of lymphoma can sometimes be difficult and should always be clinicopathological. For discussion of cutaneous B cell lymphoma refer to Robson (1999).

Malignant Melanoma

1. Gross description

Specimen

— curettage/punch biopsy/excision biopsy.
— size: length × width × depth (cm).

Tumour

Site

— anatomical location – trunk, limbs, head/neck, perineum, mucosal, ocular, multifocal (1–5%).
— epidermal/dermal/subcutaneous.

Size

— length × width × depth (mm) or maximum dimension (mm).

Appearance

— verrucous/nodular/sessile/ulcerated/pigmented or non-pigmented/halo/satellite lesions/scarring.

Edge

— circumscribed/irregular.

2. Histological type

Malignant melanoma in-situ

— intraepidermal.

Lentigo maligna melanoma

— face/Hutchinson's melanotic freckle.

Superficial spreading melanoma
— radial phase of spread.[1]

Nodular melanoma
— vertical phase of spread.[2]

Acral/mucosal/lentiginous melanoma
— sole of foot, nail bed, mucosae.

Others
— e.g. desmoplastic, neurotropic, verrucous, balloon cell, signet ring cell, minimal deviation, metastatic, malignant blue naevi.

3. Differentiation/cell type

— epithelioid.
— spindle cell.
— mixed.

4. Extent of local tumour spread

Border: pushing/infiltrative.
Lymphocytic reaction: prominent/sparse – the number of tumour infiltrating lymphocytes has a positive association with survival.

The TNM classification of malignant melanoma considers three features: tumour thickness, anatomical Clark levels and the absence or presence of tumour satellites within 2 cm of the primary tumour.

Breslow depth or thickness (mm)

— eyepiece graticule measurement of tumour maximum vertical diameter from the top of the granular layer or ulcerated tumour surface to the deepest

---

[1]Radial growth phase includes melanoma in-situ (i.e. intraepidermal) ± microinvasion of the papillary dermis. The radial phase may be indolent and the dermal component (usually<1 mm thick) can have morphologically bland cell nests (usually<10 cells across) of uniform size and cytological appearance. This may be accompanied by signs of regression. The radial phase potentially progresses by clonal expansion to the vertical phase.

[2]Vertical growth phase tumour comprises expansive nests, nodules or plaques of cytologically atypical melanoma cells in the dermis; it implies a biological potential for metastatic spread and is the main determinant of prognosis. The cell nests are usually ≥ 25 cells in dimension, show variation throughout the lesion, mitoses and a host dermal lymphocytic response.

point of invasion; melanoma cells in adjacent pilosebaceous unit epithelium do not count. S100 or melan-A immunostains can help highlight melanoma cells in the dermis that might otherwise be obscured by a heavy lymphocytic infiltrate at the base of the lesion.

Anatomical Clark level

I   intraepithelial
II papillary dermis

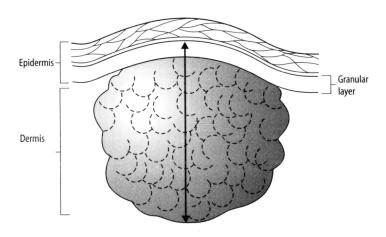

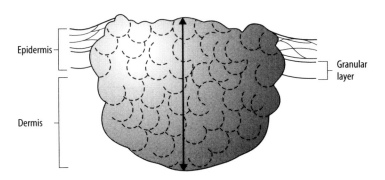

Breslow Depth or thickness (mm) = the maximum vertical depth from the top
of the granular layer or ulcerated surface to
the deepest point of invasion

Figure 78. Malignant melanoma.

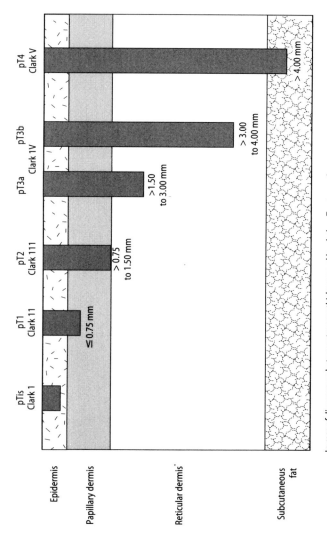

In case of discrepancy between tumour thickness and level, the pT category is based on the less favourable finding

Figure 79. Malignant melanoma.

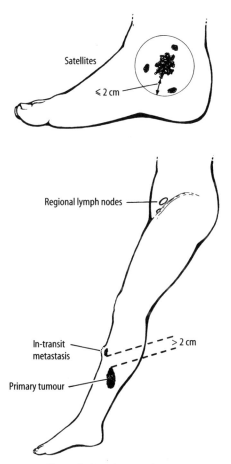

Figures 80, 81. Malignant melanoma.

III   papillary-reticular interface
IV   reticular dermis
V   subcutaneous fat.

Thickness

Thin
Low-risk: < 0.76 mm, level II.   pT1.

Intermediate
Moderate-risk: 0.76–1.5 mm, level III.   pT2.

Thick

High-risk: > 1.5 mm to 3 mm (pT3a) or > 3 mm   pT3
to 4 mm (pT3b), level IV.
> 4 mm, level V (pT4a) and/or satellite(s)   pT4
within 2 cm of the primary (pT4b).

If there is discrepancy between tumour thickness and level, base pT category on the less favourable finding.

Definition: MIN (melanocytic intraepithelial neoplasia)
= melanocytic dysplasia and melanoma in-situ (level I)   pTis.
± microinvasion.

5. Lymphovascular invasion

Present/absent.
Intra-/extratumoural.

6. Lymph nodes

Site/number/size/number involved/limit node/extracapsular spread.
Regional nodes: those appropriate to the site of the primary tumour

pN0   no regional lymph nodes involved
pN1   metastases ≤ 3 cm in regional node(s)
pN2   a. metastases > 3 cm in regional node(s), and/or
b. cutaneous deposit > 2 cm from the primary tumour but not beyond the regional nodes (in-transit metastasis)
c. both.

Spread of malignant melanoma is to regional nodes, skin (satellite nodules and in-transit metastases), liver, lungs, gastrointestinal tract, bone and CNS.

7. Excision margins

Distances (mm) to the nearest painted excision margins – either of quadrant blocks if specimen size allows or serial slices (toast racked) – of the vertical and radial disease phases and any in-situ change.

Minimum recommended margins of clearance vary according to the tumour depth of invasion:

depth   *minimum margin*
<0.76 mm   5 mm
0.76–2 mm   10 mm
> 2 mm   20 mm.

Adequate treatment is based on successful complete primary excision or, if there is initial margin involvement, secondary re-excision. This is supplemented by regional node dissection and systemic therapy for metastatic disease.

8. Other pathology

— pigmentation: none/light/moderate/heavy.
— mitoses: number/high-power field (×40 objective) or absent, low (< 6/mm²) or high.
— ulceration: present/absent.
— elastosis: present/absent.
— regression: present/absent – inflammation/fibrosis/telangiectasia/ melanophages.
— pre-existing lesion: present/absent – less common than de-novo melanoma.
— Satellite lesions: present/absent; distance (mm) from primary.

Primary versus secondary/recurrence: secondary tumour tends to be nodular and dermal/subcutaneous ± vascular invasion with no epidermal component. Occasionally secondary melanoma may show epidermal changes but usually the dermal disease is more extensive in width. Some melanomas can develop multiple locoregional cutaneous recurrences over many years and do not develop metastatic disease, although such satellite nodule and in-transit metastases are an indicator of potential systemic dissemination – they are regarded as tumour emboli arrested in lymphatics which then grow to form a tumour mass. They are seen in about 5% of malignant melanomas > 1 mm thick.

Markers
— S100 protein, HMB-45 and melan-A.
— Masson Fontana for pigment.
— Ki-67 proliferation index.

Dysplastic naevus: variable reports of predisposition to malignant melanoma. Strict criteria (clinical and pathological) must be adhered to (see below) as there is a range of benign naevi with active junctional components that can mimic dysplastic naevus or melanoma, e.g. junctional/pagetoid Spitz naevus, pigmented spindle cell naevus, halo naevus, traumatised and irradiated naevus, acral and genital naevi. Age, anatomical site, lesion type and clinical history must all be considered along with the morphology.

— single or multiple (dysplastic naevus syndrome).
— ≥ 4 mm with variable pigmentation and irregular borders.
— nested and lentiginous melanocytic proliferation.
— architectural and cytological atypia.
— elongation/fusion of rete ridges.

— dermal lamellar fibroplasia with vascularisation and chronic inflammation in the dermis.

Morphological clues to a diagnosis of malignant melanoma are: lesion asymmetry, extension of atypical melanocytes up into the epidermis and lateral to the lesion, melanocytic atypia and lack of dermal maturation, mitoses and a dermal lymphocytic infiltrate. Melanocytic cell nests also vary in size, shape and cytological atypia within a lesion.

Prognosis

Prognosis of melanoma is unpredictable but relates strongly to the vertical component or thickness/depth of invasion and adequacy of excision with the width of margins tailored accordingly. Estimated overall 5 year survival rates are about 60% but tumour stage/thickness is the most powerful prognostic determinant:

	5 year disease free survival	*regional metastases at 3 years*
pT1 (< 0.76 mm)	> 95%	0%
pT3 (> 1.5 mm)	40–60%	50–60%

Other adverse indicators are patient age (> 50 years), sex (male), histological regression, histological type (nodular), vascular invasion, tumour phase (vertical), satellitosis, necrosis, ulceration, mitotic activity and anatomical site (sole of foot, head, neck and back are worse). One study found that a prognostic index of tumour thickness multiplied by the number of mitoses/mm^2 was the most accurate method of predicting patients who would remain disease free. Occasionally malignant melanoma may present as metastatic disease, e.g. axillary nodes due to complete regression of a cutaneous lesion leaving no obvious primary tumour on examination. Other possible occult sources are the eye and mucosal surfaces of the oesophagus, vagina and anal canal. These mucosal, acral lentiginous and subungal melanomas have poor prognosis due to late presentation. In general, factors such as age, pregnancy, lesion diameter, histological type and inflammatory infiltrate are outweighed by tumour thickness and stage. However, even in thick (> 5 mm) melanomas there is a subset of patients who may survive 10 years or more; their tumours tend to be of spindle cell or Spitz-like cell type with a lack of mitoses and vascular invasion.

Balloon cell malignant melanoma tends to develop multiple cutaneous and subcutaneous metastases. The inter-related desmoplastic (myofibroblastic differentiation) and neurotropic (Schwann cell differentiation) variants arise mostly on the head and neck of elderly patients and show a high incidence of recurrence and metastases. Diagnosis requires an index of suspicion, recognition of tumour infiltrate in the deep dermis and accompanying clues in the form of an epidermal component. Immunocytochemistry (S100) is important in confirmation although it may be negative. Perineural invasion is a feature.

Breast Cancer

Breast Carcinoma

Breast Carcinoma

1. Gross description

Specimen

— fine needle aspirate/wide bore (14 gauge) needle core biopsy and imprint cytology/localisation biopsy/open biopsy/segmental excision/partial mastectomy/mastectomy.
— axillary nodes: sentinel biopsy/sampling/clearance.
— size (cm) and weight (g).

Male breast carcinoma (1% of cases) occurs in older men, presents late and has a poor prognosis. It shows the same range of morphological characteristics as female breast cancer.

Tumour

Site

— right/left/bilateral.
— quadrant: 50% UOQ, 15% UIQ, 10% LOQ, 17% central, 3% diffuse (massive or multifocal). Some estimates of multicentricity are up to 13% of cases and more frequently seen in lobular carcinoma than ductal. A general rule of thumb for multicentricity and bilaterality is 10–15%.
— distances (cm) from the nipple and resection limits.

Size

— maximum dimension of invasive lesion (cm).
— maximum dimension of whole tumour (invasive +DCIS) (cm).

Appearance

— scirrhous/fleshy/mucoid/cystic/diffuse thickening.

Ductal carcinoma tends to form a discrete mass lesion whereas lobular carcinoma can be difficult to define clinically, radiologically, cytologically and at the laboratory dissection bench. This has obvious implications for completeness of excision in patients treated with breast-conserving surgery and the pathological assessment of the surgical margins.

Edge

— circumscribed/irregular.

2. Histological type

In-situ carcinoma

Ductal carcinoma in-situ

— bound by basement membrane involving ≥ 2 ducts or 2–3 mm diameter; epithelial proliferation of lesser extent is designated atypical ductal hyperplasia unless of high cytological grade or with comedo necrosis.

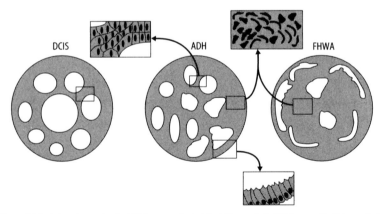

Figure 82. Ductal carcinoma in-situ (DCIS) versus atypical ductal hyperplasia (ADH) versus florid hyperplasia without atypia (FHWA): cytology and histology. DCIS features smooth, punched-out luminal borders within involved basement-membrane-bound space. The cytological features are regular and present throughout the entire population of at least two basement-membrane-bound spaces. FHWA is the most densely cellular and extensive of the proliferative disease without atypia lesions, also called "papillomatosis". There are ragged, often slit-like luminal borders. The nuclei throughout the involved area show variability and tendency to a swirling pattern, as illustrated. ADH has features predominantly of non-comedo, cribriform DCIS, but also some features of proliferative disease without atypia or normally polarised cells within the same basement-membrane-bound space. (Page DL, Rogers LW. Combined histologic and cytologic criteria for the diagnosis of mammary atypical ductal hyperplasia. Hum Pathol 1992;23:1095–1097.)

- nuclear grade: low, intermediate, high.
- necrosis: comedo or punctate; comedo = central eosinophilic necrosis containing 5 or more pyknotic nuclei.
- cell polarisation: present or absent.
- architectural patterns: comedo
                                         cribriform
                                         papillary
                                         micropapillary
                                         solid.

Lobular carcinoma in-situ

- uniform cells populating the lobule.
- no lumen in the acini.
- ≥ 50% of the acini in the lobule expanded and filled
- ± pagetoid spread into ducts.
- potentially multifocal (70%) and bilateral (30–40%).
- epithelial proliferation of lesser extent (e.g. with preservation of lumina) is designated atypical lobular hyperplasia.

Distinction between DCIS and LCIS is not always easy, e.g. lobular cancerisation by low-grade DCIS and, rarely, mixed lesions occur.

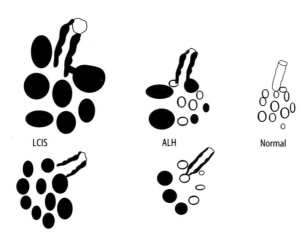

Figure 83. Schematic demonstration of diagnostic criteria for lobular carcinoma in-situ (LCIS). There is distention and distortion of more than half the acini, and an absence of central lumina. When these changes are less well developed (i.e.<50% of acini involved) atypical lobular hyperplasia (ALH) is diagnosed. Note that the pagetoid spread into adjacent ducts is more common in LCIS, but may be seen in ALH. (Page DL, Kidd TE, Dupont WD, Simpson JF, Rogers LW. Lobular neoplasia of the breast: higher risk for subsequent invasive cancer predicted by more extensive disease. Hum Pathol 1991;22:1232–1239.)

Microinvasion

— ≤ 1 mm from the adjacent basement membrane with infiltration of non-specialised interlobular/interductal stroma.

Minimal invasive cancer

— variably defined as<0.5 cm or<1 cm maximum dimension.

Invasive carcinoma

Ductal
— no specific type (NST): 70–75% of breast cancer.

Lobular
— 15% of breast cancer.
— classical: 40%; single files of small cells/targetoid periductal pattern/AB-PAS positive intracytoplasmic lumina.
— alveolar: nested pattern.
— solid: sheets.
— trabecular: bands of cells two to four across.
— pleomorphic: classical pattern but with cytological atypia.
— mixed: 40%; more than one component of these types but each is<80% of the tumour area.
— tubulolobular: classical pattern with focal microtubules which are less distinct than in tubular carcinoma.

Special types
— tubular: round,ovoid,angular tubules/single cell layer/cytoplasmic apical snouts/fibrous stroma.
— cribriform: invasive cords and islands with the morphology of cribriform DCIS – punched out lumina and cytoplasmic apical snouts.
— colloid (mucinous): extracellular mucin with small clusters (10-100 cells) of epithelial cells.
— papillary: encysted in-situ or invasive. Invasion is either (a) a dominantly invasive carcinoma with a pushing margin and papillary pattern, or (b) an encysted papillary carcinoma with focal invasion; the invasive component can be papillary or ductal, NST. Note also invasive micropapillary carcinoma (micropapillae without cores set in clear spaces) which is considered aggressive.
— medullary, classical: circumscribed margin, tumour cell syncytium with grade 3 cytology, peri-/intratumoural stromal lymphoplasmacytic infiltrate.

— medullary, atypical: contains up to 25% ductal, NST or, an irregular margin with focal infiltration, or adjacent DCIS.

Mixed types
— 10% of breast cancers.
— mixed differentiation ductal and lobular.
— tubular mixed – stellate mass, central tubules with peripheral less differentiated adenocarcinoma.

Others
— metaplastic: biphasic epithelial (ductal in-situ/invasive NST grade 2/3, or squamous) and sarcomatous elements (carcinosarcoma) or pure monophasic spindle cell carcinoma (cytokeratin/EMA positive). The sarcomatous element is either fibrosarcomatous/malignant fibrous histiocytoma-like or chondro-, osteo-, leiomyo-, rhabdomyo- or liposarcomatous. Probably represents carcinoma with a spectrum of spindle cell stromal metaplasia which can be homologous or heterologous. Behaves as a high-grade carcinoma.
— small cell: rare, aggressive, NSE/chromogranin positive.
— neuroendocrine: invasive ductal carcinoma with endocrine differentiation; carcinoid-like.
— secretory: one-third are in children, indolent, good prognosis; two-thirds are in adults, more aggressive.; tubular/solid/honeycomb patterns; PAS/AB-diastase positive luminal secretions.
— squamous cell: primary or secondary from breast skin or metastatic, e.g. lung – distinguish from metaplastic breast carcinoma.
— clear cell: glycogen rich.
— mucoepidermoid: grade determines prognosis.
— adenoid cystic: indolent with late recurrence.
— apocrine.
— adenomyoepithelioma: elderly, of low malignant potential; occasionally malignant myoepithelioma.

Pure carcinoma
— ≥ 90% of the tumour volume.

Mixed carcinoma
— ≥ 10% of the tumour volume is second component.

Metastatic carcinoma

— often solitary, upper outer quadrant at a late stage in known carcinomatosis. The majority of childhood breast malignancy is metastatic, e.g. alveolar rhabdomyosarcoma. In adults, usually lung (small cell), malignant melanoma, lymphoma/leukaemia, but also ovary, contralateral breast (usually this represents a metachronous primary), gut, kidney, thyroid carcinomas and small intestinal carcinoid tumour. A relevant clinical history, absence of in-situ change and multiple intravascular deposits are pointers to metastases. Specific antibodies (e.g. thyroglobulin, CA125, S100, HMB-45, melan-A, chromogranin) and immune markers of breast profile (e.g. ER/PR, cytokeratin 7, CEA, GCDFP-15) may be helpful in distinguishing between primary breast and non-mammary disease. Metastatic tumour should be considered in any breast lesion with unusual clinical, radiological, gross or histological features.

3. Differentiation/grade

Well/moderate/poor or grade 1/2/3.
See protocol: Grading of Invasive Breast Carcinoma.

4. Extent of local tumour spread

Border: pushing/infiltrative.
Lymphocytic reaction: prominent/sparse.
Quadrant(s):
— Paget's disease.
— skin involvement (direct extension or lymphatics).

pTis carcinoma in-situ. DCIS, LCIS or Paget's with no tumour
pT1 tumour ≤ 2 cm
     T1 mic   ≤ 0.1 cm
     T1 a   0.1 cm<tumour ≤ 0.5 cm
     T1 b   0.5 cm<tumour ≤ 1 cm
     T1 c   1 cm<tumour ≤ 2 cm
pT2 2 cm<tumour ≤ 5 cm
pT3 tumour > 5 cm
pT4 tumour any size with direct extension to chest wall (ribs, intercostal muscles, serratus anterior but not pectoral muscle) or skin
    (a) chest wall
    (b) oedema including peau d'orange, skin ulceration or satellite nodules in the same breast
    (c) a and b
    (d) inflammatory carcinoma
       sore and red due to tumour involvement of dermal lymphatics. It can be difficult to obtain tissue proof on fine needle aspiration cytology or needle core biopsy.

In-situ change
— present/absent.
— intra-/extratumoural: > 1 mm outside the main tumour mass and its extent. Pure DCIS of limited size (< 4 cm) tends to be unicentric (albeit ramifying through the involved duct system) and treated by breast-conserving surgery.

If it is mammographically extensive mastectomy is done. If it is present away from an invasive cancer in a local excision specimen it is an indication for considering proceeding to mastectomy and/or radiotherapy.

— architectural pattern.
— cytonuclear grade: shows less heterogeneity and higher inter-observer agreement than architectural pattern. It is now the favoured method for grading ductal carcinoma in-situ using either nuclear features alone (NHS Breast Screening Programme) or combined with the presence of comedonecrosis (Van Nuys classification). High-grade correlates with a greater frequency of concurrent or subsequent invasive carcinoma.

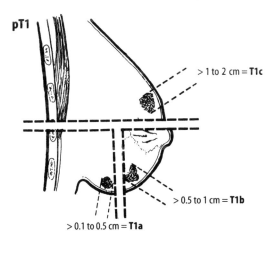

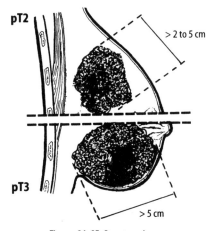

Figures 84, 85. Breast carcinoma.

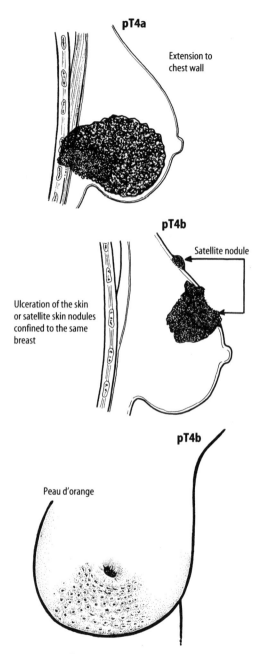

Figures 86–88. Breast carcinoma.

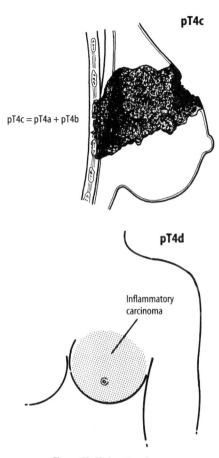

Figures 89, 90. Breast carcinoma.

Not infrequently there is correlation between DCIS architectural pattern and cytonuclear grade, e.g. comedonecrosis is high-grade and cribriform low-grade. However, this is not always the case, e.g. solid or micropapillary although usually low to intermediate-grade can be high-grade.

5. Lymphovascular invasion

Present/absent.
Intra-/extratumoural: > 1 mm outside the main tumour mass.
The commonest site for vascular invasion is at the tumour edge and it is present in about 25–35% of cases.

6. Lymph nodes

Site/number/size/number involved/apical node/extracapsular spread.
Regional nodes: axillary (levels I, II, III), internal mammary. Any other nodal metastasis is regarded as a distant metastasis pM1.

Axillary lymph nodes
Level 1: low axilla. Nodes lateral to the border of pectoralis minor muscle
Level 2: mid-axilla. Nodes between the medial and lateral borders of the pectoralis minor muscle
Level 3: apical axilla. Nodes medial to the medial margin of the pectoralis minor muscle

The regional lymph nodes are:
1. *Axillary* (ipsilateral): interpectoral (Rotter) nodes and lymph nodes along the axillary vein and its tributaries which may be divided into the following levels:
   i)   *Level I* (low-axilla): lymph nodes lateral to the lateral border of pectoralis minor muscle
   ii) *Level II* (mid-axilla): lymph nodes between the medial and lateral borders of the pectoralis minor muscle and the interpectoral (Rotter) lymph nodes
   iii) *Level III* (apical axilla): lymph nodes medial to the medial margin of the pectoralis minor muscle including those designated as subclavicular, infraclavicular or apical

   Note: Intramammary lymph nodes are coded as axillary lymph nodes

2. *Internal mammary* (ipsilateral): lymph nodes in the intercostal spaces along the edge of the sternum in the endothoracic fascia (2)

Any other lymph node metastasis is coded as a distant metastasis (M1), including supraclavicular, cervical or contralateral internal mammary lymph nodes

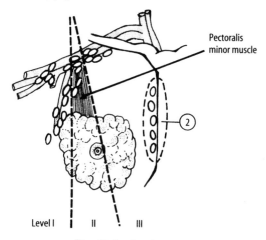

Figure 91. Breast carcinoma.

pN0   no regional lymph nodes involved
pN1   movable ipsilateral axillary nodes involved
            a. micrometastasis ≤ 0.2cm
            b. metastasis >0.2 cm
            further subdivided by the size of metastasis and number of involved
            nodes (pN1bi–pN1biv)
pN2   fixed ipsilateral axillary nodes involved
pN3   ipsilateral internal mammary nodes involved.

Cytokeratin markers are useful where the morphological appearances are suspicious, but not diagnostic of metastatic carcinoma, e.g. sinusoidal lobular carcinoma cells versus sinus histiocytosis. The significance of nodal micrometastasis remains uncertain with some regarding it as an adverse prognostic indicator but others less convinced. From a practical viewpoint it does influence choice of systemic adjuvant chemotherapy and hormonal therapy and should be reported. Histological levels and cytokeratin immunostaining may be necessary particularly if sentinel node biopsy alone is used for staging purposes in clinically node-negative patients. Other recommended approaches to axillary disease are axillary node sampling (for staging only) or axillary node clearance (for staging and treatment). Axillary node involvement is seen in 40–50% of cases; of these patients with axillary nodal disease there can also be involvement of the internal mammary chain (22%), and supraclavicular nodes (20%). Distant metastases are to the skeleton, lung and pleura, liver, ovary, adrenal gland and CNS. Presentation with metastatic tumour in axillary nodes is usually due to either breast carcinoma or malignant melanoma and this can be resolved with immunostaining. The source of the breast carcinoma is usually the ipsilateral breast or axillary tail of breast and the lesion can be clinically difficult to locate as its size is often less than 2 cm in diameter. Interestingly invasive lobular carcinoma has a greater tendency than ductal tumours to metastasise to retro-(peritoneum), meninges, gastrointestinal tract and female genital tracts.

7. Excision margins

Measure the distances (mm) to the nearest and other painted margins (superficial, deep, lateral, medial, inferior, superior). Differential block labelling and use of multi-coloured inks are important.

Adequate clearance of margins is:

— invasive carcinoma 5 mm.

— in-situ carcinoma 10 mm (ductal only as lobular can be multifocal).

Involved margins may be an indication for either radiotherapy (deep, superficial margins) or further surgery as a local re-excision or conversion to a mastectomy (other margins). Note that they can be particularly difficult to define and assess in lobular carcinoma.

8. Other pathology

Assess breast tissue away from the tumour for:

Atypical hyperplasia, carcinoma in-situ, satellite invasive foci, lymphovascular invasion (LVI).
Carcinoma in-situ and LVI away from (> 1 mm) the tumour are strong prognostic indicators of local and nodal recurrence and are important in selecting appropriate postoperative adjuvant therapy or further surgical excision. Relationship of satellite invasive foci to margins must also be assessed; they occur more frequently in infiltrating lobular carcinoma.

Atypical hyperplasia (ductal and lobular) is regarded as having ×4–5 increased risk of subsequent carcinoma and in-situ change ×10–11 increased risk over control populations. The precancerous nature of atypical hyperplasia is illustrated by its shared molecular abnormalities (e.g. loss of allelic heterozygosity) with carcinoma in-situ. LCIS is usually an incidental microscopic finding eg. adjacent to a simple cyst or present (60%) in the vicinity of invasive lobular cancer; it is potentially multifocal and bilateral. Ductal carcinoma in-situ may present as Paget's disease ± nipple discharge, a tumour-forming mass (especially comedo type with a greater propensity for invasive carcinoma), adjacent to a symptomatic invasive breast cancer, as an incidental finding on open biopsy or as a lesion detected on radiological screening (15–20% of screening cancers). This can be either as linear, branching calcifications or within the context of a radiologically suspicious but histologically benign lesion, e.g. radial scar/complex sclerosing lesion. Immunomarkers S100 and smooth muscle actin are useful in demonstrating a myoepithelial cell layer as an aid to distinction from invasive carcinoma.

It is essential to correlate the clinical mammographic abnormality with the excised specimen. This requires dissection guided by the postoperative specimen radiograph demonstrating the lesion in question with or without an in-situ localisation needle. The histological slides must contain the abnormality, e.g. carcinoma or microcalcification and, if not, all of the residual tissue processed or further blocks selected according to radiographic study of the specimen serial slices. Usual calcification (calcium phosphate) is easily recognisable as basophilic in routine sections; a minority (10%) is oxalate in character, can be partially removed by tissue processing and is recognised by being doubly refractile on polarisation. It is usually seen in benign disease, e.g. fibrocystic disease.

Paget's disease (2% of breast cancer patients) is distinguished immunohistochemically from malignant melanoma and Bowen's disease by being mucin, CEA, EMA and cytokeratin 7 positive, and S100, HMB-45 and melan-A negative. DCIS of large cell type is nearly always identified in the subareolar duct system and there is associated invasive breast carcinoma in 35–50% of cases.

Microinvasion, defined as<1 mm from the nearest basement membrane (infiltration of nonspecialised interlobular/interductal stroma), must be distinguished from the more frequent cancerisation of lobules (lobular architecture/intact basement membrane) and clinically is managed as DCIS as the incidence of axillary lymph node metastases is very low. The likelihood of invasion increases with the grade of DCIS, e.g. comedocarcinoma; extra blocks and levels should be assessed. Usually the type of invasive carcinoma correlates with the type of DCIS but LCIS can be associated with invasive carcinoma of ductal or lobular type.

Neoadjuvant chemo-/radiotherapy effects include tumour cell necrosis, degeneration, apoptosis, vacuolation, inflammation and fibrosis, and tends to be reserved for pT3/pT4 tumours which may then be followed by surgical resection. It improves resectability and may have a role to play in downstaging of the tumour although this is not yet clarified. Postoperative radiotherapy is used for the control of local recurrence in the presence of positive deep or superficial margins of excision and can result in diagnostically confusing cytological atypia in native ductulolobular unit epithelium. The presence of widespread metastatic disease should be clinically determined prior to surgical resection so that palliative systemic therapy can be considered. Localised disease is treated by wide local excision ensuring 10-20 mm palpable margins of clearance around the tumour. Conversion to mastectomy (10–15% of cases) is undertaken in the following combination of circumstances: if the patient is<50 years of age, has a tumour diameter > 2 cm, has lymphovascular invasion or involvement of the surgical margins. Otherwise the intact breast receives radiotherapy. Mastectomy is indicated as initial treatment if the tumour is centrally situated (behind the nipple), > 3 cm in diameter and/or associated with radiological evidence of extensive DCIS, or if it is the patient's preference.

Triple assessment and concordance of its three modalities (clinical examination, radiology, fine needle aspiration cytology (FNAC) ± wide bore needle core biopsy) have replaced frozen section and the majority of open biopsies in the diagnosis of breast carcinoma. This allows a one-stop assessment and progression to definitive breast-conserving or more radical surgery. Open biopsy may still be required where there is discordance between the parameters. FNAC cannot accurately distinguish between in-situ and invasive malignant cells and supplementary core biopsy is advantageous, e.g. high-grade ductal carcinoma in-situ. Note that diagnostic core biopsy can underestimate cancer grade and may not accurately reflect tumour subtype compared with the resection specimen, e.g. for reasons of tumour heterogeneity in both cellularity and differentiation. Core biopsy is also advantageous when FNAC is either insufficient (e.g. scirrhous or lobular carcinoma) or inconclusive (e.g. some well-differentiated grade I cancers).

Prognosis

Nottingham Prognostic Index (NPI) = 0.2 × size (cm) + stage + grade.

		Score	
Stage	A	No nodes	1
	B	≤ 3 low axillary nodes	2
	C	≥ 4 nodes and/or the apical node	3

NPI score	*Prognosis*	*5 year survival*
< 3.4	Good	88%
3.4–5.4	Intermediate	68%
> 5.4	Poor	21%.

Dutch workers advocate a morphometric index based on tumour size, mitotic activity index and lymph node status as giving practical clinical prognostic data.

Overall 5 year survival is 60% for clinically localised disease and 34% for regional disease.

Prognosis according to histological type (10 year survivals)

excellent (> 80%)	tubular, cribriform, mucinous, tubulolobular, encysted in-situ papillary
good (60–80%)	tubular mixed, alveolar lobular, mixed ductal NST/special type
intermediate (50–60%)	classical lobular, medullary, invasive papillary
poor (< 50%)	ductal (no special type), mixed ductal and lobular, solid and pleomorphic lobular, metaplastic.

Oestrogen/progesterone receptor expression

Most postmenopausal patients receive the anti-oestrogen tamoxifen but positive oestrogen receptor (ER) status in premenopausal patients is important so that consideration can be given to hormonal treatment. Progesterone receptor expression is a prognostic marker and may also indicate hormone responsiveness.

— tissue for staining: choose block (formalin fixed) with tumour and normal breast elements (internal control).

— staining method: strep. ABC Duet immunohistochemistry with 2 min pressure cooking heat-mediated antigen retrieval.

— monoclonal antibody: ER – DAKO 1D5/NOVOCASTRA 6F11; PR – DAKO PgR 636.

Scoring system: "Category Score"

Staining characteristics	Microscopic assessment	ER status
Negative	No staining	ER –
Weak	×25, ×40 objective	ER +
Moderate	×10 objective	ER +
Strong	×10 objective	ER +

Scoring system: "Histo Score"

In the Histo score, each cell is assessed as:

   0 – no staining
   1 – weak staining
   2 – moderate staining
   3 – strong staining.

The percentage of cells showing each intensity of staining is estimated over as much of the section as possible and the Histo Score is calculated by multiplying the intensity score by the percentage of tumour cells showing that intensity: e.g. a tumour with 50% of cells strongly stained, 25% moderately stained and 25% weakly stained would score $(50 \times 3) + (25 \times 2) + (25 \times 1) = 225$. Histo Scores less than 75 are considered to be ER negative and those above 75 are considered to be ER positive.

Individual cancers can show heterogeneity of ER receptor expression and in some respects the Histo Score can take this into account. Carcinoma in-situ, infiltrating lobular carcinoma, low-grade invasive ductal carcinoma and post-menopausal cancers tend to be ER positive while high-grade invasive ductal lesions and a significant number of premenopausal carcinomas (grade-related) are ER negative.

Miscellaneous markers

— Ki-67 proliferation index (percentage positive cells), c-erbB2, p53, DNA ploidy.

— decreased survival is associated with tumours that are ER/PR negative, DNA aneuploid, overexpress p53/c-erbB2 and have a high proliferation index.

— cytokeratin (CAM 5.2, AE1/AE3, CK7), GCDFP-15, EMA, CEA positive. Variably positive for HMB-45, S100 and vimentin.

— cytokeratin 7 positive/20 negative: the reverse of this is seen in intestinal tract tumours and this can be useful in metastatic carcinoma of uncertain origin, e.g. signet ring cell carcinoma.

— c-erbB2 overexpression indicates potential resistance to Tamoxifen and CMF chemotherapy but benefit from high dose adriamycin therapy.

9. Other malignancy

Leukaemia

— single/multiple, uni-/bilateral.

— during the course of known disease or as a primary clinical presentation.

— ALL/CLL/myeloma (κ,λ light chain restriction and clinical evidence of systemic disease).

— granulocytic sarcoma (CD 68/chloroacetate esterase positive) can mimic infiltrating lobular carcinoma (cytokeratins, cellular mucin) and lymphoma (CD 45, CD 20, CD 3).

Lymphoma

— usually secondary to known nodal/systemic disease and not biopsied.

— 0.5% of malignant breast tumours.

— may present clinically and radiologically as a carcinoma and immunos-taining of aspirate and/or biopsy material will be necessary.

Primary lymphoma (by exclusion of systemic lymphoma after staging):

1. commonest:	aggressive large B cell lymphoma usually unilateral in elderly women.
2. secondly:	aggressive Burkitt's/Burkitt's-like lymphoma in young pregnant or lactating women. Bilateral with CNS and ovarian involvement.
3. rarely:	indolent low grade MALToma (?prior lymphocytic lobulitis).

4. differential diagnosis: infiltrating lobular carcinoma, medullary carcinoma; immuno-cytokeratins, CD 45, CD 20, CD 3. ER can be positive in carcinoma and lymphoma.

5. prognosis: overall 48% 5 year survival; Burkitt's, poor.

Phyllodes tumour

— benign/borderline/malignant comprising a biphasic proliferation of hyperplastic epithelium and abundant, cellular mesenchymal elements with a leaf-like architecture.

Designation is based on:

1. circumscribed or infiltrative margins
2. stromal cellularity
   overgrowth
   atypia
   mitoses > 5–10/10 high-power fields = probably malignant when combined with overgrowth and atypia
   mitoses >10/10 high-power fields = malignant
   overexpression of p53.

At the benign end of the spectrum the differential diagnosis is cellular fibroadenoma and at the malignant end metaplastic breast carcinoma and sarcoma. Mammography and fine needle aspiration cytology are not particularly accurate at diagnosing phyllodes tumour; wide (1 cm margins) local excision is needed for histological designation and prevention of local recurrence, which can occur even with benign and borderline lesions. Those classified as malignant have metastatic potential.

Sarcoma

Sarcoma (< 1% of breast malignancies), e.g. angiosarcoma (± post radiotherapy) and other primary soft tissue sarcomas (in decreasing order of frequency): malignant fibrous histiocytoma, fibrosarcoma, rhabdomyosarcoma, liposarcoma, leiomyosarcoma. Prognosis relates to high histological grade, mitotic counts and infiltrating margins. Important and more common differential diagnoses are metaplastic breast carcinoma (identify epithelial component, cytokeratin positive) and malignant phyllodes tumour (biphasic and typical architecture). Angiosarcoma is the commonest primary breast sarcoma, occurs in middle-aged to elderly women and is on average 5 cm in diameter with poorly defined margins. Grade 1 lesions (40%) must be distinguished from haemangioma and pseudoangiomatous hyperplasia and have an 81% 10 year survival. Grade 3 lesions (40%) mimic poorly differentiated carcinoma and have 10% 10 year survival with metastases to lungs, liver, skin, bone and brain. Diagnosis can be difficult on fine needle aspiration cytology and biopsy is required. Angiosarcoma is variably factor VIII, CD 34 and CD 31 positive.

Other spindle cell lesions of the breast to be considered in a differential diagnosis are: metastatic malignant melanoma and sarcomatoid renal cell carcinoma, fibromatosis and myofibroblast-related lesions (inflammatory myofibroblastic tumour, myofibroblastoma).

Reporting categories for breast fine needle aspirates and wide bore needle core biopsies

Fine needle aspiration cytology (FNAC) is highly efficient and accurate at diagnosing a wide range of breast disease when interpreted in conjunction with the patient's age, clinical history, clinical features of the lesion and its radiological appearances. Two basic patterns are encountered:

1. Benign   a biphasic pattern of cohesive breast epithelium and background bare nuclei

low to moderate cellularity (except fibroadenoma, which is of high cellularity)

2. Malignant   dyscohesive clusters and singles of variably atypical epithelial cells

cytoplasmic preservation in dispersed cells

absence of bare nuclei

stripped (bare) malignant nuclei

moderate to high cellularity for the patient's age.

FNAC reporting categories are:

C1   an inadequate specimen: insufficient epithelial cells, epithelial cell content obscured by inflammation or a technically poorly prepared smear

C2   an adequate benign specimen: of sufficient cellularity and showing a benign biphasic pattern

C3   atypia, benign: showing some mild nuclear change or cellular dissociation but within an essentially benign pattern

C4   atypia, suspicious: a pattern and cell constitution suspicious but not diagnostic of malignancy for quantitative (inadequate cellularity) or qualitative (insufficient atypia) reasons

C5   malignant: a cellular specimen showing an unequivocally malignant pattern and individual malignant cells.

FNAC is supplemented by wide bore needle core biopsy in certain circumstances, e.g. the diagnosis of phyllodes tumour, infiltrating lobular carcinoma (which may be scanty on FNAC) and the distinction between in-situ and invasive malignancy (the latter being an indication for axillary lymph node staging/resection).

Wide bore needle core biopsy reporting categories are:

B1   unsatisfactory/normal tissue only

B2   benign: e.g. fibroadenoma, sclerosing adenosis

B3   benign but of uncertain malignant potential: benign lesions associated with the presence of cancer and/or the risk of developing it, e.g. radial scar, atypical hyperplasia

B4   suspicion of malignancy: epithelial proliferation suspicious but not diagnostic of malignancy for quantitative or qualitative reasons

B5   malignant: a. in-situ
                     b. invasive.

Reporting categories are a useful tool in the day-to-day management of individual cases and crucial for clinicopathological audit purposes. It is imperative that FNAC and wide bore needle core biopsy material are closely correlated with their respective surgical specimens.

Grading of invasive breast carcinoma

Grading is most relevant to infiltrating duct carcinoma, no specific type and special types. Infiltrating lobular carcinoma tends to be given grade 2 although the classical and pleomorphic variants score as grades 1 and 3 respectively.

Three parameters are assessed and scored:

1. Tubule formation	*Score*
Majority of tumour (> 75%)	1
Moderate (10–75%)	2
Little or none (< 10%)	3

2. Nuclear pleomorphism	
Regular, uniform	1
Larger with variation	2
Marked variation (± multiple nucleoli)	3

3. Mitoses (tumour periphery rather than the paucicellular centre)
The mitotic count (number of mitoses per 10 high-power fields) is related to the objective field diameter:

Leitz Diaplan ×40 obj.	*Leitz Ortholux* ×25 obj.	*Nikon Labophot* ×40 obj.	
0–11	0–9	0–5	1
12–22	10–19	6–10	2
> 22	> 19	> 10	3

Total score	*Grade*	
3–5	1	Well differentiated.
6–7	2	Moderately differentiated.
8–9	3	Poorly differentiated.

Gynaecological Cancer

- Ovarian Carcinoma (with comments on fallopian tube carcinoma)

- Endometrial Carcinoma

- Cervical Carcinoma

- Vaginal Carcinoma

- Vulval Carcinoma

- Gestational Trophoblastic Tumours

Ovarian Carcinoma
(with comments on fallopian tube carcinoma)

1. Gross description

Specimen

— fine needle aspirate/wedge biopsy/oophorectomy and/or cystectomy/uni-/bilateral salpigooophorectomy ± hysterectomy/omentectomy.
— weight (g) and size (cm).

Tumour

Site

— ovarian (cystic, cortical or serosal)/paratubal/broad ligament.
— unilateral/bilateral (15–40% of serous epithelial lesions).

Size

— length × width × depth (cm) or maximum dimension (cm).

Appearance

Capsule: intact/deficient, smooth/rough.

Cut surface:
— cystic: uni-/multilocular
            warty growths/nodules
            fluid contents: serous/mucoid
            sebaceous content: hair/teeth/colloid
            (struma ovarii)
— solid: partially/totally (cm)
           necrosis/haemorrhage.

Edge

— circumscribed/irregular.

Fallopian tube: length (cm); infiltration of paratubal connective tissue.

Omentum: weight (g) and size (cm); tumour nodules: number/maximum dimension (cm).

2. Histological type

Epithelial and sex cord stromal lesions form 60–70% of ovarian tumours (75% of which are benign) and 90–95% of primary ovarian malignancy, the vast majority of which arises from the surface (coelomic) epithelium. Epithelial tumours are classified according to their cell type, growth pattern (solid, cystic, surface), amount of fibrous stroma and neoplastic potential of the constituent epithelium (benign, borderline or malignant/invasive). Germ cell tumours comprise 25% of ovarian tumours and the vast majority of these are benign. They form 60–70% of childhood ovarian tumours and while the majority of these are benign (cystic teratoma) there is a greater proportion of malignant germ cell tumours (immature teratoma, yolk sac tumour) than in adults.

Epithelial

— serous	40%	
— mucinous	20%	
— endometrioid	20%	benign, borderline or malignant
— clear cell	10%	
— Brenner	2%	

— mixed: e.g.
  mucinous/Brenner
  mucinous/endometrioid: each component at least 10% and mixed differentiation of the common epithelial subtypes is relatively frequent (20–30% of cases).
  endometrioid carcinoma with squamous differentiation (benign or malignant cytology).

— undifferentiated: small cell ± hypercalcaemia
  non-small cell
  osteoclast-like
  trophoblastic differentiation.

Sex cord/stromal

— 8% of ovarian neoplasms.

— granulosa (12%):
  adult: micro-(macro)follicular (Call-Exner bodies), trabecular, insular, watered-silk, solid, sarcomatoid patterns, longitudinal nuclear grooves.
  juvenile: solid or cystic, follicular patterns of small cells ± mitoses.

— thecoma-fibroma (85%): fibroma is one of the commonest ovarian tumours; thecomatous elements are fat stain positive.

— Sertoli-Leydig: well/moderate/poor differentiation ± heterologous elements.
— mixed variants.
— gynandroblastoma: equimixed android/gynaecoid elements.
— gonadoblastoma: mixed germ cell/sex cord cell elements.
— sex cord tumour with annular tubules (SCTAT): Peutz-Jeghers syndrome; adenoma malignum cervix.
— ± α inhibin positive, CA125/CK7 negative.

Malignant mixed mesodermal (carcinosarcoma)

— old age, poor prognosis,<1% of ovarian tumours.
— homologous: cytokeratin positive, therefore a metaplastic endometrioid adenocarcinoma.
— heterologous: cartilage, striated muscle, osteoid.

Steroid cell tumours

— rare (0.1%), hormonally active with virilisation (75%).
— 30% are malignant based on size (> 7 cm), mitoses, atypia, necrosis.

Germ cell tumours

— teratoma: mature/cystic.
immature/solid.
monodermal, e.g. carcinoid, struma ovarii (thyroid tissue).
malignant transformation, e.g. squamous carcinoma (80% of malignant cases).
— dysgerminoma (seminoma analogue), yolk sac tumour, embryonal carcinoma.
— choriocarcinoma
primary: primary prepubertal or as part of a mixed germ cell tumour.
secondary: to gestational uterine, tubal or ovarian lesion (better prognosis).

Metastatic carcinoma

— 6-7%; especially stomach, appendix, colorectum, pancreas, breast (infiltrating lobular).
— Krukenberg – classically bilateral signet ring cell metastases from stomach – mucin positive with a reactive fibrous ovarian stroma ± luteinisation. Spread is peritoneal and differential diagnosis is primary ovarian signet ring cell carcinoma.
— direct spread: colorectal carcinoma, carcinoma of fallopian tube, endometrium and cervix.
— distant spread: lung, malignant melanoma, breast, kidney, thyroid. Small cell ovarian tumours (juvenile granulosa, small cell ± hypercalcaemia) must be distinguished from metastatic small cell carcinoma of lung.

Seventy per cent of secondary carcinomas are bilateral. Other clues are solid, discrete, corticomedullary nodular deposits, surface deposits and prominent lymphovascular invasion. Prognosis of metastatic ovarian carcinoma is poor. A number of metastases mimic primary ovarian carcinoma, e.g. gut (mucinous), renal cell (mesonephroid/clear cell), thyroid (struma ovarii) and hepatocellular (yolk sac tumour) carcinomas.

3. Differentiation

Adenocarcinoma

— well/moderate/poor.
— based on the degree of tubule/organoid differentiation, cellular pleomorphism and mitotic activity ± overt invasion of the stroma or capsule. The presence and extent of stromal invasion is a strong prognostic indicator.
NB: micropapillary serous carcinoma requires no demonstrable invasion but is designated on the degree of epithelial complexity. It is an exophytic lesion often associated with invasive peritoneal implants, bilaterality and advanced stage and is of worse prognosis than usual serous borderline tumours.

Borderline (low malignant potential)

— excellent prognosis regardless of stage; bilateral in 20–25%, younger age group (40–50 years); 5–10% of epithelial tumours; epithelial complexity with budding, atypia, mitoses and nuclear layering (≤3 nuclei deep in mucinous lesions); no destructive stromal invasion.

Sex cord/stromal

— well/moderate/poor differentiation; weak correlation with prognosis.

Functional: e.g. oestrogenic drive to endometrium in thecoma, granulosa cell tumour; virilisation in Sertoli-Leydig tumour.

Prognosis relates to size (< or > 5 cm), an intact or deficient capsule, bulk of extraovarian disease, atypia, mitoses, necrosis, bilaterality.

Recurrence (30%) tends to be local: it may be extra-pelvic and after a considerable lag period of 10-20 years although recurrent juvenile granulosa and Sertoli-Leydig tumours recur within 3 years. Raised serum inhibin levels may be useful in detecting recurrent granulosa cell tumour.

Germ cell

— mature: cystic (95% of cases), common tissues are skin and appendage structures, muscle, fat, ganglia, glial tissue, respiratory, gastrointestinal and pancreatic glandular tissue, retinal elements, cartilage and bone.
— immature: solid with histologically identifiable immature tissues especially cartilage, neuroepithelium, striated muscle and immature cellular mesenchyme.
— grade 1: mostly mature tissue, loose mesenchyme, immature cartilage, focal (<1 low-power field/slide) immature neuroepithelium.
— grade 3: scant mature tissue, extensive (>3 low-power fields/slide) immature neuroepithelium ± peritoneal implants which can be mature (e.g. gliomatosis peritonei) or immature and, are graded separately.

— ± carcinoma (e.g. squamous) or sarcoma (e.g. rhabdomyosarcoma, sarcoma of no specific type) in mature or immature lesions.

4. Extent of local tumour spread

Border: pushing/infiltrative.
Lymphocytic reaction: prominent/sparse.
Capsule/serosa/paratubal connective tissue/contiguous fallopian tube.

Extensive sampling of ovarian epithelial cystic lesions is necessary (1 block/cm diameter) as there can be marked heterogeneity and coexistence of benign, borderline and malignant features, e.g. mucinous lesions. Microinvasion ≤ 10 mm^2 (or approximately 3 mm diameter) can be difficult to distinguish from crypt epithelial complexity and invagination into stroma (desmoplasia is a useful feature in carcinoma); it is occasionally seen in otherwise borderline serous tumours but does not alter the prognosis. Invasion > 5 mm may help to discriminate between mucinous borderline and carcinoma lesions with a worse clinical outcome.

Invasion of stroma and/or capsule remains the hallmark of carcinoma but not infrequently its presence is difficult to assess or it is not evident. This is particularly problematic in mucinous lesions, where a designation of non-invasive carcinoma or intraepithelial carcinoma may be made on the basis of epithelial complexity with a confluent glandular pattern and cellular atypia alone, e.g. nuclear stratification ≥ 4 deep, cribriform epithelial pattern or stroma-free papillae of epithelial cells. Further sampling is necessary to exclude frankly invasive areas warranting the more usual designation of adenocarcinoma.

Minimal staging requires removal of the ovarian primary lesion, biopsy of the contralateral ovary, biopsy of omentum and peritoneal surfaces, and peritoneal washings for cytology if ascitic fluid is not present.

FIGO/TNM
pT1   growth limited to the ovaries
       a. one ovary, capsule intact, no serosal disease or malignant cells in ascites or peritoneal washings
       b. two ovaries, capsule intact, no serosal disease or malignant cells in ascites or peritoneal washings
       c. one or both ovaries with any of: capsule rupture, serosal disease or malignant cells in ascites or peritoneal washings
pT2   growth involving one or both ovaries with pelvic extension
       a. uterus, tubes
       b. other pelvic tissues
       c. 2a or 2b plus malignant cells in ascites or peritoneal washings
pT3   growth involving one or both ovaries with metastases to abdominal peritoneum, and/or regional nodes
       a. microscopic peritoneal mestastasis beyond pelvis
       b. macroscopic peritoneal metastasis ≤ 2 cm in greatest dimension beyond pelvis
       c. peritoneal metastasis > 2 cm in greatest dimension and/or regional lymph node metastasis (N1)

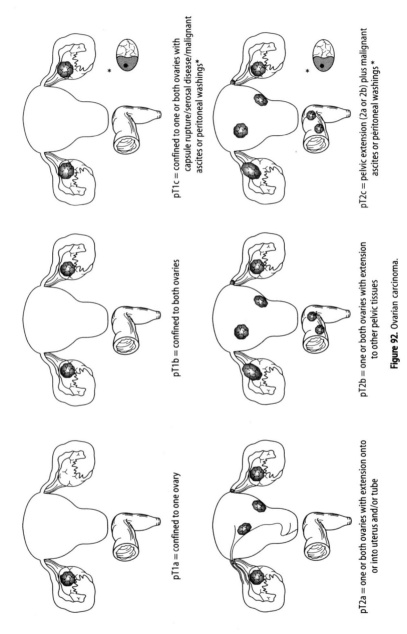

pT1a = confined to one ovary

pT1b = confined to both ovaries

pT1c = confined to one or both ovaries with capsule rupture/serosal disease/malignant ascites or peritoneal washings*

pT2a = one or both ovaries with extension onto or into uterus and/or tube

pT2b = one or both ovaries with extension to other pelvic tissues

pT2c = pelvic extension (2a or 2b) plus malignant ascites or peritoneal washings *

Figure 92. Ovarian carcinoma.

pT4/M1   growth involving one or both ovaries with distant metastases, e.g. liver parenchyma or positive pleural fluid cytology.

The commonest pattern of spread is the contralateral ovary, peritoneum, para-aortic and pelvic lymph nodes and liver. Lung is the preferred extra-abdominal site.

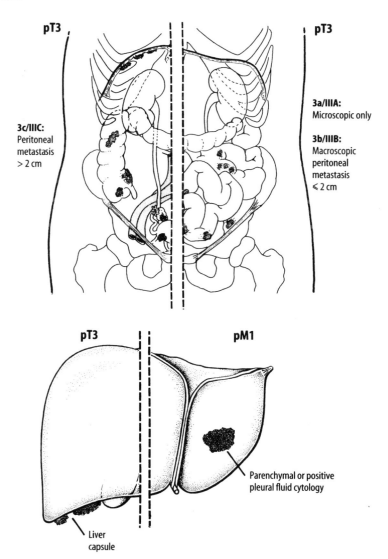

pT3

3c/IIIC:
Peritoneal metastasis
> 2 cm

pT3

3a/IIIA:
Microscopic only

3b/IIIB:
Macroscopic peritoneal metastasis
⩽ 2 cm

pT3

pM1

Parenchymal or positive pleural fluid cytology

Liver capsule

Figures 93, 94. Ovarian carcinoma.

5. Lymphovascular invasion

Present/absent.
Intra-/extratumoural.

6. Lymph nodes

Site/number/size/number involved/extracapsular spread.
Regional nodes: obturator, common iliac, external iliac, lateral sacral, para-aortic, inguinal.

pN0   no regional lymph node metastasis
pN1   metastasis in regional lymph node(s).

7. Omentum/peritoneum

Fifty per cent of serous borderline tumours are associated with foci of peritoneal serous epithelial proliferation.

Endosalpingiosis
— no atypia: ± a benign or borderline ovarian lesion.
— a metaplastic process in serosal epithelial inclusions.

Implants
— atypia: + borderline ovarian serous lesion.
  The implants are assessed independently of the ovarian tumour as:
  non-invasive or invasive (infiltration of underlying tissue disrupting the omental lobular architecture); epithelial (proliferative) or stromal (desmoplastic).
  Probably represent multifocal neoplasia arising in peritoneal inclusions. Endosalpingiosis, desmoplastic and non-invasive proliferating implants should be noted and follow-up recommended; invasive proliferating implants should be regarded as low-grade carcinoma as they progress in 80% of cases. Non-invasive proliferating implants are distinguished from surface serous carcinoma by greater nuclear atypia and epithelium comprising > 25% of the lesion area in carcinoma.

Pseudomyxoma peritonei
Pseudomyxoma peritonei is strongly associated with borderline ovarian mucinous lesions (especially of intestinal type) and/or concurrent appendiceal neoplasia. The peritoneal cavity fills with abundant mucin ± a component of proliferating or malignant epithelium. Prognosis is poor as it is refractory to treatment, slowly progressive and leads to bowel obstruction. It arises due to either rupture or spread from an ovarian/appendiceal lesion or from metaplasia in peritoneal endosalpingiosis. Appendiceal and ovarian lesions in

pseudomyxoma coexist in 90% of cases and some consider the latter to be metastatic from the former. Irrespective of the current debate each lesion should be assessed individually as benign, borderline or malignant. In addition comment should be made as to whether pseudomyxoma peritonei is free mucinous ascites, organising mucin fluid or mucin dissection with fibrosis. The latter, abundant mucin in the peritoneal cavity, and the presence of epithelial cells in the mucin and atypical cytological appearances are also adverse prognostic parameters. Because of the strength of association appendicectomy should be considered particularly when ovarian tumours are bilateral and there is extraovarian disease.

Primary peritoneal carcinoma

— young to middle-age females.
— serous adenocarcinoma in type.
— extensive peritoneal disease ± an ovarian serosal component with otherwise normal ovaries (any ovarian invasion<5 mm^2).

Metastatic adenocarcinoma.

8. Other pathology

Hereditary factors are responsible for 5–10% of ovarian carcinoma. Mutations in the BRCA1 and BRCA2 genes carry a 20–50% risk of ovarian cancer up to the age of 70 years. The tumours occur 5 years earlier than sporadic ovarian carcinoma, are mainly of serous histological type, have a strong association with breast cancer (BRCA1: 87% risk) and to a lesser extent (9% risk) hereditary non-polyposis colorectal cancer. Prognosis is similar to that of sporadic ovarian carcinoma.

— Meig's syndrome: ascites, ovarian fibroma and right sided pleural effusion.
— Contralateral ovary and tube: synchronous/metastatic disease of parenchyma or serosa (e.g. serous papillary lesions – 40%).
— Uterus: synchronous/metastatic disease of endometrium, endocervix or serosa (e.g. endometrioid carcinoma) i.e. multifocal Müllerian neoplasia.

Concurrent ovarian endometriosis (± atypical hyperplasia) and endometrial carcinoma is seen in up to 25% of ovarian endometrioid adenocarcinomas; the frequency of associated disease is lower in ovarian clear cell (mesonephroid) carcinoma, which is regarded as a variant of endometrioid carcinoma and may also be related to foci of ovarian endometriosis (10–20%) which is now considered as a potentially premalignant lesion. Clear cell carcinoma should be distinguished from yolk sac tumour, dysgerminoma and metastatic renal cell carcinoma.

DNA aneuploidy can sometimes help to distinguish borderline ovarian epithelial lesions from ovarian adenocarcinoma, and is an adverse prognostic indicator in borderline lesions. Mucinous borderline tumours are intestinal (85%; ± associated with pseudomyxoma peritonei) or Müllerian (endocervical; 30% are associated with endometriosis) in type with differing pathological and clinical features. A wide spectrum of intestinal differentiation can be seen and metastases from appendix, stomach, pancreas and colon need to be excluded. Mucinous tumours can also rarely show a spectrum of mural nodules of varying size and appearances ranging from anaplastic carcinoma (aggressive) and sarcoma (fibrosarcoma, rhabdomyosarcoma) to benign behaving sarcoma-like lesions. Pseudomyxoma ovarii is commoner in borderline and malignant lesions, particularly those with pseudomyxoma peritonei.

Mucinous (intestinal type) and endometrioid ovarian carcinomas and Sertoli-Leydig tumours can closely mimic or be imitated by colorectal and other gut adenocarcinomas. These secondaries can occur after, concurrently or even predate by up to several years (e.g. gastric carcinoma) the detection of the primary tumour.

Gut metastases to the ovary tend to be bilateral, solid with areas of necrosis, show crescentic garland-type strips of tumour with segmental and dirty necrosis on microscopy and diffuse cellular staining with CEA. CA19-9 may be positive and CA125 is usually negative. Ovarian carcinomas tend to be cystic with solid areas, uni- or bilateral, show cell apex CEA staining, ± CA125 and variable CA19-9. Mucin is scanty in endometrioid variants and negative in Sertoli-Leydig tumours. Anatomical distribution of disease is important. Despite this the differential diagnosis between ovarian and colorectal cancer can still be difficult and in any ovarian mucinous or endometrioid tumour the possibility of a gastrointestinal origin must be excluded clinically. Differential cytokeratin expression may be of use with intestinal tumours showing a different profile (cytokeratin 20 positive/7 negative) to ovarian tumours (cytokeratin 7 positive/20 negative). Gut cancers are also usually p53 positive – note that gastric, pancreatic and biliary cancers are variably cytokeratin 7/20 positive and may even express CA 125 as do some endometrial cancers. Metastatic breast carcinoma shows a similar cytokeratin profile (CK7+/CK20–)but may also be ER/PR and GCDFP-15 positive.

Serum levels and tissue expression of various antigens are detectable in a range of ovarian neoplasms but characteristically strong associations are:

CA125	ovarian carcinoma (serous type)
AFP	ovarian yolk sac tumour, immature teratoma
βHCG	ovarian choriocarcinoma, immature teratoma
α–inhibin, MIC-2	granulosa cell tumour
HPL/PLAP	dysgerminoma.

Prognosis

Prognosis of ovarian carcinoma relates to morphological features such as histological type and grade, volume percentage epithelium and mitotic activity index as well as large volume of disease after cytoreduction, high-volume ascites and high postoperative CA125 levels. Overexpression of cerb–B2 may also be adverse but the predominant factor is stage of disease. Early stage disease confined to the ovary or pelvis has a 5 year survival rate of 80% whereas the majority of patients present late with widespread metastatic disease and 10–20% survival at 5 years. Undoubtedly there are different types of ovarian adenocarcinoma according to their origins and behaviour – e.g. cystadenocarcinoma arising from a cystic ovarian neoplasm, or adenocarcinoma arising from a thin rim of outer cortex and showing aggressive behaviour with disproportionately extensive local spread and involvement of adjacent structures. Overall survival probability at 5 years is about 35–40%. Serum CA 125 levels are useful for monitoring disease progression and response to treatment but will be elevated in only 50% of early, curable disease. A suggested screening strategy is a combination of clinical examination, serum CA125 levels and abdominopelvic ultrasound examination. Fine needle aspiration cytology has a role to play in the distinction between functional (e.g. granulosa/luteal) cysts and benign or malignant epithelial lesions. Accurate surgical assessment is needed to avoid understaging of ovarian cancer, with surgical excision the mainstay of treatment. Cytoreductive surgery is also used for extensive disease with adjuvant therapy. Borderline ovarian epithelial neoplasms are uniformly of excellent prognosis (95–100% 5 year survival), even if microinvasion (<1–3 mm diameter) is present, with uni- or bilateral adnexectomy as effective as radical surgery. Prognosis is poor for intestinal-type borderline mucinous lesions associated with pseudomyxoma peritonei. Stage I mucinous adenocarcinoma has a good prognosis but may metastasise if extensive stromal invasion is present. Clear cell carcinoma has a worse outlook than the other usual types of ovarian cancer and is closer to that of undifferentiated carcinoma, e.g. 5 year survival 70% for stage I disease. The vast majority of sex cord/stromal tumours are stage I with 85–95% 5 year survival. Higher stage and tumour rupture are adverse indicators but only about 10–30% subsequently recur. Malignant ovarian germ cell tumours are unusual and occur mainly in children, adolescents and young adults. 60% present with stage I disease (5 year survival 90%) with a 5 year survival rate of 70–80% for all stages of disease. Serum βHCG and AFP levels are useful in postoperative monitoring and postoperative chemotherapy is used for tumours other than stage I, grade I immature teratoma.

9. Other malignancy

Lymphoma
— primary or more commonly secondary to systemic disease, particularly if low-grade B cell lymphoma.
   Burkitt's/Burkitt's-like: childhood, young adults, associated with bilateral breast lymphoma in young women.
   non-Hodgkin's: B cell, diffuse large cell, average survival 3 years, often shows sclerosis.
— differential diagnoses: granulosa cell tumour and dysgerminoma; confirm by immunohistochemistry for lymphoid markers.

Leukaemia
— granulocytic sarcoma (CD 68/chloroacetate esterase positive).
— 10–20% of acute and chronic leukaemias; site of relapse for ALL during bone marrow remission.

Sarcoma

— leiomyo-/rhabdo-/angio-/chondro-/osteo-/neurofibro-sarcoma: all rare and more often part of a malignant mixed mesodermal tumour or (immature) teratoma.
— endometrioid stromal sarcoma: low/high-grade.

Malignant melanoma

— secondary: present in 20% of fatal cases.
— primary: within the wall of a dermoid cyst.

Secondary involvement by peritoneal mesothelioma (well-differentiated papillary/multicystic or of no specific types), intra-abdominal desmoplastic small round cell tumour (with divergent differentiation; cytokeratin, EMA, vimentin, desmin positive; pelvis and abdomen of young people), Ewing's sarcoma/PNET, neuroblastoma and rhabdomyosarcoma.

10. Comments on fallopian tube carcinoma

Primary carcinoma of the fallopian tube is rare(< 1% of primary genital tract malignancy) and greatly outnumbered by direct tubal extension from ovarian carcinoma (where the bulk of tumour is in the ovary) and uterine carcinoma (where the bulk of tumour is in the uterus). The uterus and ovaries should be grossly normal with any malignancy conforming to features of metastases or, alternatively, in keeping with the size and distribution of an independent primary. In primary fallopian tube carcinoma the tube is distended by a solid or papillary tumour and histologically the cancer is invasive papillary adenocarcinoma usually similar to ovarian serous papillary carcinoma. However, the full spectrum of Müllerian subtypes has been reported, e.g. endometrioid, mucinous, clear cell, transitional. Prognosis depends mostly on the stage of disease, with 5 year survival rates of 77% for stage I and 20% for stage III. Tumour recurrence is intra-abdominal and spread is similar to that of ovarian carcinoma. Other rare malignant tumours recorded are malignant mixed mesodermal tumour, leiomyosarcoma and gestational choriocarcinoma.

FIGO/TNM
For details see ovarian carcinoma.

pT1   tumour limited to the fallopian tube(s)
pT2   tumour involving tube(s) with pelvic extension
pT3   tumour involving tube(s) with metastases to abdominal peritoneum, and/or regional nodes
pT4   tumour involving tube(s) with distant metastases, e.g. liver parenchyma or positive pleural fluid cytology.

Endometrial Carcinoma

1. Gross description

Specimen

— curettage/pipelle sample (on an outpatient basis: some cases are also detected by routine cervical smear).
— subtotal/total/radical hysterectomy/bilateral salpingo-oophorectomy/limited pelvic node dissection.
— size (cm) and weight (g).

Tumour

Site
— fundus, body, isthmus.

Size
— length × width × depth (cm) or maximum dimension (cm).

Appearance
— polypoid/papillary/solid/ulcerated/necrotic/haemorrhagic.

Edge
— circumscribed/irregular.

Extent
— infiltration endometrium, myometrium, serosa, endo/ectocervix.

Adjacent endometrium

— atrophic, hyperplastic, polypoid.

2. Histological type (ISGP/WHO)

The vast majority are adenocarcinoma.

Endometrioid adenocarcinoma

— 60–80% of cases.
— typical: low-grade, perimenopausal, due to unopposed oestrogenic drive ± adjacent endometrial hyperplasia, well-differentiated lesions; *or*, older age, non-oestrogen related, adjacent atrophic endometrium, less frequently well-differentiated lesions.
— variants: with squamous differentiation – up to 30% of cases: the tumour is graded on the glandular component as it can be difficult to tell if the squamous element is benign or malignant.
secretory carcinoma – cells resemble secretory endometrium.
ciliated carcinoma – rare.
villoglandular carcinoma – well differentiated and papillary, exclude high-grade serous papillary carcinoma (high-grade nuclear characteristics).
sertoliform carcinoma.

Serous papillary adenocarcinoma

— 5–10% of cases.
— high grade; elderly; de novo with no adjacent hyperplasia.
— lymphovascular/myometrial invasion and omental spread often disproportionate to the amount of endometrial disease.
— potentially multifocal with extrauterine lesions, e.g. ovary, tube.
— necrosis and psammoma bodies are often seen; overexpresses p53.

Clear cell adenocarcinoma

— 1–5% of cases; postmenopausal; not related to diethylstiboestrol; aggressive with myometrial invasion.

Mucinous adenocarcinoma

— > 50% cells have stainable mucin.
— distinguish from cervical adenocarcinoma by differential biopsy/currettage and exclude a gastrointestinal primary.

Squamous cell carcinoma

— old age; exclude spread from cervical carcinoma.

Mixed

— second component > 10%: adenocarcinoma with squamous differentiation is excluded. Adenosquamous carcinoma (where both components are malignant) has a poor prognosis.

Undifferentiated carcinoma

— small cell/not otherwise specified: aggressive.

— Cervical primary and lung primary must be excluded in small cell carcinoma.

Malignant mixed mullerian tumours (MMMT)

— low-grade malignancy: adenosarcoma; carcinofibroma.
— high-grade malignancy: carcinosarcoma (syn. metaplastic endometrioid adenocarcinoma as it can contain cytokeratin positive spindle cells).
  Lesions can be either homologous or heterologous (containing tissues alien to the uterus, commonly cartilage, striated muscle, bone). Carcinosarcoma is the commonest malignant mixed tumour and 50% contain heterologous elements.

Metastatic carcinoma

— direct spread: cervix, bladder, rectum.
— distant spread: infiltrating lobular breast carcinoma, kidney, malignant melanoma, stomach, pancreas. The commonest are breast, stomach, colon, pancreas. Often myometrial with an endometrial component, metastases can mimic primary endometrial disease, e.g. infiltrating lobular breast carcinoma (stromal sarcoma), renal carcinoma (clear cell carcinoma) and colorectal carcinoma (mucinous carcinoma).

3. Differentiation

Well/moderate/poor.

— 80–85% are well to moderately differentiated.

Grade I/II/III

The glandular component of endometrioid adenocarcinomas is graded I<5%, II 6–50%, and III > 50% non-squamous, non-morular solid growth pattern. Serous, clear cell and undifferentiated carcinomas are considered high grade. Nuclear grading can also raise the architectural grade, e.g. II→ III: grade 1 (oval nuclei, even chromatin, inconspicuous nucleolus, few mitoses) and grade 3 (irregular, rounded nuclei, prominent nucleoli, frequent mitoses). Grade 2 nuclear grade is intermediate between grades 1 and 3.

4. Extent of local tumour spread

Border: pushing/infiltrative.
Lymphocytic reaction: prominent/sparse.

Endometrium

— intra-endometrial carcinoma, in-situ carcinoma, EIN (endometrial intraepithelial neoplasia) – present in 90% of serous papillary carcinoma cases and overexpresses p53.

Myometrium

— proportion of wall involved<50%, > 50%.
— if > 50% on MRI scan a radical hysterectomy is indicated.

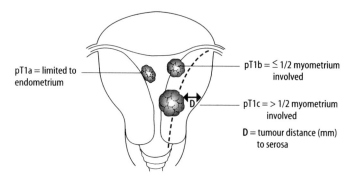

pT1a = limited to endometrium

pT1b = ≤ 1/2 myometrium involved

pT1c = > 1/2 myometrium involved

D = tumour distance (mm) to serosa

pT1 = confined to corpus uteri

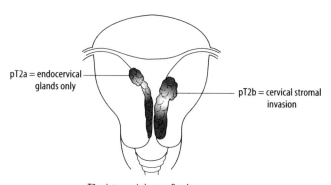

pT2a = endocervical glands only

pT2b = cervical stromal invasion

pT2 = into cervix but confined to uterus

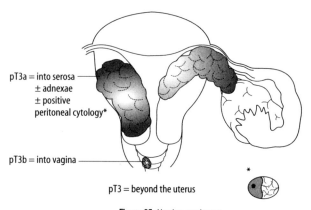

pT3a = into serosa ± adnexae ± positive peritoneal cytology*

pT3b = into vagina

pT3 = beyond the uterus

Figure 95. Uterine carcinoma.

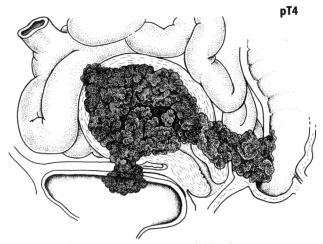

pT4

Tumour invades bladder mucosa and/or bowel mucosa

Figure 96. Uterine carcinoma.

Extent of myometrial invasion relates to the histological type and grade of carcinoma. True myometrial invasion must be distinguished from expansion of the endo-/myometrial junction (look for a continuous line of myometrial vascular structures in a compressed myometrium) and abnormal epithelium in pre-existing adenomyosis (look for periglandular endometrial stroma). Invasive stromal desmoplasia and inflammation are useful diagnostic clues although often not present in carcinoma. Endometriosis and endometrial–myometrial junction containing carcinoma usually have a broad front and smooth outline.

Serosa
— distance (mm) of the deepest point of invasion from the nearest serosal surface.

Endocervix/exocervix
— 10% of cases usually by direct invasion, occasionally by implantation following curettage. Distinction between an endometrial and cervical origin can be difficult clinically and histologically in curettage samples; some reliance is placed on the nature of the tissue from which the carcinoma appears to be arising, e.g. normal or neoplastic cervix, or hyperplastic endometrium.

Fallopian tubes/ovaries

Omentum

pTis carcinoma in-situ

pT1 tumour confined to the corpus:
   a. limited to the endometrium
   b. invades less than half of myometrium
   c. invades more than half of myometrium

pT2 tumour invades corpus and cervix:
   a. endocervical glands only
   b. cervical stroma

pT3 outside the uterus but not outside the true pelvis:
   a. serosa and/or adnexae, and/or malignant cells in ascites/peritoneal washings
   b. vaginal disease (direct extension or metastasis)

pT4 extends outside the true pelvis or has obviously involved the mucosa of the bladder or rectum.

5. Lymphovascular invasion

Present/absent.
Intra-/extratumoural.

— particularly serous papillary carcinoma.

6. Lymph nodes

Site/number/size/number involved/extracapsular spread.
Regional nodes: pelvic (obturator and internal iliac), common and external iliac, parametrial, sacral and para-aortic.

pN0 no regional lymph nodes involved

pN1 metastases in regional lymph node(s).

The commonest sites of extrauterine spread are the regional nodes and ovaries. Nodal disease relates to the tumour grade, type, depth of invasion and lymphovascular involvement. Recurrences are in the pelvis and vaginal vault; distant metastases go to lung, liver, bone, CNS and skin of the scalp.

7. Excision margins

Distances (mm) to the serosa, tubal and inferior vaginal limits.

8. Other pathology

Uterus

— polyp(s), hyperplasia (simple or complex with architectural ± cytological atypia), adenomyosis.

The regional lymph nodes are:

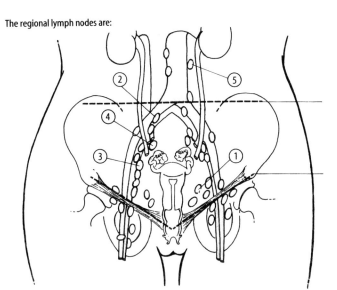

1 hypogastric; *2* common iliac; *3* external iliac; *4* lateral sacral; *5* para-aortic

Figure 97. Uterine carcinoma.

Carcinoma only rarely develops within a preexisting endometrial polyp although this is increased in tamoxifen therapy.

Twenty-five per cent of untreated atypical hyperplasias progress to adenocarcinoma. Features favouring adenocarcinoma over complex hyperplasia with cytological atypia are: intraglandular epithelial bridges, intraglandular polymorphs and necrosis, cytological atypia, mitoses and stromal invasion. The latter and superficial myometrial invasion are useful in distinguishing between intraendometrial and invasive adenocarcinoma in curettage specimens.

Ovary

— thecoma, granulosa cell tumour, endometrioid carcinoma, endometriosis. Accompanying ovarian carcinoma is seen in 5–10% of endometrial carcinomas. Distinction between synchronous primary lesions and ovarian secondaries rests on the latter being bilateral, multinodular, often serosal and with ovarian stromal lymphovascular invasion. There is a higher frequency of concurrent primaries in endometrioid carcinoma of ovary (25%).

Tamoxifen-related polyps, hyperplasia, adenocarcinoma, carcinosarcoma (MMMT): tamoxifen is an anti-oestrogen but has paradoxical oestrogenic effects on the endometrium leading to an increased frequency of a range of endometrial neoplasms some of which are prognostically adverse. Polyps can be large, multiple, necrotic, have areas of glandular, papillary or clear cell metaplasia and may even harbour carcinoma.

Carcinosarcoma is often polypoid at the fundus of an elderly patient and 30% present with stage III/IV disease. The carcinomatous component is usually high-grade glandular (endometrioid, clear cell or papillary serous) and the sarcomatous element homologous (cf. endometrial stroma, leiomyosarcoma, fibrosarcoma) or heterologous (striated muscle, cartilage, bone, fat). Immunohistochemistry for epithelial and mesenchymal markers, e.g. desmin may be necessary for diagnosis. Five year survival is 20–40% in this aggressive neoplasm.

The majority (80%) of adenosarcomas arise in the postmenopausal endometrium. They are polypoid with proliferative type glands and usually homologous stromal type sarcoma distributed in a condensed periglandular cambium layer. Recurrence (30%) relates to mitoses, stromal overgrowth and myoinvasion in this intermediate-grade malignancy.

Endometrial carcinoma usually co-expresses cytokeratins (7, 8, 18, 19) and vimentin. Oestrogen and progesterone marking is common relating to histological grade. High-grade endometrioid and papillary serous carcinomas overexpress p53. CEA stains weaker than in cervical carcinoma. DNA aneuploidy is an index of high-grade, advanced-stage tumours.

Radical hysterectomy is considered for endometrial carcinoma if there is > 50% myometrial invasion with grade II or III histology, invasion of the cervix, mucinous, clear cell or papillary serous carcinoma, lymphovascular invasion or suspicious nodes on CTscan. Preoperative adjuvant chemo-/radiotherapy is also used in these circumstances. Intraoperative frozen section of suspect nodes is an important prequel to radical resection.

Prognosis

Overall 5 year survival for endometrial carcinoma is 80–85% with oestrogen-related cases arising from a background of hyperplasia doing better than non-oestrogen-dependent lesions. Serous, undifferentiated, mucinous and clear cell carcinomas are more aggressive than equivalent stage endometrioid tumours. Lymphovascular invasion, which correlates with progressing tumour grade, myometrial invasion and stage (cervical and extra-uterine spread), is an adverse prognostic factor (70–75% 5 year survival). Prognosis also relates strongly to tumour stage: I, 82–95% 5 year survival; II, 50–60%; III, 15–25%. Grade I tumours (87% 5 year survival) fare better than grade III cancers (58% 5 year survival).

9. Other malignancy

Endometrial stromal lesions can be benign (stromal nodule) or malignant, the latter having infiltrating margins. Curettings impose limitations in making this assessment, which is more appropriately done on a hysterectomy specimen.

Endometrial stromal sarcoma

— low-grade malignancy; resembles endometrial stroma; infiltrative margins; variable mitoses (usually<5/10 high-power fields), characteristic lymphovascular invasion (previously called endolymphatic stromal myosis); prone to local pelvic recurrence (30%) after many years have elapsed; may cause pressure effects, e.g. hydronephrosis.

Undifferentiated uterine sarcoma

— previously high-grade stromal sarcoma; pleomorphism; mitoses (> 10/10 high-power fields), infiltrating margins; aggressive behaviour. Size of tumour (> 4 cm) and extrauterine extension are adverse indicators in low- and high-grade lesions. Treatment is surgical although there is some evidence for partial response to chemotherapy and hormonal manipulation in metastatic disease.

Stage:

I   tumour confined to the uterine corpus
II   tumour confined to the corpus and cervix
III   extrauterine pelvic extension
IV   extrapelvic extension.

Endometrial stromal sarcomas are vimentin positive ± actin/desmin and low-grade lesions preserve a pericellular reticulin pattern. Differential diagnosis is undifferentiated carcinoma (cytokeratin, EMA positive) and leiomyomatous tumour (strongly desmin positive).

Leiomyomatous tumours

— malignancy relates to a combination of:
  infiltrative margins.
  cellular atypia.
  coagulative tumour cell necrosis.
  mitoses > 10/10 high-power fields.

— uncertain malignant potential:
  cellular atypia and mitoses 5–10/10 high-power fields indicate probable malignancy if the atypia is moderate or severe.

— cellular leiomyoma:
  benign; identify thick-walled vessels and strong desmin positivity to distinguish from an endometrial stromal tumour.

— mitotically active leiomyoma:
  benign if no significant cell atypia, abnormal mitoses or coagulative tumour cell necrosis.

— cell type:
  myxoid and epithelioid leiomyosarcomas have less cellular atypia and mitotic activity.

— beware pseudomalignancy:
  (1) bizarre symplastic leiomyoma. Benign if the symplastic nuclear change is focal, the mitotic count is low (< 3/10 high-power fields) and coagulative tumour cell necrosis is absent.
  (2) changes after gonadotrophin analogue treatment, viz. haemorrhage and necrosis, symplastic type nuclear atypia and apparent hypercellularity
  (3) intravenous leiomyomatosis with vascular invasion and "metastases" but not malignant.

Choriocarcinoma/placental site trophoblastic tumour (PSTT)

— after abortion, normal or molar pregnancy.
— see Chapter 28.

Lymphoma/leukaemia

— see Chapter 25.

Others

— haemangiopericytoma, angiosarcoma, soft tissue sarcomas and germ cell tumours are all rare.

Cervical Carcinoma

1. Gross description

Specimen

— cervical smear/punch or wedge biopsy/diathermy (hot) or knife (cold) cone biopsy/LLETZ (large loop excision of transformation zone)/hysterectomy/ radical (Werdheim's) hysterectomy with vaginal cuff and lymph nodes/pelvic (anterior/posterior/ total) exenteration (bladder, ureters, uterus, vagina, tubes and ovaries, rectum)

— size (cm) and weight (g).

Tumour

Site

— endocervix/exocervix.

— anterior/posterior.

— lateral (right/left).

Size

— length × width × depth (cm) or maximum dimension (cm).

— stromal invasion: breech of basement membrane with scant stromal penetration<1 mm in depth.

— microinvasion:
depth – ≤ 3 mm (FIGO IA1) or 5 mm (FIGO IA2) depth of invasion from the nearest (superior or lateral) basement membrane, usually involved by CIN/CGIN.
volume – ≤ 500 mm^3 (Burghardt) or ≤ 5mm depth × 7 mm horizontal axis (FIGO).
vessels – venous or lymphatic permeation does not alter the staging.

Appearance

— polypoid/papillary/nodular/solid/ ulcerated/burrowing.

Edge

— circumscribed/irregular.

Extent

— infiltration cervical wall, parametria, corpus uteri, vagina.

2. Histological type

Squamous cell carcinoma

— 80% of cases.
— classical: keratinising
                non-keratinising – large cell/small cell.

Squamous cell carcinoma variants

— verrucous: exophytic and locally invasive; may recur after excision and radio-therapy; bland cytology; deep bulbous processes.
— warty: surface koilocytosis and deep invasive margin.
— spindle cell: low-grade malignancy with tumour cell fibroplasia.
— papillary: papillary neoplasm with dysplastic/in-situ type epithelium, late metastases and recurrence.
— basaloid: aggressive; nests of basaloid cells with necrosis.
— lymphoepithelioma-like: circumscribed margin, lymphocytic infiltrate, large uniform cells with prominent nucleolus, good prognosis, radiosensitive.

Adenocarcinoma

— 10–15% of cases.
— endocervical: glandular/mucinous –varies with differentiation.
— endometrioid: exclude uterine carcinoma extending to cervix; typically at the junctional zone arising from endometriosis/endometrial metaplasia and may coexist with usual endocervical type adenocarcinoma: a minimal deviation variant exists.
— minimal deviation (adenoma malignum): late presentation, poor prognosis, bland epithelium with mitoses and gland extension deep (> 50%) into the cervical stroma; Peutz-Jeghers syndrome.
— villoglandular: good prognosis, young females; papillary with CGIN type epithelium and connective tissue cores; indolent invasion at base; more aggressive moderately differentiated variants occur.
— clear cell: clear, hobnail cells, glycogen PAS positive, solid, tubules, papillae; in utero exposure to diethylstilboestrol (50%).
— serous papillary: poor prognosis; potentially multifocal in endometrium and ovary; high-grade cytological appearances ± psammoma bodies – exclude villoglandular carcinoma.

- mesonephric: from mesonephric duct remnants deep in the lateral cervical wall; small glands; eosinophilic secretions.
- non-Müllerian mucinous: enteric; signet ring cell; poor prognosis; exclude gut secondary.

Poorly differentiated carcinoma
- scirrhous, undifferentiated.

Mixed tumours
- mixed type (e.g. squamous/adenocarcinoma) and differentiation (e.g. endo-cervical/endometrioid adenocarcinoma).
- adenosquamous, solid with mucus production: from well-differentiated adenoacanthoma with a good prognosis to poorly differentiated squamous with PAS positive mucin production (up to 30% of cases); more aggressive than usual squamous carcinoma.

Miscellaneous carcinoma
- glassy cell: a poorly differentiated adenosquamous carcinoma in young women.
- adenoid basal: indolent; often an incidental finding at hysterectomy or cone biopsy; organoid lobules and nests of cells with punched-out lumina.
- mucoepidermoid and adenoid cystic: low-grade, indolent behaviour, although recurrence/metastasis if incompletely removed.

Small cell undifferentiated carcinoma
- primary or secondary; chromogranin positive; poor prognosis.

Neuroendocrine carcinoma
- atypical carcinoid-like of intermediate-grade malignancy.

Metastatic carcinoma
- direct spread: endometrium (commonest), colorectum, bladder.
- distant spread: breast (especially infiltrating lobular), stomach, ovary.

3. Differentiation

Well/moderate/poor.
Varies according to lesion type, e.g. keratinising squamous carcinoma is well to moderately differentiated, non-keratinising large cell moderate and non-keratinising small cell poorly differentiated. Tumour grade does not reliably predict prognosis and is only broadly indicative. However, grade 1 (small amount of solid growth with mild nuclear atypia) has a better prognosis than grade 3 (solid pattern with severe nuclear atypia) adenocarcinoma.

4. Extent of local tumour spread

Border: pushing/infiltrative.
Lymphocytic reaction: prominent/sparse.

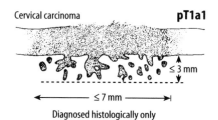

Cervical carcinoma **pT1a1**

≤ 3 mm

≤ 7 mm

Diagnosed histologically only

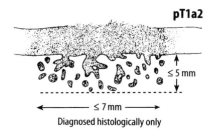

pT1a2

≤ 5 mm

≤ 7 mm

Diagnosed histologically only

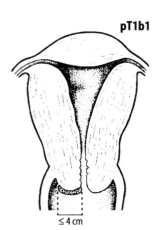

pT1b1

≤ 4 cm

Tumour confined to the uterus ≤ 4 cm

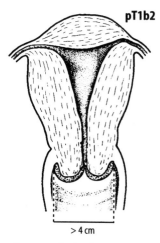

pT1b2

> 4 cm

Tumour confined to the uterus > 4 cm

Figures 98–103. Cervical carcinoma.

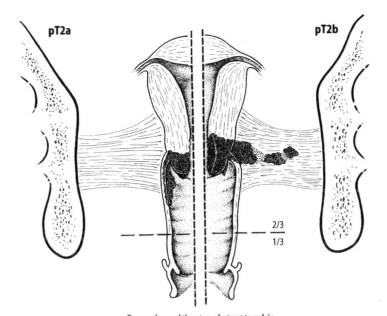

Tumour beyond the uterus but not to pelvic
wall or lower third of vagina

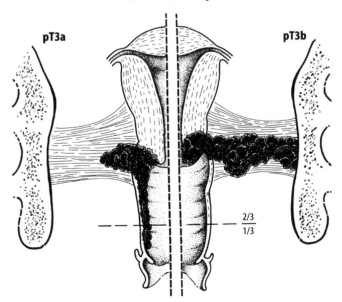

Tumour extends to pelvic wall and/or lower third vagina
and/or causes hydronephrosis or non-functioning kidney

Cervical Carcinoma   243

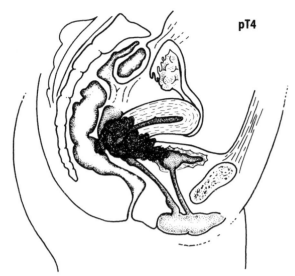

pT4

Tumour invades mucosa of bladder or
rectum and/or extends beyond true pelvis

Figure 104. Cervical carcinoma.

Infiltration

— cervical wall, parametria, endometrium, myometrium, vagina.

— depth through the cervical stroma and parametrium and distance to the nearest parametrial resection margin (mm).

FIGO/TNM

pTis   carcinoma in-situ (= CIN III or adenocarcinoma in-situ/high-grade CGIN)

pT1   carcinoma confined to the uterus

    1A   lesions detected only microscopically; maximum size 5 mm deep and 7 mm across; venous or lymphatic permeation does not alter the staging

          IA1 $\leq$ 3 mm deep, $\leq$ 7 mm horizonal axis

          IA2 3 mm<tumour depth $\leq$ 5 mm, $\leq$ 7 mm horizontal axis

    IB   clinically apparent lesions confined to the cervix or preclinical lesions larger than stage IA (occult carcinoma)

          IB1 clinical lesions no greater than 4 cm in size

          IB2 clinical lesions greater than 4 cm in size

pT2   invasive carcinoma extending beyond the uterus but has not reached either lateral pelvic wall. Involvement of upper two-thirds of vagina, but not lower third

    a. without parametrial invasion

    b. with parametrial invasion

pT3   a. invasive carcinoma extending to either lower third of vagina and/or
         b. lateral pelvic wall and/or causes hydronephrosis/non-functioning kidney
pT4   invasive carcinoma involving urinary bladder mucosa and/or rectum or
         extends beyond the true pelvis.

Spread is typically to vagina, uterine corpus, parametria, lower urinary tract
(ureters) and uterosacral ligaments. Involvement of regional nodes relates to the

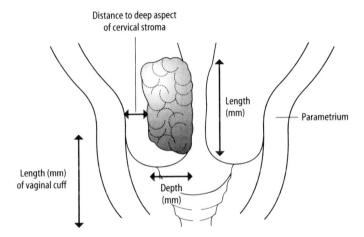

Width (mm) = sum of involved serial blocks of standard thickness
Tumour volume (mm³) can be estimated by length x depth x width

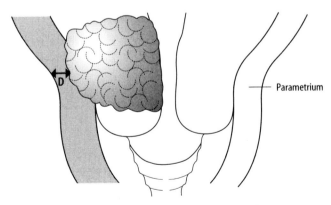

D = tumour distance (mm) to the Circumferential
Radial Margin (CRM) of excision of
the parametrium

Figure 105. Cervical carcinoma.

The regional lymph nodes are:

(*1*) paracervical nodes
(*2*) parametrial nodes
(*3*) hypogastric (internal iliac) including obturator nodes
(*4*) external iliac nodes
(*5*) common iliac nodes
(*6*) presacral nodes
(*7*) lateral sacral nodes

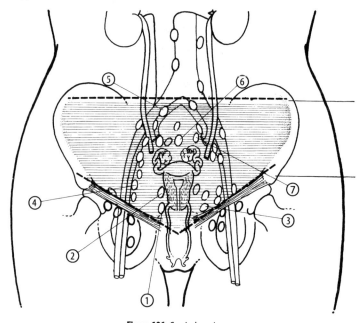

Figure 106. Cervical carcinoma.

stage of disease with lungs and bone the commonest (5–10%) sites of distant metastases.

5. Lymphovascular invasion

Present/absent.
Intra-/extratumoural.
Lymphovascular invasion should be noted on biopsy material as it may influence the choice of more extensive surgical resection.

6. Lymph nodes

Site/number/size/number involved/extracapsular spread.
Regional nodes: paracervical, parametrial, hypogastric (internal iliac, obturator), common and external iliac, presacral, lateral sacral.
pN0   no regional lymph nodes involved
pN1   metastasis in regional lymph node(s).

7. Excision margins

Distances (mm) to the nearest deep cervical (anterior and posterior), lateral parametrial and inferior vaginal resection margins.

8. Other pathology

HPV
— human papilloma virus: anogenital field change of viral infection, intraepithelial neoplasia and carcinoma.

CIN
— cervical intraepithelial neoplasia.

SIL
— squamous intraepithelial lesion.

AIS/CGIN
— adenocarcinoma in-situ and lesser changes of glandular dysplasia (cervical glandular intraepithelial neoplasia); low-grade/high-grade CGIN.

VAIN
— vaginal intraepithelial neoplasia

VIN
— vulval intraepithelial neoplasia.

AIN
— anal intraepithelial neoplasia.

Bowenoid papulosis
— brown perineal patches in young women; HPV induced; histology of VIN III; negligible risk of progression to carcinoma.

Evidence indicates that "high"-risk HPV infection results in high-grade CIN (SIL) with a higher rate of progression to carcinoma. "Low"-risk HPV and low-grade CIN may potentially regress. HPV infection is also an aetiological factor in cervical glandular dysplasia (CGIN), which often coexists with squamous epithelial dysplasia (CIN, SIL).

Low- and high-grade CGIN also potentially progress to microinvasive and invasive disease with a strong association between high-grade CGIN and invasive lesions. CGIN should also be distinguished from benign changes, e.g. tuboendometrial metaplasia. CGIN shows an abrupt junction with normal epithelium, nuclear atypia, mitoses and apoptosis. Ciliation is less frequent than in metaplasia.

"low"-risk HPV	types 6, 11	condylomas, CIN I
"high"-risk HPV	types 16, 18, 31, 33, 35, 39, 51	CIN II/III
		squamous carcinoma
	typing by in-situ hybridisation	
CIN (SIL)	low-grade	CIN I, SIL I
	high-grade	CIN II, CIN III, SIL II.

Cervical squamous cell carinoma and adenocarcinoma are cytokeratin and CEA positive.

Microinvasion: The larger the CIN lesion the more likely it is to show microinvasion. Microinvasive carcinoma is not diagnosed on small, limited biopsy samples but rather on a large biopsy specimen, e.g. cone biopsy which allows removal and assessment of the whole lesion. Five year survival rates are about 95%. Risk factors for progression to frankly invasive carcinoma are increasing depth of invasion, increasing lateral extent (horizontal axis) of the lesion, lymphovascular invasion and incomplete removal by LLETZ/cone biopsy. Adverse factors in occult carcinoma (i.e. bigger than microinvasion but not clinically detectable) are a depth > 5 mm and lymphovascular invasion. Very occasional cases, where the CIN lesion has focal areas suspicious of penetrating the stroma but lacking definite evidence of invasion, warrant a designation of "questionable stromal invasion". Tangential cutting and extension of CIN into endocervical crypts must be excluded.

The first stage of microinvasive squamous cell carcinoma is recognised by budding of invasive cells with morphology similar to that of the overlying CIN lesion through the basement membrane. With lesion progression the tongues of tumour may be more differentiated with cytoplasmic eosinophilia and nuclear clearing; a stromal fibro-inflammatory reaction is also seen. The distinction between adenocarcinoma in-situ and early invasive adenocarcinoma is more difficult to define and measure with features such as depth, complexity and budding of glandular architecture and stromal reaction of use. Measurement of tumour extent in cervical carcinoma is readily obtained in the longitudinal and deep axes, whereas the transverse dimension depends on summation of the number of involved adjacent blocks of known thickness. Microinvasive carcinoma may be treated with loop or cold knife cone biopsy (ensuring a minimum 3 mm clearance of margins) or simple hysterectomy, whereas radical hysterectomy is indicated for larger tumours or where there is lymphovascular invasion. Radiotherapy produces tumour cell necrosis, degeneration, pleomorphism, maturation, inflammation and fibrosis. Combination radio-/chemotherapy is used to augment radical surgery or on its own for palliative control in high-stage disease.

Prognosis

Prognosis relates to tumour type and volume, invasion of endometrium, parametrium and vessels, and most importantly stage of disease. Overall 5 year survival rate is 55%, with stage I carcinoma 85–90% and 35%/10% for stage III/IV. Tumours with a glandular component, lymphovascular invasion and young age at diagnosis (< 30 years) are more aggressive and more often positive for pelvic node metastases. The incidence of cervical adenocarcinoma is increasing and presents on average 5 years younger than squamous carcinoma. Since it has a worse prognosis than equivalent squamous cell tumours more radical surgery is undertaken. Mixed differentiation tumours, and the coexistence of CIN and CGIN particularly on the surface and in crypts respectively, are not uncommon. High-grade CGIN or adenocarcinoma in-situ is usually treated by hysterectomy although conservative conisation may be used if the patient is young (< 36 years) and wishes to remain fertile.

9. Other malignancy

Malignant melanoma
— usually metastatic.
— primary lesion rare: 40% 5 year survival.

Embryonal rhabdomyosarcoma
— infancy/childhood.
— syn. sarcoma botryoides.
— cellular subepithelial cambium zone/myxoid zone/deep cellular zone.
— small cells/rhabdomyoblasts/desmin positive.
— ± heterologous elements.

Leiomyosarcoma
— 40–60 years.
— Cellular atypia/> 5 mitoses/10 high-power fields.
— >10 mitoses/10 high-power fields if no atypia.

Adenosarcoma
— polypoid.
— 25% have heterologous elements (striated muscle, cartilage, fat).
— low-grade malignancy.

Stromal sarcoma and malignant mixed mesodermal tumour are more likely to represent spread to the cervix from an endometrial lesion rather than a primary tumour.

Lymphoma

— more often secondary spread from systemic/nodal disease.

— primary: 70% are intermediate grade of large B cell type.

— 5 year survival about 75%.

Leukaemia

— granulocytic sarcoma as a presentation of chronic myeloid leukaemia.

— CD 68/chloroacetate esterase positive.

— relapse of AML, blast transformation of CML.

Vaginal Carcinoma

1. Gross description

Specimen

— vaginal smear/biopsy/partial/subtotal vaginectomy/ radical vaginectomy (with hysterectomy, salpingo-oophorectomy and lymphadenectomy)
— weight (g) and size (cm), number of fragments.

Tumour

Site

— anterior/posterior/lateral (right or left). Usually anterior/lateral and upper third (50–60%).

Size

— length × width × depth (cm) or maximum dimension (cm).

Appearance

— polypoid/verrucous/papillary/sessile/ulcerated/ pigmented.
— exophytic lesions are commoner than endophytic.

Edge

— circumscribed/irregular.

2. Histological type

Squamous cell carcinoma

— 90–95% of primary vaginal carcinomas.
— keratinising/non-keratinising.

- large cell/small cell.
- mainly moderately differentiated.

Squamous cell carcinoma variants
- verrucous: exophytic, bland cytology with deep bulbous processes, locally invasive.
- warty (condylomatous).
- spindle cell: cytokeratin positive.

Adenocarcinoma
- clear cell, PAS positive for glycogen, solid/tubules/papillae; 14–25 years, in utero exposure to diethylstilboestrol (DES).
- non-DES cases in the older age group are rare; clear/hobnail cells ± vaginal adenosis.
- differential diagnosis: vaginal adenosis with microglandular hyperplasia and Arias-Stella reaction in pregnancy or hormone therapy.
- endometrioid.
- mucinous: endocervical; intestinal.

Adenosquamous carcinoma

Adenoid cystic carcinoma
- indolent, late local recurrence, potential for metastases.

Adenoid basal carcinoma
- indolent

Small cell carcinoma
- primary or secondary from cervix or lung.

Undifferentiated carcinoma

Transitional cell carcinoma
- primary (rare) or in association with concurrent bladder/urethral carcinoma.

Carcinoid tumour
- chromogranin positive.

Endodermal sinus tumour
- yolk sac spectrum of appearances, AFP positive; infants.

Malignant melanoma
- 3%; mucosal junctional activity indicates a primary lesion; poor prognosis.

Metastatic carcinoma

— comprises 80% of malignant vaginal tumours, far outnumbering primary lesions.
— direct spread: cervix, endometrium, rectum, vulva, bladder, urethra.
— distant spread: kidney, breast, gut, ovary.
  The commonest metastases (cervix and endometrium) are usually in the upper third of the vagina.

3. Differentiation/grade

Well/moderate/poor.
WHO I/II/III: transitional carcinoma.

4. Extent of local tumour spread

Border: pushing/infiltrative.
Lymphocytic reaction: prominent/sparse.

FIGO/TNM
Category of microinvasive carcinoma is not established.
pTis   carcinoma in-situ

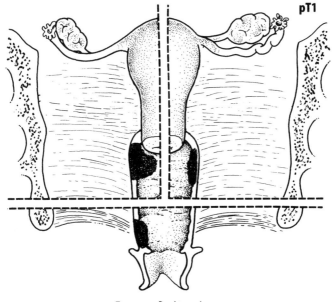

Tumour confined to vagina

Figure 107. Vaginal carcinoma.

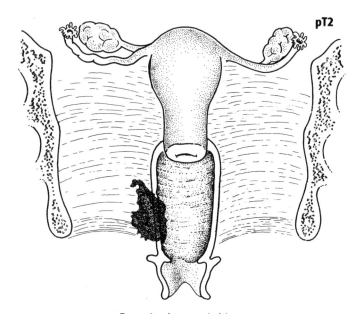

Tumour invades paravaginal tissues

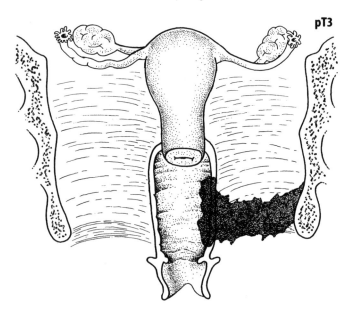

Tumour extends to pelvic wall

Figures 108, 109. Vaginal carcinoma.

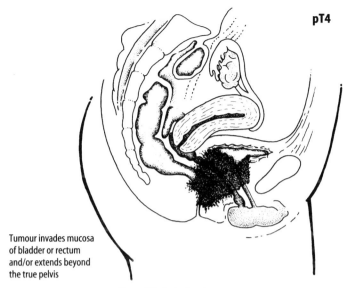

pT4

Tumour invades mucosa
of bladder or rectum
and/or extends beyond
the true pelvis

Figure 110. Vaginal carcinoma.

pT1 tumour confined to the vagina
pT2 tumour invades paravaginal tissues but does not extend to pelvic wall
pT3 tumour extends to pelvic wall
pT4 tumour invades mucosa of bladder or rectum, and/or extends beyond the
true pelvis.

Spread is mainly by early direct invasion and lymph node metastases, with 50%
beyond the vagina (pT2) at presentation and 25% in the rectum or bladder (pT4).

5. Lymphovascular invasion

Present/absent.
Intra-/extratumoural.

6. Lymph nodes

Site/number/size/number involved/extracapsular spread.
Regional nodes: upper two-thirds – pelvic nodes; lower third – inguinal nodes.

pN0 no regional lymph node metastasis
pN1 metastasis in regional lymph node(s).

7. Excision margins

Distances (mm) to the nearest longitudinal resection limit and deep circumferential radial margin.

The presence of epithelial (squamous or glandular) dysplasia or atypical adenosis at a mucosal resection margin may increase the frequency of recurrent tumour.

8. Other pathology

Vaginal intraepithelial neoplasia (VAIN): grades I/II/III
— rarer and less well established than the CIN or VIN/cancer sequences.

Cervical intraepithelial neoplasia (CIN)

Anal intraepithelial neoplasia (AIN)
HPV 16/18 is a common aetiology in CIN, VAIN, AIN and VIN (vulva) and is instrumental in the field change effect of carcinogenesis in the female genital tract which results in synchronous or metachronous cancers in the vulva, cervix and vagina. The vagina is also a common site of direct spread from vulva and cervix carcinomas and it should be noted that the commonest vaginal malignancies are secondary cervical and endometrial carcinoma.

Initial treatment of vaginal carcinoma is by irradiation, with better response for squamous cell carcinoma than adenocarcinoma, malignant melanoma and sarcoma. Surgery is used for non-responsive cases or local recurrence.

Prognosis

Prognosis relates strongly to disease stage, e.g. 43% 5 year survival with 66% for stage I and 25% for stage III. Vaginal malignant melanoma spreads early to pelvic soft tissues, lymph nodes, peritoneum, lung and bone with 5 year survival rates of 21%.

9. Other malignancy

Lymphoma/leukaemia
— lymphoma is usually secondary to systemic disease: rare primary lesions are intermediate-grade B cell in type.

Embryonal rhabdomyosarcoma (sarcoma botryoides)
— infants/children.
— superficial subepithelial cambium layer, intermediate myxoid zone, deep cellular zone, desmin positive, ± sarcomeric actin.
— locally aggressive necessitating surgery, irradiation and chemotherapy.

Leiomyosarcoma

— usually > 3 cm, with cell atypia and ≥ 5 mitoses/10 high-power fields.

Müllerian stromal sarcomas and other sarcomas, e.g. alveolar soft part, malignant fibrous histiocytoma, synovial sarcoma.

Vulval Carcinoma

1. Gross description

Specimen

— biopsy/partial/simple/radical vulvectomy/uni-/bilateral groin node dissection.
— size (cm) and weight (g).

Tumour

Site

— anterior/posterior.
— lateral (right/left).
— labia majora/labia minora/clitoris.
— labia majora is the commonest site.

Size

— length × width × depth (cm) or maximum dimension (cm).

Appearance

— polypoid/verrucous/ulcerated/necrotic/satellite lesions/pigmented.
— 50% are ulcerated, 30% exophytic.

Edge

— circumscribed/irregular.

2. Histological type

Squamous cell carcinoma

— 80–90% of malignant vulval neoplasms.

— classical: 65% of cases; large cell/small cell; keratinising/non-keratinising.

Squamous cell carcinoma variants

— basaloid: 28% of cases, younger age (< 60 years), association with HPV, cervical and vaginal lesions; nests of basaloid cells and mitoses.
— warty: association with HPV and koilocytosis.
Prognosis intermediate between usual squamous carcinoma and verrucous carcinoma. Distinguish from pseudoepitheliomatous hyperplasia overlying lichen sclerosus, Crohn's disease or granular cell tumour.
— adenoid: pseudoglandular/acantholytic.
— verrucous: may become aggressive after radiotherapy; pushing deep margin of cytologically bland bulbous processes; local recurrence.
— spindle cell: cytokeratin positive.

Basal cell carcinoma

— 20% local recurrence rate; metastases are rare.
Distinguish from basaloid squamous carcinoma, Merkel cell tumour and secondary small cell tumour by its lobulated margins and peripheral palisading.

Adenocarcinoma

— appendage origin/Bartholin's gland/mesonephric duct remnants, or metastatic.

Paget's disease

— 2% of vulval malignancy.
— intraepithelial adenocarcinoma cells with, in 20%, a locoregional or extra-genital malignancy, e.g. vulval appendage tumour or bladder carcinoma, anorectal carcinoma, breast carcinoma.
— multifocal: check margins histologically as there is a 40% recurrence rate.
Mucin stains and immunohistochemistry (EMA, CEA, cytokeratin 7) may be necessary to distinguish from bowenoid VIN and superficial spreading malignant melanoma (S100, HMB-45, melan-A).
Paget's disease without an associated neoplasm has a very good prognosis but it may also, per se, progress to invasive carcinoma.

Merkel cell tumour

— exclude secondary small cell carcinoma from lung.
— aggressive neuroendocrine carcinoma.
— CAM 5.2, cytokeratin 20, chromogranin positive.

Malignant melanoma

— 3–10% of malignant vulval neoplasms.
— usually mucosal and cutaneous involvement; Breslow depth and clinical stage are prognostic indicators.

Metastatic carcinoma

— 10% of malignant vulval neoplasms.

— direct spread: cervix, endometrium, vagina, urethra, bladder.

— distant spread: ovary, kidney, rectum, breast, lung, malignant melanoma, choriocarcinoma.

3. Differentiation

Well/moderate/poor.

— well > 50%; moderate 20–40% of cases.

4. Extent of local tumour spread

Border: pushing/infiltrative.
Lymphocytic reaction: prominent/sparse.
Microinvasion ≤ 3 mm: use of this nomenclature should be avoided as some of these carcinomas will have nodal metastases and invasive lesions > 1 mm in depth should probably have radical surgery.
Distance (mm) to the nearest painted surgical margin.
Involvement of vagina, urethra, perineum, anus.

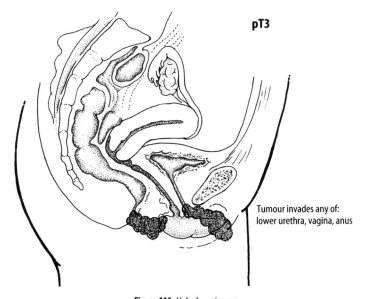

pT3

Tumour invades any of:
lower urethra, vagina, anus

Figure 111. Vulval carcinoma.

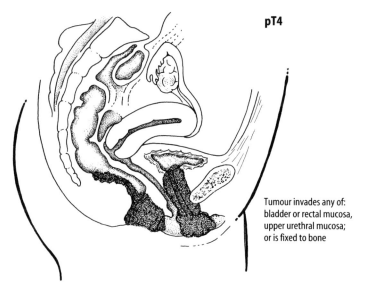

Figure 112. Vulval carcinoma.

pTis   carcinoma in-situ
pT1   tumour confined to vulva/perineum ≤ 2 cm in greatest dimension
         a. stromal invasion ≤ 1 mm
         b. stromal invasion > 1 mm
pT2   tumour confined to vulva/perineum > 2 cm in greatest dimension
pT3   tumour invades lower urethra/vagina/anus
pT4   tumour invades any of: bladder mucosa/rectal mucosa/upper urethral mucosa/pubic bone.

Spread is direct to the vagina, urethra, anus, inferior pubic and ischial rami and ischiorectal fossae.

5. Lymphovascular invasion

Present/absent.
Intra-/extratumoural.

6. Lymph nodes

Site/number/size/number involved/extracapsular spread.
Regional nodes: femoral and inguinal

pN0 no regional lymph node metastasis
pN1 unilateral regional lymph node metastasis
pN2 bilateral regional lymph node metastasis.

Labial tumours go initially to inguinal nodes whereas clitoral lesions may go directly to deep nodes. Ulcerated tumours can produce reactive regional lymphadenopathy mimicking metastatic disease.

7. Excision margins

Distances (mm) to the nearest painted cutaneous and subcutaneous excision margins and anal, vaginal, urethral limits.

8. Other pathology

Lichen sclerosus
— atrophic/hyperplastic.
— associated with (5–25% of cases) but low risk (5%) of progression to carcinoma.

Bowenoid papulosis
— brown perineal patches in young women.
— HPV induced.
— histology of VIN III.
— negligible risk of progression to carcinoma.

Vulval intraepithelial neoplasia (VIN) grades I/II/III
— typically multifocal and present in the adjacent epithelium of 60–70% of cases of squamous carcinoma.
— progression to carcinoma is in the order of 10–20%
— bowenoid type: young; HPV; associated cervical/anal disease.
— basaloid type: old; de novo; greater risk of carcinoma.

Squamous carcinoma
— in the older age group may also arise from hyperplastic epithelium with no obvious preceding HPV or VIN.

Prognosis

Nearly 30% of vulval squamous carcinomas have metastasised to inguinal or pelvic nodes at presentation. Prognosis relates to tumour size, an infiltrative tumour margin, depth of invasion, vascular involvement and nodal disease. Stage I lesions have a 5 year survival of 85%, stage II 60%, stage III 40%, stage IV 20% and overall 50–75%. Treatment is by radical vulvectomy with bilateral inguinal lymph node dissection. A limited local excision with wide (1 cm) surgical margins may be used in early-stage disease or medically unfit patients. Prognosis of malignant melanoma relates to tumour thickness and depth of invasion at the time of presentation, with average 5 year survival of 30–35%.

9. Other malignancy

Lymphoma/leukaemia
— secondary to systemic disease.

Adnexal/Bartholin's gland carcinomas
— rare; arising from eccrine or apocrine glands when distinction from metastatic ductal carcinoma of the breast can be problematic.
Bartholin's gland carcinoma forms 1–5% of vulval neoplasms and shows a range of differentiation: squamous cell, adenocarcinoma, mixed adenoid cystic/mucoepidermoid carcinoma. Ideally an origin from adjacent Bartholin's gland structures should be demonstrable. Five year survival rates vary from 40% to 80% depending on the stage at presentation.

Aggressive angiomyxoma
— myxoid stroma, prominent vessels, spindle cells – locally infiltrative and recurrent.

Sarcomas
— leiomyo-/rhabdo-/liposarcoma.
— leiomyosarcoma: > 5 cm diameter, infiltrating margins, > 5–10 mitoses/10 high-power fields, cellular atypia.
— rhabdomyosarcoma occurs in childhood and young adults with vaginal disease, being embryonal in type and vulval alveolar; desmin positive.

Others
— dermatofibrosarcoma protuberans, epithelioid sarcoma, malignant rhabdoid tumour.

Gestational Trophoblastic Tumours

1. Gross description

Specimen

— curetting/hysterectomy.
— weight (g) and size (cm), number of fragments, villous diameter.

Tumour

Site

— endometrial/myometrial/extrauterine: serosa
                                           parametria
                                           adnexae.
— fundus, corpus, isthmus – cavity.

Size

— length × width × depth (cm) or maximum dimension (cm).

Appearance

— haemorrhagic/necrotic/vesicular/nodular/polypoid masses.

Edge

— circumscribed/irregular.

2. Histological type

Choriocarcinoma

— suspect on curettings if: abundant necrotic/haemorrhagic decidua, bilaminar aggregates of exuberant syncytiotrophoblast and cytotrophoblast and *no* chorionic villi.

— 50% are preceded by a molar gestation: also seen after normal pregnancy (20%) or spontaneous abortion (30%).

— 2–3% of complete moles progress to choriocarcinoma.

— destructive myometrial and vascular invasion are common, leading to haematogenous spread.

— 5 year survival > 90% with chemotherapy (uterine disease > 95%, metastatic disease 83%).

Invasive hydatidiform mole (chorioadenoma destruens)

— 16% of complete moles.

— penetration into the myometrium or uterine vasculature ± adjacent structures of molar villi associated with variable degrees of trophoblast hyperplasia: haemorrhage and perforation can occur.

— haematogenous transport of "metastatic" nodules to vagina, lung and CNS: they do not affect the prognosis but may present with per vaginum bleeding or haemoptysis and respond well to chemotherapy.

Placental site trophoblastic tumour (PSTT)

— mostly following a normal term pregnancy (75%).

— polypoid mass composed of monomorphic intermediate trophoblast-mononuclear cytotrophoblast ± multinucleated cells, dissecting myofibres without necrosis or haemorrhage.

— HCG negative, HPL (human placental lactogen) positive.

— 10–15% malignant (mitoses > 2/10 high-power fields, deep invasion, clear cells): not chemoresponsive.

3. Differentiation

See above.

4. Extent of local tumour spread

Border: pushing/infiltrative.
Lymphocytic reaction: prominent/sparse.

TNM (FIGO)

pT1 (I)	tumour confined to the uterus
pT2 (II)	tumour extends to other genital structures: vagina, ovary, broad ligament, fallopian tube by metastasis or direct extension
pM1a (III)	metastasis to the lung(s)
pM1b (IV)	other distant metastasis with or without lung involvement (brain, liver, kidney, gut).

FIGO stages I–IV are subdivided according to risk factors:

A   no risk factors
B   one risk factor
C   two risk factors.

Risk factors are:

1.   HCG > 100 000 IU/24 h urine
2.   detection of disease > 6 months from termination of antecedent pregnancy.

5. Lymphovascular invasion

Present/absent.
Intra-/extratumoural.
Physiological trophoblast in placental site reaction is frequently endovascular with potential for myometrial invasion and this must not be over interpreted as malignancy.
Choriocarcinoma typically shows *destructive* myometrial and vascular invasion.

6. Lymph nodes

Usually tertiary metastases from a large extrauterine lesion.

7. Excision margins

Distances (mm) to the serosa and parametrial resection limits.

8. Other pathology

Complete hydatidiform mole
— androgenetic 46XX.
— diffuse villous vesicular swelling.
— central cistern formation.
— circumferential/multifocal trophoblast; grading the degree of trophoblast proliferation is not of prognostic value.
— absence of fetal red blood cells and tissues.
— volume of placental tissue often abundant > 100 g.
— early moles: lobulated villi but diagnosis can be problematic.

The vast majority regress but 8% develop persistent trophoblastic disease representing either incomplete removal of molar tissue, residual invasive mole within the myometrium or its vasculature, or choriocarcinoma.

Partial hydatidiform mole

— biparental; triploid 69XXY, a minority are trisomy.
— ± fetus (usually abnormal).
— a mixture of focal villous vesicular swelling with central cisterns and normal-sized villi.
— "Norwegian fjord" scalloped outline with trophoblast inclusions.
— circumferential/multifocal trophoblast.
— volume of placental tissue normal.
— persistent disease in up to 5% of cases.

In molar change vesicles of 2–3 mm diameter are usually seen grossly.

Hydropic degeneration

— often trisomy or triploid.
— villi <2–3 mm and rounded.
— no cisterns.
— trophoblast polar in distribution and/or attenuated.

Placental site reaction is a common localised phenomenon in curettings from abortions and must not be confused with gestational trophoblastic tumours. It comprises an exaggerated response of decidua, altered myometrial smooth muscle cells and intermediate trophoblast without myometrial destruction or invasion. Placental site nodules or plaques are characterised by small size, circumscribed margins and hyalinisation.

Trophoblast is unlikely to be neoplastic if the last known pregnancy was recent, of short duration, aborted, and characterised by a mixture of villous and placental site trophoblast. The differential diagnosis between hydropic degeneration, partial and complete moles is often difficult and monitoring serum β sub-unit HCG levels is useful to ensure that they revert to normal in time. Trophoblastic disease is associated with persistently abnormal levels and if this is present after 60 days with a previous diagnosis of hydatidiform mole consideration is given to use of chemotherapy. Another differential diagnosis for choriocarcinoma is non-gestational carcinoma with trophoblast metaplasia, e.g. ovary, endometrium.

In curettage specimens trophoblast can be categorised as:

a. Villous trophoblast: the usual post abortion finding.
b. Simple non-villous trophoblast: distinction between syncytio- and cytotrophoblast cannot be made and usually occurs after abortion.
c. Suspicious non-villous trophoblast: no villi, a bilaminar arrangement of syncytio- and cytotrophoblast but no tissue invasion.
d. Non-villous trophoblast diagnostic of choriocarcinoma: myometrial fragments with demonstrable invasion by bilaminar trophoblast.

Urological Cancer

- Renal Cell and Renal Pelvis/Ureter Carcinoma
- Bladder Carcinoma
- Prostate Carcinoma
- Urethral Carcinoma
- Testicular Cancer
- Penile Carcinoma

Renal Cell and Renal Pelvis/Ureter Carcinoma

1. Gross description

Specimen

— fine needle aspirate/partial nephrectomy/ nephrectomy ± ureterectomy/radical nephrectomy (kidney, pelvis, perirenal fat out to Gerota's fascia, adrenal gland, and a length of ureter).
— right/left.
— weight (g) and size (cm).
— length of attached ureter.
— adrenal gland: present/absent.

Tumour

Site

— upper/lower pole, midzone, hilum, medullary, cortical, subcapsular, extracapsular, pelvic/ peripelvic.
— single/multiple – bilateral (1%).

Size

— length × width × depth (cm) or maximum dimension (cm).

Appearance

— cystic/solid: renal cell carcinoma.
— necrotic/haemorrhagic/yellow/white/scirrhous: renal cell carcinoma.
— tan/central scar: oncocytoma and chromophil/ chromophobe carcinomas.
— papillary/sessile/scirrhous: renal pelvis carcinoma.

Edge

— circumscribed/irregular.

Compression/infiltration structures

— perinephric fat, capsule, cortex, medulla, pelvis, peripelvic fat, adrenal gland.

2. Histological type

Renal cell carcinoma

Adenocarcinoma

— 90% of cases
— cell type: clear (70%), chromophil (15% – eosinophil, basophil), mixed (10%), chromophobe (5%).
— pattern: papillary (15%): unilateral/bilateral, solitary/multifocal. non-papillary: (not otherwise specified) solid, trabecular, alveolar, cystic, tubulo-acinar with a prominent, branching vascular stroma. sarcomatoid (2–5%): poorly differentiated carcinoma of various subtypes characterised by spindle cells with high nuclear grade. It is not a specific variant but an indication of disease progression.

The commonest renal cell cancers are non-papillary and of clear cell to eosinophilic granular cell type with variable nuclear morphology. Mixed patterns and cell types are not unusual and undifferentiated forms (unclassified) occur.

Oncocytoma

— 5% of renal cell neoplasms (occasionally multifocal/bilateral).
— oncocytes (small round central nucleus, abundant eosinophilic cytoplasm in tubules, sheets and nests),central radial scar, benign.

Differential diagnosis is well-differentiated (grade 1) renal cell carcinoma with eosinophilic cells; oncocytoma is excluded by necrosis, mitoses, clear cells, spindle cells, papillary areas, gross vascular invasion or gross extension into perirenal fat.

Renal collecting duct carcinoma

— 1%
— medulla; irregular tubules; hobnail cells; desmoplastic stroma; aggressive.

Neuroendocrine carcinoma

— carcinoid/small cell/large cell.
— NSE, chromogranin positive.

Small cell carcinoma may arise from the pelvic mucosa as part of a transitional cell carcinoma secondarily involving the kidney parenchyma.

Renal pelvis/ureter carcinoma

Transitional cell carcinoma
— ± calculi.
— single/multifocal.
— 20% of upper renal tract neoplasms.
— frequently low-grade and papillary giving hydroureter/hydronephrosis with a non-functioning kidney and a radiological filling defect in the pelvis/ureter. Sessile high-grade forms can infiltrate the medulla and cortex with a scirrhous gross appearance and squamoid or spindle cell morphology.

Squamous cell carcinoma
— calculi/infection/squamous metaplasia of the pelvic mucosa.
— mostly high-grade and locally advanced/metastatic at presentation. Prognosis is poor.

Adenocarcinoma
— pure: mucin secretion/glands/signet ring cells; adjacent pyelitis cystica/ glandularis secondary to chronic inflammation, e.g. calculi.
— mixed: as part of a transitional cell carcinoma.

Sarcomatoid carcinoma
— spindle cell carcinoma with high nuclear grade, cytokeratin positive.

Metastatic carcinoma

— often small and bilateral (50%).
— direct spread: cervix, prostate, bladder (distal ureter), gut, retroperitoneal metastases, e.g. lung and breast.
— distant spread: lung, malignant melanoma (skin), breast, stomach, pancreas, ovary, testis.

3. Differentiation/grade
Renal cell carcinoma

Well/moderate/poor.
Differentiation and nuclear grade are not infrequently heterogeneous within a lesion; the malignant cell typically has a low nuclear/cytoplasmic ratio.

Nuclear grade (Fuhrman)
1. Round, uniform, 10 μm, nucleoli absent
2. Slightly irregular, 15 μm, nucleoli visible
3. Moderately to markedly irregular, 20 μm, large nucleoli

4. Bizarre multinucleated forms, ≥ 20 μm, prominent nucleoli, clumped chromatin.

Grades 2 (35%) and 3 (35%) account for the majority of cases. Prognostic significance of nuclear grade also varies according to tumour type, e.g. metastatic papillary renal carcinoma is usually high grade whereas metastatic clear cell renal carcinoma is often of low nuclear grade.

Transitional cell carcinoma

Well/moderate/poor.
WHO I/II/III.
Low-grade (WHO I) or high-grade (WHO II/III).

4. Extent of local tumour spread

Border: pushing/infiltrative.
Lymphocytic reaction: prominent/sparse.
Adjacent mucosa: dysplasia or carcinoma in-situ.

Capsule, perirenal fat
The capsule is often elevated and compressed by the lobulated margin of renal cell adenocarcinoma and this must be distinguished from actual histologically proven invasion of perirenal fat. In this respect the capsule and fat should not be stripped from the kidney prior to sectioning it otherwise the cortex/capsule/fat interface is lost. Extension to the renal pelvis occurs late in the course of the disease.

Pelvis, ureter
Renal pelvic transitional cell carcinoma is not infrequently multifocal (40%) with concurrent ureteric lesions ± bladder tumour. The adjacent urothelium is abnormal ranging from hyperplasia through dysplasia to carcinoma in-situ.

Renal vein
Renal cell adenocarcinoma has a propensity for venous invasion.

Renal cell carcinoma

pT1 tumour ≤ 7 cm in greatest dimension, limited to the kidney
pT2 tumour > 7 cm in greatest dimension, limited to the kidney
pT3 tumour invades:
    a. perinephric fat, adrenal gland
    b. renal vein, IVC below diaphragm
    c. IVC above diaphragm
pT4 tumour invades neighbouring organs, abdominal wall, beyond Gerota's fascia.

Involvement of renal vein and ipsilateral adrenal gland is seen in 10% and 5% of cases respectively. Metastases occur in the lung, skeleton and skin and to almost any site where they can mimic primary clear cell tumour in the involved organ, e.g. thyroid, ovary. Preferential metastatic sites are seen with various subtypes of carcinoma, e.g. papillary carcinoma has fewer lung metastases and more lymph node deposits than clear cell carcinoma, and chromophobe carcinoma tends to spread to liver.

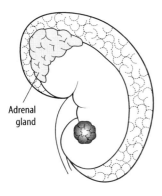

pT1 = ≤ 7 cm dia, confined to kidney

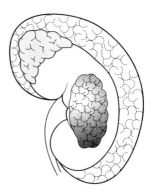

pT2 = > 7 cm dia, confined to kidney

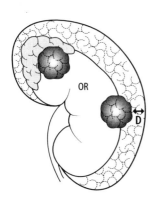

pT3a = into adrenal gland or perirenal fat
pT3b = into renal vein or IVC below diaphragm
pT3c = into IVC above diaphragm
   D = tumour distance (mm) to the
      Circumferential Radial Margin (CRM)
      of excision of perinephric fat

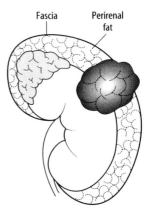

pT4 = beyond Gerota fascia, into
abdominal wall or adjacent organs

Figure 113. Renal cell carcinoma.

The surface component may be exophytic/papillary or sessile

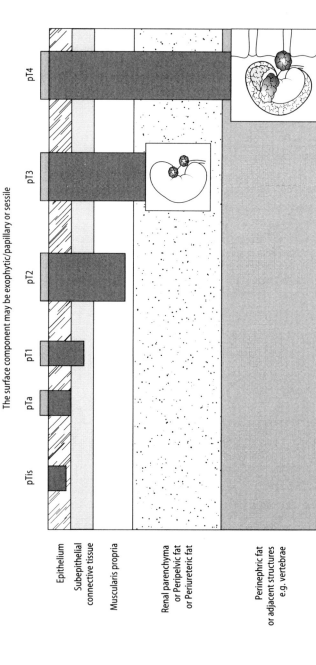

Figure 114. Renal pelvis and ureter carcinoma.

Pelvis/ureter carcinoma

pTis   carcinoma in-situ
pTa   papillary non-invasive
pT1   tumour invades subepithelial connective tissue
pT2   tumour invades muscularis propria
pT3   tumour invades beyond muscularis into peripelvic fat or renal parenchyma
       (pelvis)
       tumour invades beyond muscularis into periureteric fat (ureter)
pT4   tumour invades adjacent organs, perinephric fat.

Pelvis/ureter carcinoma: single/multifocal lesion(s); hydroureter/hydronephrosis.

5. Lymphovascular invasion

Present/absent.
Intra-/extratumoural.
Renal cell carcinoma has a tendency to involve the main renal vein while infiltrating pelvic transitional cell carcinoma often shows invasion of small lymphovascular channels in the cortex and medulla; however, it can also subsequently involve the renal vein.

6. Lymph nodes

Site/number/size/number involved/limit node/extracapsular spread.
Regional nodes: hilar, abdominal para-aortic, paracaval (ureter-intrapelvic)

Renal cell carcinoma

pN0   no regional lymph nodes involved
pN1   metastasis in a single regional node
pN2   metastasis in more than one regional node.

Regional node metastases occur in 10–15% of cases.

Pelvis/ureter carcinoma

pN0   no regional lymph node metastasis
pN1   single regional node metastasis ≤ 2 cm
pN2   single regional node metastasis > 2 cm to 5 cm, multiple ≤ 5 cm
pN3   regional node metastasis > 5 cm.

7. Excision margins

Distances (mm) to the distal ureteric limit, renal vein limit, perirenal fat resection margin.

8. Other pathology

There is a degree of correlation between cell type and architectural pattern in renal cell carcinoma, e.g. clear cell is non-papillary while chromophil is papillary. Chromophil and chromophobe (cell nests, prominent cytoplasmic membranes, pale flocculent cytoplasm, positive with Hale's colloidal iron and alcian blue) lesions have slightly better prognosis than equivalent grade and stage renal clear cell carcinoma of usual type. Sarcomatoid carcinoma (aggressive) is usually pale and scirrhous in appearance while renal cell adenocarcinoma may become totally cystic with only residual mural nodules of viable tumour.

Chromosomal analysis characterises various morphological subtypes, e.g. papillary versus non-papillary renal carcinoma; papillary carcinoma is well differentiated with uniform cells covering stromal cores containing macrophages, can be multifocal and bilateral and associated with precursor cortical adenomas. The papillary pattern, which forms at least 70% of the tumour area, is striking and although the cytology is usually uniform with a high nuclear/cytoplasmic ratio it can vary. Cytogenetically these tumours show a gain on chromosomes 7 and 17 rather than the 3p13 deletion of usual renal cell carcinoma.

Von Hippel Lindau syndrome has an increased incidence (40–50%) of renal cell carcinoma as do acquired and congenital polycystic disease (5–10%). Occasionally renal cell carcinoma can spontaneously regress and also be host to cancer metastasising to within cancer, particularly from lung carcinoma. Other associated characteristics are fever, hepatic dysfunction, hypercalcaemia, hypertension (secretion of renin), polycythaemia (secretion of erythropoietin) and hormonal effects (secretion of ACTH-like substance).

Amyloid renal interstitium adjacent to renal cell carcinoma and systemic in distribution.

Xanthogranulomatous pyelonephritis and malakoplakia can mimic pelvic/renal cell carcinoma grossly and on needle biopsy. Percutaneous fine needle aspiration cytology is useful in the diagnosis of simple renal cysts versus cystic or solid renal cell carcinoma. Carcinoma is cellular, shows nuclear atypia with a low nuclear/cytoplasmic ratio, nucleolar enlargement and variable fat/glycogen positive cytoplasmic vacuolation. Pelvic carcinoma also shows cytological features of malignancy.

Renal cell carcinoma is positive with markers for cytokeratin, EMA and vimentin. Sarcomatoid variants also retain vimentin and cytokeratin positivity. Papillary carcinoma is characteristically EMA and cytokeratin 7 positive in contrast to other renal epithelial tumours with papillary areas that are cytokeratin 7 negative.

A solid, clear cell lesion of any size (even if<2.5 cm) should probably be regarded as carcinoma. Adenoma should be reserved for small (<0.5–1 cm) lesions with a papillary pattern of acidophil cells. Renal cell carcinoma is treated by heminephrectomy (nephron sparing surgery) or radical nephrectomy depending on the size and location of the tumour. Indications for nephron sparing surgery are: tumour <4cm diameter, location at a renal pole and of non-papillary type. Renal pelvis/ureter carcinoma requires nephrectomy with ureterectomy, often including resection of the ureteric orifice because of multifocality and involvement of its terminal, vesical (intramural) portion. Resection of solitary pulmonary metastases can be of benefit.

Prognosis

Up to 30% of renal cell carcinomas present with spread beyond the kidney and 10% involve renal vein with a tendency to solitary distant metastases, e.g. lung, skin and bone with pathological fracture. Overall 5 year survival is 70% relating to tumour grade, type (e.g. grade III and sarcomatoid lesions are aggressive), vascular invasion and stage:

pT1   60–80%
pT2   40–70%
pT3   20–40%
pT4   5%.

Carcinoma of the renal pelvis/ureter is predominantly transitional cell in type with occasional squamous cell, adenocarcinoma and sarcomatoid carcinoma. Typically there are multifocal, synchronous pelvi-ureteric (25%) and bladder (15%) lesions with a 50% risk of subsequent metachronous tumours at these sites. The majority (75%) are WHO I, pT1 but invasive lesions form poorly differentiated nests, sheets and cords of tumour in a desmoplastic stroma often assuming a squamoid appearance. Retrograde involvement of medullary collecting ducts (mimicking adenocarcinoma) and lymphovascular invasion are not uncommon. Most are of good prognosis but critical invasion of ureteric muscle coat, renal pelvis or parenchyma results in 5 year survival rates of 35%.

9. Other malignancy

Lymphoma/leukaemia
— usually secondary to systemic/nodal disease and present in up to 50% of cases. If established as a primary lymphoma it is usually large B cell in type.

Leiomyosarcoma, liposarcoma, malignant fibrous histiocytoma, rhabdomyosarcoma
— all rare and important to exclude more common diagnoses, i.e. sarcomatoid renal cell carcinoma and primary retroperitoneal sarcoma with secondary renal involvement.

Angiomyolipoma with malignant transformation
— tuberose sclerosis in 30%, multifocal (30%), bilateral (15%).
— HMB-45 positive spindle cells with variable cellularity and pleomorphism ± mitoses, mature fat and thick-walled vessels.
— capsular invasion and nodal disease may be seen and is often regarded as multicentricity rather than malignancy. Rarely true malignant change can occur.
— prone to catastrophic/potentially fatal haemorrhage.
— rarely associated with concurrent renal cell carcinoma.

Bladder Carcinoma

1. Gross description

Specimen

— urine cytology/bladder washings/cystoscopic biopsy/transurethral resection bladder (TURB)/ cystectomy/cystourethrectomy/cystoprostatectomy (including seminal vesicles)/cystoprostatourethrectomy/anterior or total exenteration (including uterus and adnexae ± rectum).
— weight (g) and size (cm).
— length (cm) of ureters and urethra.

Tumour

Site

— fundus/body/trigone/neck/ureteric orifices.
— anterior/posterior/lateral (right or left).
— single/multifocal.
— diverticulum.

Size

— length × width × depth (cm) or maximum dimension (cm).

Appearance

— papillary/sessile/ulcerated/mucoid/keratotic/calcification.
— bladder mucosa – erythematous/oedematous (carcinoma in-situ).

Edge

— circumscribed/irregular.

2. Histological type

Transitional (urothelial) cell carcinoma

— 90% of cases.
— usual type: papillary or sessile.
  Variants:
— microcystic type: intraurothelial microcysts containing protein secretions.
— nested type: uniform cell nests in the lamina propria.
— with pseudosarcomatous stroma or trophoblastic cells (HCG positive).
— inverted type: architecturally similar to inverted papilloma but has WHO II/III cytology.
— also clear cell, plasmacytoid, micropapillary, lipid cell variants.

Squamous cell carcinoma

— 5% of cases.
— classical/verrucous.
— old age; ± calculi; ± schistosomiasis; ± diverticulum and chronic infection. Prognosis is poor: 13–35% 5 year survival with two-thirds pT3/pT4 at presentation.

Adenocarcinoma

— 2% of bladder malignancy.
— mucinous, signet ring, enteric, clear cell types.
— can arise either from from intestinal metaplasia/cystitis glandularis (60%), extrophy, diverticula or bladder dome wall urachal remnants (30%); usually muscle invasive and of poor prognosis (particularly signet ring cell carcinoma).

Carcinoma with mixed differentiation

— squamous cell carcinoma/adenocarcinoma components are seen in 20–30% of high-grade invasive transitional cell carcinoma emphasising a capacity for divergent differentiation.

Spindle cell carcinoma

— "sarcomatoid carcinoma" or carcinosarcoma.
— old age; large and polypoid; poor prognosis (50% dead within 1 year); recognisable in-situ or invasive epithelial (transitional, glandular, squamous or undifferentiated) component and cytokeratin/vimentin positive spindle cells with varying degrees of stromal metaplasia, from non-specific fibrosarcoma-like to specific heterologous, mesenchymal differentiation, e.g. rhabdomyosarcoma, chondrosarcoma, osteosarcoma.

Small cell carcinoma

— primary or secondary from lung; aggressive with early metastases to nodes, liver, bone and peritoneum; may be pure or mixed with other in-situ or invasive bladder cancer subtypes; there is coexistent prostatic disease in 50% of cases.

Malignant melanoma
— primary or secondary (commoner).
— note there can be spread to bladder from a primary urethral lesion.

Metastatic carcinoma
— metastases should be considered in any bladder tumour with unusual histology, e.g. adenocarcinoma or squamous cell carcinoma.
— direct spread: from adjacent pelvic organs (> 70% of cases): prostate, cervix, uterus, anus, rectum, colon. To distinguish primary adenocarcinoma from secondary colorectal carcinoma look for an origin at the dome from urachal remnants, or areas of adjacent mucosal intestinal metaplasia cystitis glandularis in a primary lesion.
Prostatic cancer is PSA/PSAP positive.
— distant spread: breast, malignant melanoma, lung, stomach.

3. Differentiation/cytological grade

Well/moderate/poor.
Based on the degree of nuclear stratification, crowding, atypia and hyperchromasia.

WHO	I	least anaplastic	low-grade:<5% risk of progression to invasion
	II	↓	
	III	most anaplastic	high-grade: 15–40% risk of progression to invasion.

Poorly differentiated invasive urothelial carcinoma often assumes a squamoid appearance in addition to actual squamous or glandular differentiation (20–30% of cases).

4. Extent of local tumour spread

Border: pushing/infiltrative.
Lymphocytic reaction: prominent/sparse.

pTis carcinoma in-situ: potential multifocal urinary tract field change
pTa   papillary non-invasive
pT1   invasion of subepithelial connective tissue
pT2a invasion of superficial muscle (inner half)
pT2b invasion of deep muscle (outer half)
pT3   invasion of perivesical fat:
    a. microscopically
    b. extravesical mass (macroscopically)

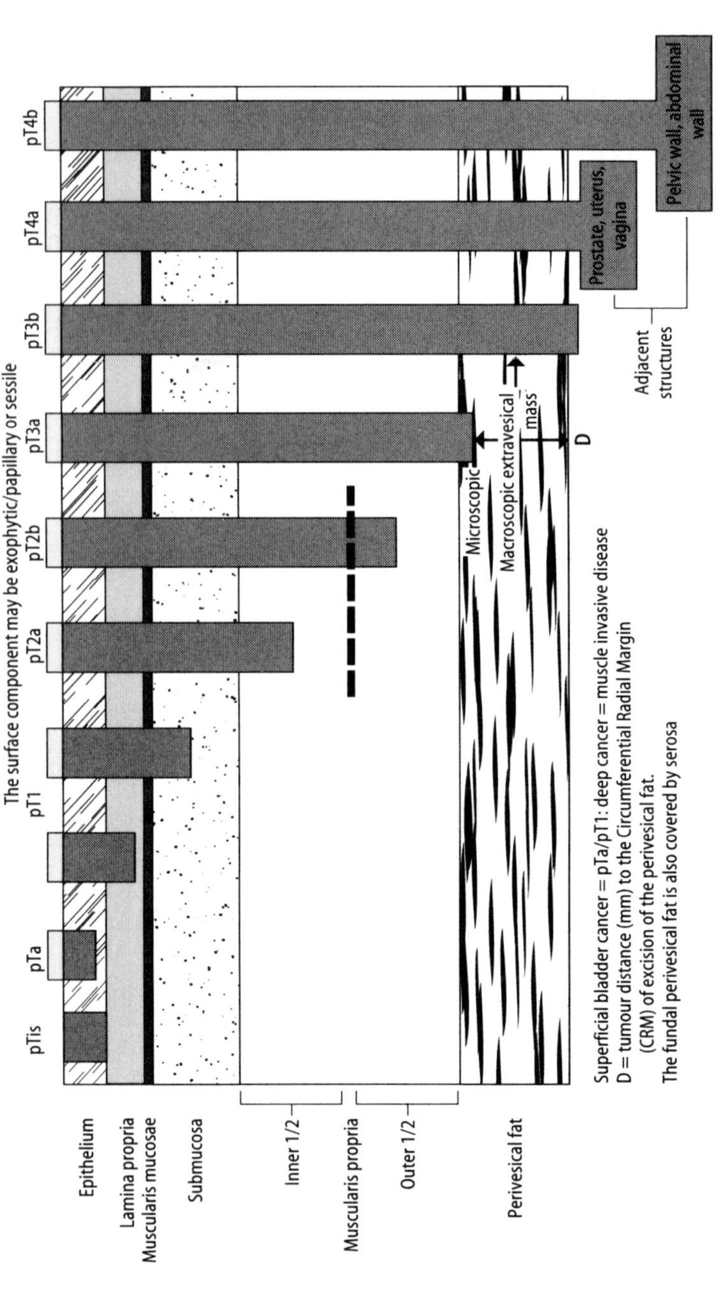
Epithelium
Lamina propria
Muscularis mucosae
Submucosa
Inner 1/2
Muscularis propria
Outer 1/2
Perivesical fat
pTis
pTa
pT1
pT2a
pT2b
pT3a
pT3b
pT4a
pT4b
The surface component may be exophytic/papillary or sessile
Microscopic
Macroscopic extravesical mass
D
Adjacent structures
Prostate, uterus, vagina
Pelvic wall, abdominal wall
Superficial bladder cancer = pTa/pT1: deep cancer = muscle invasive disease
D = tumour distance (mm) to the Circumferential Radial Margin
(CRM) of excision of the perivesical fat.
The fundal perivesical fat is also covered by serosa

Figure 115. Urinary bladder carcinoma.

pT4   invasion of:
      a. prostate, uterus, vagina
      b. pelvic wall, abdominal wall.
Superficial tumours are regarded as either pTa or pT1 and are usually histological grade I or II.

Deeply (muscle) invasive tumours are pT2 or pT3 and more often grade III. They are prognostically adverse requiring more radical treatment and assessment of invasion of the muscularis propria is of crucial importance.

5. Lymphovascular invasion

Present/absent.
Intra-/extratumoural.
Invasion into the lamina propria may result in prominent retraction artefact spaces around tumour cells and nests mimicking lymphovascular invasion. For true vascular involvement identify an endothelial lining/± factor VIII, CD 31 positivity/± red blood cells/± adherence of the tumour plug to the endothelial lining. Vascular invasion is associated with an increased rate of recurrence.

6. Lymph nodes

Site/number/size/number involved/limit node/extracapsular spread.
Regional nodes: pelvic nodes below the bifurcation of the common iliac arteries.

pN0   no regional lymph nodes involved
pN1   metastasis in a single regional node ≤ 2 cm
pN2   metastasis in a regional node > 2 cm but ≤ 5 cm or multiple regional nodes each ≤ 5 cm
pN3   metastasis in a regional node > 5 cm.

Nodal metastases are present in 25% of invasive transitional cell carcinomas. Common sites of distant metastases are lungs, liver, bone and CNS.

7. Excision margins

Distances (mm) to the limits of the urethra, ureters, perivesical fat and fundal serosa.

8. Other pathology
Diagnostic criteria for TCC

Carcinoma in-situ (CIS)
— flat urothelium of variable thickness (3–20 layers).
— marked cytological abnormality of usually (but not always) the whole epithelial thickness.

- note unusual patterns such as the pagetoid variant, or clinging CIS resulting from dyscohesion and shedding of cells.
- CIS equates to severe dysplasia and is by its nature a high-grade lesion.
- present adjacent to invasive carcinoma in 50–60% of cases.
- beware of overcalling dysplasia or in-situ change, as normal urothelium often partially denudes on biopsy leaving a thin covering of basal cells which can then appear hyperchromatic.
- note that a biopsy diagnosis of dysplasia with no previous history may progress to CIS or invasive malignancy in up to 19% of cases over the course of several years.

Papillary TCC
> 7 cell layers thick.
- papillae with fine stromal cores which are not true lamina propria (a distinguishing factor from polypoid cystitis).
- variable nuclear grade of abnormality – similar lesions without cytological atypia are classified as papillary urothelial neoplasm of low malignant potential in the 2nd edition WHO classification.

Growth pattern

Papillary, exophytic

Sessile
- tends to be associated with high-grade lesions.

Endophytic and non-invasive, or invasive
- differentiate from inverted papilloma (covering of normal urothelium, no atypia or mitoses, inversion of the epithelial layers).
- non-invasive lesions have an intact, round basement membrane and no desmoplastic or inflammatory stromal response and often represent a complex crypt pattern to the lesion base or extension of malignant epithelium into Brunn's nests. Invasive endophytic lesions can have a rounded deep border with no inflammatory reaction making assessment of invasion difficult – look for atypical urothelim present in relation to muscularis propria.

Pathological predictors of prognosis

- number of tumours/multifocality: both within the bladder and extravesical, e.g. ureters and renal pelvis.
- size of tumour.
- depth of invasion.
- histological grade.

— coexistent carcinoma in-situ/dysplasia adjacent to or away from the tumour: markers of higher risk for recurrence and progression.
— progression of grade and stage with time.
— poor initial response to chemo-/radiotherapy

Additional comments

Biopsies

Assess material from: the base (for pT stage), and adjacent and distant mucosa (for pTis). Clear distinction between superficial and deep muscle cannot be made on biopsy material (unless submitted separately by the clinician), so that muscle-invasive carcinoma should be reported as at least pT2a in depth. The muscle bundles should be coarse indicating the detrusor layer or muscularis propria rather than the fine fibres of the poorly defined lamina propria.

Resection blocks

— urethral limit.
— ureteric limits.
— prostate, seminal vesicles.
— normal bladder.
— tumour and wall.

Post-operative necrobiotic granuloma

— post-TURP fibrinoid necrosis with palisading histiocytes.

Post-operative spindle cell nodule and pseudosarcomatous fibromyxoid tumour

These are reactive fibroproliferative processes histologically resembling sarcoma. Spindle cell nodule is small (5–9 mm) and has a history of recent genitourinary tract instrumentation. It comprises a proliferation of cytologically bland spindle cells in which normal mitoses are readily seen and it occurs at the operative site. Pseudosarcomatous fibromyxoid tumour occurs de novo, can be several centimetres in diameter and could be regarded as a visceral form of nodular fasciitis. The atypical fibro/myoblastic proliferation is associated with prominent inflammation and granulation tissue-type vasculature. Mitoses can be seen, and are not prominent or abnormal. Both lesions are benign and must be distinguished from sarcoma although some cases of pseudosarcomatous fibromyxoid tumour have been reported to recur and even progress with local infiltration. Cytokeratin is positive in spindle cell nodule but usually negative in fibromyxoid tumour (a useful discriminator from spindle cell carcinoma); actin and desmin are variably positive.

Diverticulum ± calculus: squamous cell carcinoma.

Transitional cell carcinoma is positive for cytokeratins 7, 8, 18 and 20, CEA, CA19-9, Leu M1 and Lewis X antigen. Overexpression of p53 correlates with the likelihood of progression in superficial disease.

Treatment of bladder transitional cell carcinoma is usually by transurethral resection and cystoscopic follow-up. Refractory superficial disease (i.e. confined to the mucous membrane) may also need radiotherapy and/or intravesical chemotherapy/BCG. The latter are also useful for transitional cell carcinoma in-situ. Non-responsive superficial or deep (muscle-invasive) cancer necessitates surgery. In follow-up note that intravesical agents such as mitomycin lead to urothelial atypia and these changes must not be confused with dysplasia or carcinoma in-situ. The nuclei are focally enlarged and have a "smudged" chromatin appearance rather than the angular, ink blank hyperchromasia of in-situ change. BCG often results in inflammation and superficial non-caseating granulomas but tubercle are usually not seen.

Prognosis

Muscle-invasive cancer often starts as carcinoma in-situ or a flat/sessile rather than a papillary lesion and relates strongly to histological grade (WHO I = 2% invasive; WHO III = 40% invasive). Invasive cancer will develop in up to 30–50% (or more) of patients with untreated carcinoma in-situ but 85–90% 5 year survival rates can be achieved by radical surgery which is also targeted at multifocal field change in the urothelium (bladder, prostatic ducts, urethra, ureters, seminal vesicles). Up to 80% of urothelial carcinomas are non-invasive at the time of presentation and although tumour recurrence is common (single lesion 30–45%, multiple 60–90%) tumour progression (10%) relates strongly to histological grade, tumour size, non-tumour dysplasia of bladder mucosa and depth of invasion. Overexpression (> 20% of tumour cells) of p53 and cerb-B2 may also be another indicator. Five year survival rates also vary according to these parameters:-

transitional cell carcinoma	superficial invasion	
	grade I	70%
	grade III	60%
	deep muscle invasion	40–55%
squamous cell carcinoma		15%
adenocarcinoma		15–35%

As can be seen, squamous cell carcinoma and adenocarcinoma are of worse prognosis.

9. Other malignancy

Lymphoma/leukaemia

— usually secondary to systemic disease.

Primary lymphoma varies from low-grade MALToma with indolent behaviour to diffuse large B cell lymphoma. Leukaemic involvement is seen in 15–30% of cases.

Carcinoid tumour

— rare.

Phaeochromocytoma

— local recurrence and metastases can occur.

Leiomyosarcoma

— commonest sarcoma in adults, bladder dome, infiltrates muscle.

Other sarcomas

— rhabdomyosarcoma, malignant fibrous histiocytoma, osteosarcoma: all rare and must exclude sarcomatoid carcinoma (carcinosarcoma).

Rhabdomyosarcoma

— embryonal variant in children, sarcoma botryoides.
— cellular subepithelial cambium layer, loose myxoid zone, cellular deep zone ± rhabdomyoblasts, ± myoglobin/desmin positive.

Choriocarcinoma and yolk sac tumour

— choriocarcinoma: exclude urothelial carcinoma with trophoblastic differentiation.
— yolk sac tumour: rare; childhood.

Prostate Carcinoma

1. Gross description

Specimen

— fine needle aspirate/needle core biopsy (18 gauge) transurethral resection (TUR) chippings/ radical prostatectomy (including seminal vesicles).
— weight (g) and size (cm).
— number and length of cores (cm).

Tumour

Site

— inner (transitional)/outer (central and peripheral) zones
— medial/lateral (right or left) lobes.
— posterior/subcapsular.

The majority of carcinomas are posterior and peripheral; multicentricity is present in up to 75% of cases.

Size

— length × width × depth (cm) or maximum dimension (cm).
— tumour volume (cm^3).

Appearance

— soft/firm
— pale/yellow/granular

Similar changes are seen in tuberculosis, infarction, granulomatous prostatitis and acute and chronic prostatitis, i.e. histological assessment is necessary.

Edge

— circumscribed/irregular.

2. Histological type

Acinar/proximal duct origin

Adenocarcinoma with acinar, diffuse cell infiltration, papillary, cribriform, comedo patterns

— usual types (>90–95% of cases).

Mucinous adenocarcinoma

— distinguish from secondary colorectal or bladder cancer.

— 25% of the tumour area is intra-/extracellular mucin.

— fewer bone metastases and less hormone/radioresponsive than usual prostatic carcinoma.

Signet ring cell adenocarcinoma

— rare; distinguish from secondary gastric or colorectal cancer.

— 25% of the tumour area is signet ring cells, usually coexisting with other poorly differentiated carcinoma; poor prognosis.

Adenoid basal carcinoma

— a continuum of basal cell hyperplasia/adenoma and adenoid cystic-like differentiation, variably 34βE12 positive; a tumour of low malignant potential.

Undifferentiated, small oat cell type

— chromogranin/NSE positive; immunonegative cases are classified as poorly differentiated prostatic carcinoma.

— primary or secondary from lung, pure or mixed (25%) with usual prostatic carcinoma ± bladder cancer.

— aggressive: sometimes inappropriate ACTH/ADH secretion.

— carcinoid tumour is rare: up to 33% of usual prostatic carcinomas can show neuroendocrine differentiation on immunohistochemistry and this is usually of no prognostic significance.

Undifferentiated, non-small cell type or basaloid

— similar to basaloid carcinoma of the anal canal and oesophagus; aggressive.

Adenosquamous/squamous carcinoma

— rare; poor prognosis; exclude squamous metaplasia due to infarction or hormone therapy.

Clear cell adenocarcinoma

— prostatic urethra ± diverticulum.

— papillary, clear cells, hobnail cells; exclude secondary renal cell or ovarian carcinoma.

Sarcomatoid carcinoma

— syn. carcinosarcoma or metaplastic carcinoma.
— cytokeratin positive spindle cells with variable stromal metaplasia and mesenchymal differentiation – homologous ± heterologous elements (bone, cartilage, striated muscle).
— older men, variable prognosis.

Distal (large) duct origin

Periurethral duct adenocarcinoma

— syn. endometrioid carcinoma
— old age; polypoid/villous or infiltrative on cystoscopy. Have a more advanced stage at presentation but higher short-term survival.
— papillary, clear cell, cribriform and endometrioid patterns. Prostate specific antigen/ prostatic acid phosphatase (PSA/PSAP) positive, ± oestrogen dependent.

Transitional cell carcinoma

— 2% of prostatic cancers.
— PSA/PSAP positive to exclude spread from a bladder or urethra transitional cell carcinoma.

Mixed adenocarcinoma/transitional cell carcinoma

Squamous cell carcinoma

— rare; poor prognosis.

Metastatic carcinoma

— direct spread: bladder (in 40% of radical cystoprostatectomies for bladder cancer), colorectum, anus, retroperitoneal sarcoma.
— distant spread: kidney, lung (squamous carcinoma), malignant melanoma.

3. Differentiation/grade

Well/moderate/poor.
— 50% of cases show heterogeneity of tumour grade.

Gleason score

The Gleason system proposes that any given prostate carcinoma may show one or several of five histological glandular architectural patterns ranging from the lowest grade (grade 1) to the highest grade (grade 5). Taking the two predominant patterns one can arrive at a score (e.g. 2 + 3 = 5; 3 + 4 = 7) which has prognostic significance. The following rules apply:

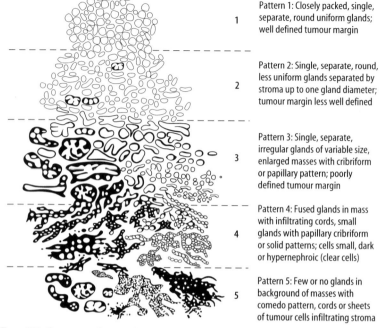

Pattern 1: Closely packed, single, separate, round uniform glands; well defined tumour margin

Pattern 2: Single, separate, round, less uniform glands separated by stroma up to one gland diameter; tumour margin less well defined

Pattern 3: Single, separate, irregular glands of variable size, enlarged masses with cribriform or papillary pattern; poorly defined tumour margin

Pattern 4: Fused glands in mass with infiltrating cords, small glands with papillary cribriform or solid patterns; cells small, dark or hypernephroic (clear cells)

Pattern 5: Few or no glands in background of masses with comedo pattern, cords or sheets of tumour cells infiltrating stroma

Figure 116. Gleason score in prostatic carcinoma. (Gleason DF. The Veterans Administration Cooperative Urologic Research Group: Histologic grading and clinical staging of prostatic carcinoma. In: Tannenbaum M (ed) Urologic pathology: the prostate. Philadelphia: Lea and Febiger, 1977.)

(a) Choose the two predominant patterns where more than two are present.

(b) When there is only one pattern, double it, e.g. 3 + 3 = 6.

(c) In limited samples (e.g. needle biopsy, TUR chippings) where there are more than two patterns and the worst grade is neither the predominant nor the second most predominant pattern, choose the main pattern and the highest grade. For example, if grade 3 is 60%, grade 1 is 30% and grade 4 is 10%, the score is 3 + 4 = 7. Note that needle biopsy samples can underestimate the Gleason score compared with the subsequent resection specimen.

4. Extent of local tumour spread

Border: pushing/infiltrative.
Lymphocytic reaction: prominent/sparse.
Weight of chippings or length of cores and proportion (%) involved.
Apex of gland, urethral limit, capsule and margins, seminal vesicles.

pT1   clinically inapparent tumour not palpable or visible by imaging
    T1a   incidental finding in ≤ 5% of tissue resected

T1b incidental finding in > 5% of tissue resected
T1c identified by needle biopsy (e.g. because of elevated PSA)
pT2 tumour confined within the prostate
T2a involves one lobe
T2b involves both lobes
pT3 tumour extends through the prostatic capsule
T3a extracapsular extension
T3b invades seminal vesicle(s)
pT4 tumour is fixed or invades neighbouring structures: bladder neck, external sphincter, rectum, levator muscles, and/or pelvic wall.

Due to the inferoposterior approach of per rectal needle biopsy there may be representation of extracapsular, capsular and seminal vesicle tissues which should be assessed for invasion (= pT3). Advanced disease manifests spread

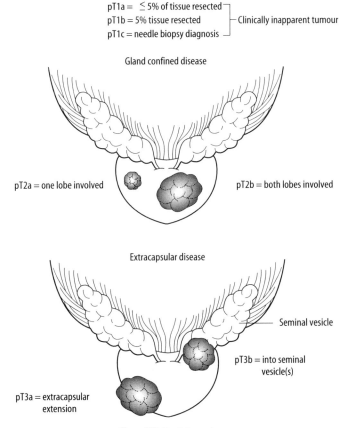

pT1a = ≤ 5% of tissue resected ⎤
pT1b = 5% tissue resected ⎬ Clinically inapparent tumour
pT1c = needle biopsy diagnosis ⎦

Gland confined disease

pT2a = one lobe involved   pT2b = both lobes involved

Extracapsular disease

Seminal vesicle

pT3b = into seminal
       vesicle(s)

pT3a = extracapsular
       extension

Figure 117. Prostatic carcinoma.

Tumour is fixed or invades adjacent structures other than seminal vesicles: bladder neck, external sphincter, rectum, levator muscles and/or pelvic wall (Figs. 118, 119)

pT4

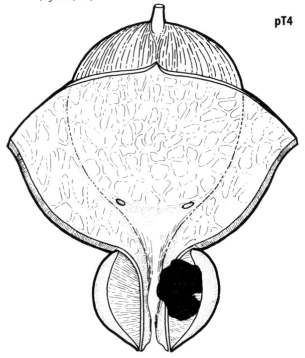

Figure 118. Prostatic carcinoma.

into seminal vesicle, prostatic urethra and bladder. Presentation can be by an anterior rectal mass or stricture and PSA staining of rectal biopsy material is of use.

5. Lymphovascular invasion

Perineural and lymphovascular space: while its positive predictive value is low perineural invasion is an independent indicator of potential extraprostatic extension and is associated with prostatic carcinoma of higher Gleason score and volume.

Present/absent.
Intra-/extratumoural.

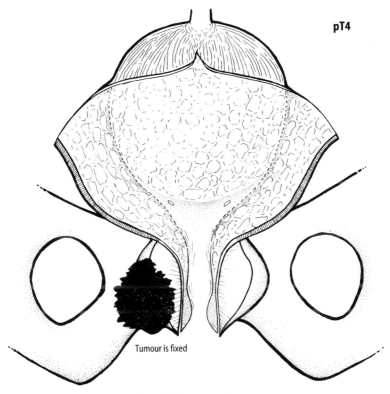

pT4

Tumour is fixed

Figure 119. Prostatic carcinoma.

6. Lymph nodes

Site/number/size/number involved/limit node/extracapsular spread.
Regional nodes: pelvic nodes below the bifurcation of the common iliac arteries.

pN0   no regional lymph node metastasis
pN1   metastasis in regional lymph node(s).

Lymph node metastases are present in up to 10–30% of radical prostatectomy specimens relating to tumour stage, volume, differentiation and serum PSA levels. Nodal tumour volume or maximum diameter is an index of metastatic potential. The next commonest sites of metastases are bone (osteoblastic in character) and lung. Occult primary disease can present with metastases to unusual sites, e.g. pleura, bronchus, mediastinal and supraclavicular lymph nodes. Bronchial biopsy and aspiration cytology coupled with PSA immunoreactivity can be useful in these circumstances.

7. Excision margins

Distances (mm) to the capsule, surgical resection margins and urethral limits. Capsular and marginal invasion are strong indicators of extraprostatic disease and potential progression. Note that the prostatic capsule is poorly defined particularly at the base and apex of the gland.

8. Other pathology

Extent of high-grade (HG) PIN (prostatic intraepithelial neoplasia) and location (usually peripheral as in carcinoma): HGPIN has malignant cytology (i.e. nuclear/nucleolar enlargement) within preserved ducts ± focal disruption of the basal cell layer with high molecular weight 34βE12 cytokeratin stain. Its intra-ductal architectural patterns are tufting, micropapillary, cribriform and flat. About 40–50% are associated with concurrent or subsequent adenocarcinoma. Its presence in biopsy cores or chippings indicates the need to process more tissue and for clinical reassessment and follow-up.

High molecular weight cytokeratin antibody 34βE12 reacts with the basal cells of prostatic glands in benign conditions but is negative in adenocarcinoma. Important morphological markers of adenocarcinoma are: nuclear/nucleolar enlargement, absence of the basal cell layer, perineural invasion (especially if circumferential and intraneural) and loss of gland architecture. Luminal crystalloids may also be seen.

34βE12 is of use in difficult differential diagnoses of prostatic adenocarcinoma, i.e. HGPIN, post-atrophic hyperplasia, sclerosing adenosis and atypical adenomatous hyperplasia (benign cytology within an abnormal glandular architecture at the edge of hyperplastic nodules). Overdiagnosis of seminal vesicle epithelium as malignant should also be borne in mind: look for cytoplasmic lipofuscin pigment and characteristic cytoarchitectural appearances. Basal cell hyperplasia/adenoma are also 34βE12 positive. About 3% of needle biopsy specimens show small acinar proliferation suspicious but not diagnostic of malignancy. Interpretation must be viewed in light of the clinical findings, e.g. serum PSA. Further biopsy may be necessary.

Radiotherapy/hormonal treatment (androgen deprivation therapy) produce glandular atrophy/nuclear apoptosis/cytoplasmic vacuolation/stromal fibrosis. These may lead to underestimation of tumour bulk in post-treatment resection specimens and difficulty in deriving a Gleason score.

Mucinous and signet ring cell carcinoma have to be distinguished from secondary colorectal carcinoma. Immune markers PSA and PSAP will be positive in 95% of primary prostatic carcinomas. If immune markers are negative absence of any obvious primary elsewhere is important in designation as a primary prostate lesion. Note that PSAP can also be positive in rectal carcinoid tumours and anal carcinoma. PSA can also stain some ovarian, salivary gland, skin and breast cancers.

Endometrioid (periurethral duct) carcinoma probably has a similar prognosis to prostatic carcinoma of usual type but may also be oestrogen sensitive. It has cribriform or papillary patterns and is PSA positive. Many coexist with typical acinar prostatic carcinoma and may be related to it.

Prostatic carcinoma has a tendency to be peripheral and posterior in distribution allowing a diagnosis to be made in a significant number of cases by multiple per rectal needle biopsies. Multiple sextant biopsies can also act as a guide to the distribution and extent of the lesion. Biopsies should be examined histologically through multiple levels (at least 3) to detect focal lesions. The weight of prostatic chippings determines the number of blocks processed for histology but it is estimated that with selection 5–8 blocks will detect 90–98% of the prostatic carcinomas that are represented in a specimen.

Postoperative necrobiotic granuloma
— post-TURP fibrinoid necrosis with palisading histiocytes.

Postoperative spindle cell nodule and pseudosarcomatous fibromyxoid tumour
See Chapter 30.

Prognosis

Prognosis in prostatic cancer is related to the volume of tumour, Gleason score and extracapsular extension. Tumour volume can only really be derived by systematic measurement of serial slices of prostatectomy specimens; however, the proportion or percentage of TURP chippings or needle biopsy cores involved gives a reasonable estimate of disease extent. Overall 10 year survival is 50% and up to 30% can be regarded as cured. Gland-confined disease (pT1, pT2) shows 80–95% 10 year survival depending on tumour volume whereas extraprostatic extension (pT3, pT4) decreases 10 year survival to 60% and a "cure" rate of only 25%. Other prognostic factors are positive surgical margins, perineural and lymphovascular invasion and serum PSA levels (an indirect indicator of tumour volume and extension). Treatment (surveillance only for localised disease, radical prostatectomy, radiotherapy, hormonal manipulation) is tailored to the patient's age, general level of health and clinicopathological stage of disease. Non-surgical modalities are of use in localised disease and as palliation in locally advanced or metastatic disease. Indications for radical prostatectomy are a younger patient (up to sixth/seventh decade) with persistent but modestly elevated serum PSA (less than 10–15 ng/ml), needle biopsy-proven adenocarcinoma and an absence of extraprostatic spread on bone scan. Serum PSA > 15 ng/ml is associated with a greater likelihood of the tumour not being gland-confined and subsequent positive surgical margins.

Serum PSA level
High levels (> 4–5 ng/ml at ≥ 50 years: > 2.8 ng/ml at<50 years: free to total ratio <15%) of PSA should prompt processing of further tissue and/or multiple levels as there is a strong correlation with the presence of adenocarcinoma (elevated in 64% of cases). Levels above 4 ng/ml and 10 ng/ml confer cancer risks of 25% and 60% respectively. There is also a significant positive correlation with Gleason grade as poorly differentiated tumours are usually of high volume. Elevated levels in inflammatory conditions (prostatitis, infarct) are usually of lesser magnitude, transitory and resolve with time and treatment.

Screening is based on digital rectal examination, transrectal ultrasonography and serum PSA levels. Tissue expression of PSA/PSAP is useful in identifying a prostatic origin for metastatic carcinoma and distinguishing it from poorly differentiated transitional cell carcinoma particularly in specimens derived from the bladder neck.

9. Other malignancy

Lymphoma/leukaemia

— especially chronic lymphocytic leukaemia (20% of cases at autopsy).
— primary MALToma (rare) or secondary to systemic/nodal lymphoma; prognosis is poor.

Leiomyosarcoma

— adults; 26% of prostatic sarcomas, local recurrence and metastases common.

Other rare sarcomas must be distinguished from sarcomatoid carcinoma with homologous or heterologous differentiation.

Embryonal rhabdomyosarcoma

— < 20 years age
— second commonest site after head and neck.
— usually extensive tumour of prostate, bladder and surrounding soft tissues with a botryoid (grape-like) appearance.
— cellular subepithelial cambium layer, loose myxoid zone, cellular deep zone, ± rhabdomyoblasts.
— vimentin, desmin, myoglobin positive; a minority are alveolar and more aggressive.

Urethral Carcinoma

1. Gross description

Specimen

— biopsy/urethrectomy or as part of cysto (prostato) urethrectomy.
— weight (g) and size/length (cm), number of fragments.

Tumour

Site

— prostatic/membranous/bulbar/pendulous urethras/meatus.

Size

— length × width × depth (cm) or maximum dimension (cm).

Appearance

— polypoid/verrucous/papillary/sessile/ulcerated/pigmented.

Edge

— circumscribed/irregular.

2. Histological type

Squamous cell carcinoma

— 60–70% of cases.
— distal.
— keratinising/non-keratinising.

— large cell/small cell.
— verrucous: exophytic, pushing deep margin of cytologically bland bulbous processes. May coexist with usual squamous carcinoma.

Transitional cell carcinoma
— 20–30% of cases.
— proximal.

Adenocarcinoma
— female > male; arising in strictures, diverticula or fistulae.
— glandular, colonic-like, papillary, hob-nail or clear cell patterns with or without urethritis cystica/glandularis.
— prostatic urethra: mesonephroid/endometrioid carcinoma (PSA positive); also known as carcinoma of the prostatic periurethral ducts. See chapter 31.

Adenosquamous carcinoma
— rare.

Small cell carcinoma
— primary or secondary from lung.

Malignant melanoma
— 4% of urethral malignancy.

Extensive radial growth is common leading to local recurrence. Spread is common to regional nodes, liver, lungs and brain. Prognosis, which is poor, relates to the tumour thickness. Mucosal junctional activity indicates a primary lesion.

Metastatic carcinoma
— multifocal/direct spread: urothelial cancer from bladder is commoner than a primary lesion. Other cancers that spread directly are rectum, vagina, cervix and endometrium.
— distant spread: ovary, kidney (distinguish from primary clear cell carcinoma).

3. Differentiation/grade

Well/moderate/poor.
WHO I/II/III.

4. Extent of local tumour spread

Border: pushing/infiltrative.
Lymphocytic reaction: prominent/sparse.

Urethra (male and female)

pTa non-invasive papillary, polypoid or verrucous carcinoma
pTis carcinoma in-situ
pT1 tumour invades subepithelial connective tissue
pT2 tumour invades any of: corpus spongiosum, prostate, periurethral muscle
pT3 tumour invades any of: corpus cavernosum, beyond prostatic capsule, anterior vagina, bladder neck
pT4 tumour invades other adjacent organs.

Transitional cell carcinoma of prostatic urethra (PSA, PSAP positive)

pTis pu: carcinoma in-situ, involvement of prostatic urethra
pTis pd: carcinoma in-situ, involvement of prostatic ducts
pT1 tumour invades subepithelial connective tissue
pT2 tumour invades any of: prostatic stroma, corpus spongiosum, periurethral muscle
pT3 tumour invades any of: corpus cavernosum, beyond prostatic capsule, bladder neck (extraprostatic extension)
pT4 tumour invades other adjacent organs (invasion of the bladder).

Distinction must be made between periurethral duct involvement by tumour and invasion into periurethral or prostatic stroma as the latter worsens the prognosis.

5. Lymphovascular invasion

Present/absent.
Intra-/extratumoural.

6. Lymph nodes

Site/number/size/number involved/limit node/extracapsular spread.
Regional nodes: inguinal, pelvic.

pN0 no regional lymph node metastasis
pN1 metastasis in a single regional lymph node ≤ 2 cm maximum dimension
pN2 metastasis in a single regional lymph node > 2 cm maximum dimension or multiple regional lymph nodes.

7. Excision margins

Distances (mm) to the nearest longitudinal and deep resection limits.

8. Other pathology

Urethral involvement by bladder carcinoma is much commoner than primary urethral carcinoma. In the female it is removed by cystectomy, which involves total urethrectomy, but there is potential for local recurrence in the residual male urethra. The histological status of the prostatic urethra is therefore assessed by biopsy prior to definitive surgical resection.

Multifocal transitional cell carcinoma of urethra, bladder, ureter, renal pelvis: either as papillary carcinoma, carcinoma in-situ or pagetoid urethral spread from a bladder lesion.

Female:male ratio 3:1.

Carcinomas arising proximally (proximal third in women; prostatic, membranous urethra in men) are generally transitional cell carcinoma while distal lesions (distal two-thirds in women; bulbous, penile urethra in men) are usually squamous cell carcinoma. In the distal third they are often well-differentiated squamous cell or verrucous in type.

Clear cell (mesonephroid) adenocarcinoma is rare, arising in either the female or prostatic urethra where it may be associated with a stricture or diverticulum. It should be distinguished from similar lesions arising in the female genital tract and metastatic renal cell adenocarcinoma by clinical history and anatomical site of disease. Another differential diagnosis is nephrogenic adenoma, which is usually small and lacks significant cellular atypia and mitoses. Endometrioid carcinoma arises from periurethral prostatic ducts (PSA, PSAP positive) and may be oestrogen sensitive.

Nephrogenic adenoma is a reactive (? metaplastic) proliferative lesion that does not predispose to but rarely may be associated with concurrent carcinoma, e.g. with adenocarcinoma in a urethral diverticulum. It usually has an exophytic, polypoid or papillary growth pattern with a tubular proliferation of cuboidal epithelium in the underlying lamina propria. Other protuberant urethral lesions than can mimic carcinoma at cystoscopy are benign prostatic urethral polyp, prominent veru montanum, fibrovascular polyp, villous adenoma and inverted transitional cell papilloma. Condyloma acuminatum may undergo malignant transformation to verrucous or infiltrating squamous cell carcinoma.

Prognosis

Distal urethral carcinoma (well-differentiated squamous/verrucous) presents early with a reasonable prognosis. Overall prognosis of urethral carcinoma (40% 5 year survival) relates to the anatomical site and stage of disease, e.g. bulbous/pendulous urethral carcinomas have 5 year survivals of 60–70% while the figure for membranous/prostatic lesions is 20%. Proximal cancers also present at a more advanced stage and with high-grade (poorly differentiated) histology in which it may be difficult to distinguish squamous from transitional cell carcinoma.

9. Other malignancy

Lymphoma/leukaemia

— as a manifestation of systemic disease.

Embryonal rhabdomyosarcoma

— sarcoma botryoides; children.
— superficial subepithelial cambium layer, intermediate myxoid zone, deep cellular zone, ± desmin, ± sarcomeric actin.

Aggressive angiomyxoma

— myxoid stroma/thick vessels.
— locally recurrent/infiltrative.

Testicular Cancer

1. Gross description

Specimen

— biopsy (open or needle)/radical orchidectomy (testis, tunica vaginalis and spermatic cord).
— weight (g) and size (cm) – overall and testicular.
— length of spermatic cord (cm).

Tumour

Site

— testicular/paratesticular.
— bilateral: 1–3% of cases, synchronous or metachronous, similar or dissimilar types. Commonest is seminoma or spermatocytic seminoma but beware lymphoma in the older age group.

Size

— length × width × depth (cm) or maximum dimension (cm).

Appearance

— pale/fleshy/nodular ± necrosis: seminoma/lymphoma.
— cysts/cartilage ± necrosis: teratoma.
— haemorrhage: choriocarcinoma, yolk sac tumour.
— fibrous/calcific scar: regression.
— tan/lobulated: Leydig cell/stromal tumour.

Edge

— circumscribed/irregular.

2. Histological type

NB: List and semi-quantify the percentage of tumour types present in a mixed germ cell tumour.

Germ cell tumours comprise 95% of testicular neoplasms (of which 40–50% are seminoma) and sex cord stromal lesions 4%.

Seminoma
— classical/anaplastic: same behaviour despite different mitotic rates and the term anaplastic is not really justified.
— spermatocytic: benign; three cell types; PLAP negative; old age.

Malignant teratoma
— differentiated, MTD.
— intermediate (a mix of MTD and MTU), MTI. ⎫ Embryonic
— undifferentiated (syn. embryonal carcinoma), MTU. ⎬ differentiation

— yolk sac (endodermal sinus) tumour, YST. ⎫ Extraembryonic
— trophoblastic/choriocarcinoma, MTT[1]. ⎬ differentiation

Teratoma differentiated (5-10% of cases) may have:
— *mature tissues*: benign in childhood (usually<4 years of age) but potentially malignant in the postpubertal patient. Somatic tissues commonly represented are: cartilage, muscle, neuroglia, enteric glands, squamous/respiratory and urothelial epithelia. Ovarian type cystic teratoma with sebum and hair is rare.
— *immature tissues*: e.g. cartilage, variably cellular mesenchymal stroma arranged concentrically around glandular epithelium, neuroectoderm, blastema and embryonic tubules. It is uncertain as to whether grading is of prognostic significance but a qualitative assessment of the amount (rare, focal, diffuse) and degree of immaturity (low/high-grade) should be made.
— *malignant transformation*: adenocarcinoma, squamous carcinoma, rhabdomyosarcoma (a designation of sarcoma requires at least one low-power field of atypical mesenchyme).

Mixed germ cell tumour
More than one germ cell type in any combination occurs in 30–50% of cases, e.g. seminoma and embryonal carcinoma, embryonal carcinoma and choriocarcinoma. Sample extensively (1 block/cm diameter and target block any unusual gross appearance, e.g. the association of choriocarcinoma with haemorrhage) to allow for this tumour heterogeneity.

---

[1]Requires additional specific chemotherapy.

Anaplastic germ cell tumour

— morphologically and immunohistochemically intermediate between semi-noma and embryonal carcinoma.

Mixed germ cell and sex cord stromal tumour

— gonadoblastoma: mixture of seminoma type cells and sex cord cells usually progressing to invasive germ cell tumour, mostly seminoma.

Sex cord stromal tumours

— Leydig: 30% hormonally active – gynaecomastia; eosinophilic or clear cells, Reinke's crystalloids (40%); α-inhibin positive, cytokeratin/alphafetoprotein (AFP)/placental alkaline phosphatase (PLAP) negative.
— Sertoli
— granulosa: adult – microfollicular (Call-Exner bodies), nuclear grooves.
        juvenile –<1 year old, cystic follicular structures, benign.
— undifferentiated or mixed.

Malignancy (10% of cases) relates to size, cellular atypia, mitoses (>3/10 high-power fields), infiltrative margins, vascular invasion and a high Ki-67 proliferation index.

Other tumours

— adenocarcinoma of the rete
    rare, poor prognosis.
— lymphoma
    diffuse large B cell non-Hodgkin's: old age, uni-/bilateral, 5% of testicular neoplasms.
    primary (2/3 of cases) or secondary to systemic/nodal disease.
    interstitial/peritubular pattern of infiltration.
    stage I 60% 5 year survival (> stage I 17%).
    children: Burkitt's lymphoma.
— leukaemia
    ALL: children, site of relapse in 5–10% and predictive of systemic relapse.
    CLL: 20–35% of patients involved.
    leukaemia can be bilateral and the presenting feature in a minority of cases.
    plasmacytoma: rare, usually secondary to an established myeloma.
— metastatic carcinoma
    prostate, lung, malignant melanoma, colon, kidney.
    bilaterality, vascular involvement and absence of intratubular germ cell neoplasia (ITGCN) favour metastatic disease.
— carcinoid tumour
    good prognosis, a monodermal teratoma, 20% have other teratomatous elements.
    exclude metastatic carcinoid (vascular invasion, extratesticular extension, bilateral).

Paratesticular: lipo-, rhabdo-, leiomyosarcoma, mesothelioma of the tunica vaginalis, lymphoma (secondary from testis)

— liposarcoma: adults; well-differentiated/sclerotic; local excision; 23% local recurrence.
— rhabdomyosarcoma: children; embryonal (± spindle cells); excision and adjuvant therapy; 80% long-term survival.
— leiomyosarcoma: adults; atypia, necrosis, mitoses.
— mesothelioma: cystic/solid/nodular masses lining a hydrocoele/hernia sac, aggressive.

3. Extent of local tumour spread

Border: pushing/infiltrative.
Lymphocytic reaction: prominent/sparse.

Lymphocytic reaction is a consistent (80%) feature of seminoma, and granulomas can also be present in up to 50% of cases. Sometimes the inflammatory infiltrate can be so intense that it partially obscures the germ cells and immunohistochemical markers are necessary. The intensity of inflammation and presence of granulomas are not prognostically significant.

Intratubular germ cell neoplasia (ITGCN))/carcinoma in-situ: sample the adjacent testis.

Intratubular spread: seminoma/embryonal carcinoma.

It can be difficult to distinguish between ITGCN and intratubular spread although in embryonal carcinoma ITGCN will be PLAP positive and intratubular spread PLAP negative. Intratubular spread of seminoma into the rete can also mimic embryonal carcinoma or carcinoma of the rete.

Rete: pagetoid or luminal spread – seminoma/embryonal carcinoma. Extratesticular extension of germ cell tumours is commoner at the rete/hilum.

Tunica albuginea/vaginalis, epididymis, spermatic cord.

pTis ITGCN (carcinoma in-situ)
pT1   tumour involves testis and epididymis or tunica albuginea, no lymphovascular invasion
pT2   tumour involves testis and epididymis with lymphovascular invasion or tunica vaginalis
pT3   tumour involves spermatic cord ± lymphovascular invasion
pT4   tumour involves scrotum ± lymphovascular invasion.

4. Lymphovascular invasion

Present/absent.
Intra-/extratumoural.

Lymphovascular invasion is correlated with a significantly elevated risk of distant metastasis and is an indication for chemotherapy. Consequently strict criteria for

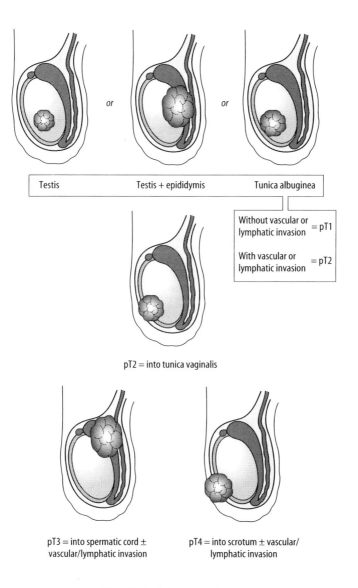

Testis | Testis + epididymis | Tunica albuginea

Without vascular or lymphatic invasion = pT1

With vascular or lymphatic invasion = pT2

pT2 = into tunica vaginalis

pT3 = into spermatic cord ± vascular/lymphatic invasion

pT4 = into scrotum ± vascular/lymphatic invasion

Figure 120. Testicular germ cell tumours.

its identification are necessary: an endothelial lined space with tumour conformed to its shape ± thrombosis or a point of attachment to the endothelium.

5. Lymph nodes

Site/number/size/number involved/limit node/extracapsular spread.
Regional nodes: abdominal periaortic and pericaval, those located along the spermatic veins.

pN0   no regional lymph node metastasis
pN1   regional lymph node metastasis ≤ 2 cm and ≤ 5 positive nodes
pN2   regional lymph node metastasis > 2 cm but ≤ 5 cm, or > 5 positive nodes, or extranodal extension
pN3   regional lymph node metastasis > 5 cm.

Seminoma tends to metastasise through lymphatics while choriocarcinoma shows haematogenous spread with presentation from metastatic disease to lung, liver, brain, bone and gut. Embryonal carcinoma spreads by a combination of these mechanisms. Nodal involvement depends on the stage of disease and laterality of the primary tumour. External iliac and inguinal node involvement may be seen if the tumour spreads to the epididymis and scrotal skin respectively. Mediastinal and left supraclavicular node metastases occur late in the disease course.

6. Clinical stage

I   tumour confined to the testis
II   nodes below the diaphragm
III   nodes above/below the diaphragm
IV   extranodal metastases.

Up to 30% of patients with seminoma have metastases at the time of diagnosis, 50–60% with embryonal carcinoma and the majority with choriocarcinoma.

Clinical staging is based on the determination of the anatomical extent of disease and the assessment of postorchidectomy serum markers lactate dehydrogenase (LDH), human chorionic gonadotrophin ß subunit (HCG) and AFP. High levels (AFP > 10 000 ng/ml, HCG > 50 000 IU/l, LDH > 10× normal) indicate worse prognosis and usually a diagnosis of non-seminomatous germ cell tumour.

7. Excision margins

Distances (mm) to the tunica, epididymis and limit of the spermatic cord.

8. Other pathology

ITGCN is the precursor lesion of all germ cell tumours except spermatocytic seminoma, and infantile teratoma differentiated and yolk sac tumours. It is usually seen in a patchy distribution within the testicular tubules away from and adjacent to the tumour in up to 80% of seminomas and malignant teratomas and may also be detected by needle biopsy as a risk factor for tumour development in the contralateral testis particularly if the testis is soft, atrophic or of low volume. It can be treated by low-dose irradiation as 50–90% of untreated ITGCN will progress to germ cell tumour over a five year period. Chemotherapeutic agents do not cross the blood/testis barrier. It comprises a proliferation of seminoma-like cells (clear cytoplasm, PAS/PLAP positive) at the base of the tubules which often have a hyalinised and thickened basement membrane. It can show intratubular or extratubular (microinvasive) extension as either seminoma or embryonal carcinoma.

Prior testicular tumour on the contralateral side (increased risk ×5–10).

Maldescent/cryptorchidism and infertility (increased risk ×3–5 and 1% incidence respectively).

"Scar" cancer (fibrosis, haemosiderin-laden macrophages, intratubular calcification) with retroperitoneal secondaries: regression of the primary and presentation with metastatic disease, especially embryonal carcinoma or choriocarcinoma.

Age is also a helpful indicator in that malignant germ cell tumours and sex cord stromal tumours present in the third and fourth decades but lymphoma and spermatocytic seminoma occur in old age. Seminoma is usually in patients 10 years older than those with non-seminomatous germ cell tumours. Yolk sac tumour is the commonest testicular neoplasm in children but also a common component of adult germ cell tumours.

Other scrotal swellings mimicking testicular cancer are: epididymo-orchitis, granulomatous orchitis, malakoplakia and peritesticular hydrocoele. Ultrasound examination is useful in delineating the last and intratesticular lesions. This, coupled with increased male health awareness, has led to an increasing proportion of small and unusual tumours being detected, e.g. sex cord stromal lesions, epidermoid inclusion cyst.

Fine needle aspiration cytology can be of use in those patients suspected of having metastatic carcinoma in the testes or testicular relapse in lymphoma and leukaemia. It is usually limited in germ cell tumours to those patients who are medically unfit for orchidectomy but in whom a tissue diagnosis is necessary for further management. Due to the considerable heterogeneity of germ cell tumours it can be subject to marked sampling error. Abdominal and thoracic aspiration cytology (± core biopsy) are useful for the assessment of germ cell metastases and should be categorised as seminomatous (requiring radiotherapy ± chemotherapy depending on the bulk of disease) or non-seminomatous; the latter is either pure teratomatous (requiring surgery) or other, e.g. embryonal carcinoma or yolk sac tumour (requiring chemotherapy). Serum HCG and AFP levels are also useful in making these management decisions.

Spermatocytic seminoma (1–2% of germ cell tumours) has indolent behaviour and is treated by orchidectomy alone. It presents in the older age group (50–70 years) and shows no evidence of adjacent ITGCN. It is lobulated ± microcystic change and comprises small, intermediate and large glycogen negative cells with indistinct cell boundaries, a "spireme" chromatin pattern and scattered mitoses. It lacks a stromal lymphocytic component and is PLAP negative. Differential diagnosis is seminoma of usual type (distinct cell boundaries, uniform polygonal cells with clear cytoplasm, an enlarged nucleolus with clumped nuclear chromatin, lymphocytic stroma, PLAP positive) and malignant lymphoma

(CD 45, CD 20, κ/λ light chain restriction, interstitial/peritubular infiltration, can be bilateral). Rarely it undergoes highly malignant (rhabdomyo-)sarcomatous change.

Anaplastic germ cell tumour: low-power: seminoma-like; high-power: cellular atypia/anaplasia/mitoses, variable PLAP/CAM 5.2 positivity.

Embryonal carcinoma (MTU) is present in 87% of non-seminomatous germ cell tumours but usually as part of a mixed germ cell tumour. It comprises primitive anaplastic epithelial cells in solid, glandular or tubulopapillary patterns.

Yolk sac tumour is the commonest prepubertal testicular germ cell tumour and is present in up to 40–50% of adult lesions. It is histologically heterogeneous assuming a spectrum of patterns, the commonest being microcystic (honeycomb, reticular, vacuolated), papillary, endodermal sinus (perivascular Duvall-Schiller bodies), solid, myxomatous and glandular (enteric or endometrioid). Other characteristics are PAS positive diastase-resistant, intra- and extracellular hyaline globules and deposition of extracellular basement membrane. AFP is present in the vast majority of cases but can be patchy in expression and is expressed in the tumour cell cytoplasm rather than the globules.

Note that there are terminological differences between the British Testicular Tumour Panel (BTTP) and the WHO systems interpreted as follows (optional):

BTTP	WHO
Malignant teratoma differentiated, MTD	Teratoma mature
MTD (with immature elements)	Teratoma immature
MTD (with malignant transformation)	Teratoma with an overtly malignant component
Malignant teratoma intermediate, MTI	Embryonal carcinoma or yolk sac tumour mixed with mature or immature teratoma ("terato-carcinoma")
Malignant teratoma trophoblastic, MTT	Choriocarcinoma
Malignant teratoma undifferentiated, MTU	Embryonal carcinoma.

Immunohistochemistry

The reactions of different tumour types with immunohistochemical markers are given in Table 33.1 and summarised below.

Table 33.1.

	PLAP	CAM 5.2	AFP	HCG
CIS/ITGCN	+	±	−	−
Seminoma	+	−	±	±
Spermatocytic seminoma	−	−	−	−
YST	±	+	+	±
MTU	±	+	±	±
MTT	±	±	−	+

CIS/ITGCN	PLAP+	CAM ±
Seminoma	PLAP+	CAM – /PAS + (glycogen)
YST	AFP+	CAM +
MTU	CAM+	PLAP ±
MTT	HCG+	

PLAP positivity in seminoma/ITGCN is membranous and not cytoplasmic as seen in some non-small cell lung carcinomas and malignant melanomas. Markers may also help distinguish metastatic embryonal carcinoma (CAM+, PLAP±, CD 30±, EMA–) from metastatic carcinoma (CAM+, PLAP–, EMA+).

Serum markers often do not show good correlation with their tumour tissue expression but are good for monitoring disease treatment response and relapse as they are raised in 70–75% of patients with non-seminomatous germ cell tumours. Seminoma rarely produces high HCG levels but may have increased serum PLAP levels (40% of cases). Seminoma and MTD rarely give elevated AFP levels. If present, other elements, e.g. yolk sac tumour or embryonal carcinoma, are identified.

Apparently aberrant tissue expression is acceptable without changing the diagnosis or prognosis, e.g. seminoma with HCG positive syncytiotrophoblastic cells (10–20% of cases) or embryonal carcinoma with elevated serum HCG. MTT (5% of cases) requires biphasic syncytio- and cytotrophoblastic differentiation for diagnosis (although the "syncytio"- element may be inconspicuous) and angioinvasion is common. Designation is dependent on the morphology and not the serum hormone levels The syncytiotrophoblast is HCG positive capping the cytokeratin 7 positive cytotrophoblast.

Prognosis

Prognosis relates to serum marker levels, stage of disease, histological type and lymphovascular invasion. Stage I disease and stage II with non-bulky (< 5–10 cm) retroperitoneal secondaries have 5 year survival rates of 90–95% for both seminoma and embryonal carcinoma whereas the rate for bulky stage II tumour is 70–80%. Yolk sac tumour presents as stage I (90%) in childhood with > 90% 5 year survivals; it can exhibit chemoresistance in adults with metastatic disease. The presence of yolk sac elements in an immature teratoma of childhood is also an indicator for potential recurrence of disease.

Prognosis of seminoma worsens with:

1. Tumour diameter ≥ 6cm.
2. Age > 34 years.
3. Vascular invasion.

Prognosis of teratoma worsens with:

1. Increasing stage.
2. Presence of MTU.
3. Absence of YST.
4. Lymphovascular invasion.

The Medical Research Council scheme scores 1 for each of: presence of MTU, absence of YST, lymphatic invasion, blood vessel invasion.

Tumour score:
0–2   surgery with follow-up only
3–4   surgery with adjuvant chemotherapy.

Low volume/percentage tumour area of MTU and low Ki-67 index are beneficial. Relapse rates are 15–20% for seminoma (80% in the retroperitoneum) and 30–35% for teratoma (66% in the retroperitoneum, 33% in the lung or meliastinum). Vascular invasion is a strong determinant of postoperative chemotherapy in stage I disease. Stage I and non-bulky stage II seminoma is treated by orchidectomy and radiation to regional node sites – bulky stage II and more advanced disease require more extensive radiotherapy and in addition chemotherapy. Non-seminomatous germ cell tumours require orchidectomy and platinum-based chemotherapy supplemented by retroperitoneal lymph node dissection for bulky stage II and more advanced disease. Postchemotherapy cytoreduction of metastases results in necrosis, xanthomatous inflammation, fibrosis and variably viable tumour tissue. Ominously carcinomatous or sarcomatous (e.g. rhabdomyosarcoma, primitive neuroectodermal tumour) differentiation may occasionally occur. Metastatic disease not infrequently changes differentiation, with treatment leaving residual masses of cystic, mature tissues in the lung or para-aortic nodes which are insensitive to adjuvant therapy, can press on local structures (the growing teratoma syndrome) and may require surgical resection. Alternatively they can be monitored by serum hormone levels and CT scan and further investigated for malignant change if growth recurs. Prognosis of metastatic disease relates to the size, site and number of metastases, the extent of tumour mass shrinkage during chemotherapy, completeness of excision, nature of the resected masses and serum HCG and AFP levels. Metastases comprising total necrosis or fully mature tissue correlate with better prognosis. Fibrosis, necrosis and undifferentiated teratoma are present in 20–70% of cases; MTU, MTT and YST in 5–25% of cases. A minority of seminomas may develop non-seminomatous germ cell tumour metastases; this may relate either to true transformation of seminoma or a focus of non-seminatous germ cell tumour in the primary lesion which was not sampled. In general, patterns of metastases are:

primary	*metastasis*
seminoma	seminoma
MTD	MTI
MTI	MTD, MTI or MTU
	MTD is usually postchemotherapy maturation
mixed germ cell tumour + MTT	MTT.

The number of chemotherapy cycles is minimised by titrating against normalisation of the serum marker levels; this is done to decrease the risk of developing a second malignancy in later life, e.g. sarcoma or lymphoma.

Penile Carcinoma

1. Gross description

Specimen

— biopsy/partial or total penile amputation/radical penectomy (including scrotum, testes, spermatic cords, groin lymph node dissection).
— size (cm) and weight (g).

Tumour

Site

— urethral meatus/glans/prepuce/coronal sulcus/shaft (dorsal/ventral/lateral).

Size

— length × width × depth (cm) or maximum dimension (cm).

Appearance

— verrucous/warty/exophytic or sessile/ulcerated and infiltrative.
— pale/pigmented.

Edge

— circumscribed/irregular.

2. Histological type

Squamous cell carcinoma

— 95% of penile malignancies, 70–80 years of age.
— exophytic (fungating/papillary) or endophytic (ulcerated/infiltrating).

- large cell/small cell.
- keratinising/non-keratinising.
- verrucous: 5–16%; verruciform with a deep pushing margin of cytologically bland bulbous processes; prone to local recurrence if incompletely excised and may dedifferentiate with radiotherapy. Can coexist with usual squamous carcinoma.
- spindle cell.

Basal cell carcinoma

Mucoepidermoid carcinoma

Adenocarcinoma
- and extramammary Paget's disease.

Transitional cell carcinoma
- ±associated bladder cancer; penile urethra.

Malignant melanoma
- < 1%; primary or secondary, glans penis; 50% have nodal metastases at presentation and prognosis is poor, being related to tumour thickness and stage.

Metastatic carcinoma
- rare; prostate, bladder, kidney, gut, testis.
- usually as a late manifestation of systemic disease; can present with priapism or as extramammary Paget's disease from an underlying adnexal tumour or distant spread, e.g. bladder.

3. Differentiation

Well/moderate/poor.
Many are exophytic and well to moderately differentiated with variable keratinisation. Grading based on the degree of keratinisation, mitoses, cellular atypia and inflammatory infiltrate correlates with prognosis. Ulcerated, infiltrating cancers of the glans penis tend to be moderately to poorly differentiated. About 50% of shaft cancers are poorly differentiated and only 10% of prepuce tumours.

4. Extent of local tumour spread

Border: pushing/infiltrative.
Lymphocytic reaction: prominent/sparse.

pTis   carcinoma in-situ
pTa   noninvasive verrucous carcinoma

pT1   tumour in subepithelial connective tissue
pT2   tumour in corpus spongiosum, cavernosum
pT3   tumour in urethra, prostate
pT4   tumour in other adjacent structures (scrotum, testis, skin).

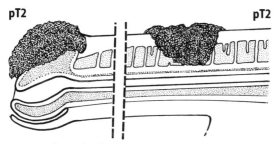

Tumour invades corpus spongiosum or cavernosum

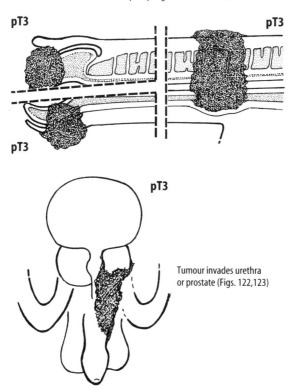

Tumour invades urethra
or prostate (Figs. 122,123)

Figures 121–123. Penile carcinoma.

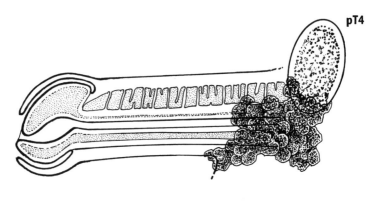

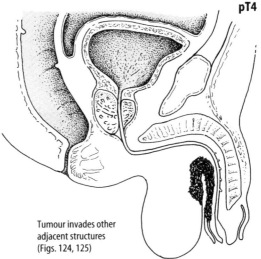

Tumour invades other
adjacent structures
(Figs. 124, 125)

Figures 124, 125. Penile carcinoma.

Initial spread is local into the prepuce and penile shaft and the extent of this
and the pattern of infiltrative spread correlate with the incidence of nodal metastases. Despite the vascularity of the structures haematogenous spread to the liver,
lung and bone is rare (2%).

5. Lymphovascular invasion

Present/absent.
Intra-/extratumoural.

6. Lymph nodes

Site/number/size/number involved/limit node/extracapsular spread.
Regional nodes: superficial and deep inguinal and pelvic.

pN0   no regional lymph node metastasis
pN1   metastasis in one superficial inguinal lymph node
pN2   metastasis in multiple or bilateral superficial inguinal lymph nodes
pN3   metastasis in deep inguinal or pelvic lymph node(s).

The incidence of nodal metastases is greater (> 80%) in deeply invasive than superficially spreading carcinomas (42%).

7. Excision margins

Distance (mm) to the proximal limit of excision.

8. Other pathology

Balanoposthitis xerotica obliterans
— similar to lichen sclerosus in the vulva it may be associated with but does not predispose to penile carcinoma.

Leukoplakia
— hyperkeratosis, epthelial hyperplasia ± dysplasia.

Erythroplasia de Queyrat/Bowen's disease/bowenoid papulosis
— progression to carcinoma is estimated as 10%/5–10%/0 respectively. All show features of carcinoma in-situ, erythroplasia being a lesion of the glans penis whereas Bowen's disease and bowenoid papulosis are abnormalities of the penile/perineal skin. The latter is caused by HPV infection in young men.

Condyloma accuminatum
— HPV 16,18.
— other possible predisposing factors for carcinoma are old age (rare<40 years of age), lack of circumcision, poor hygiene and phimosis.

Concurrent urothelial neoplasia ± pagetoid spread of transitional cell carcinoma into the penile urethra.

Prognosis

More than 95% of penile carcinomas are squamous cell carcinoma; at presentation about 40% are superficially invasive with extensive in-situ change, 30% deeply invasive, 10–20% verrucous and 5–10% multifocal. Inguinal lymph node metastases are present in 15–30%. Prognosis relates to the tumour stage, histological grade and vascular invasion with average 5 year survival rates of 70–80%.

9. Other malignancy

Sarcoma
— < 5% of penile malignancy especially:

Kaposi's sarcoma: about 20% of AIDS male patients on the skin of the shaft or glans; it is usually associated with other systemic lesions.

Leiomyosarcoma: 50–70 years; superficial and subcutaneous has a good prognosis; deep with early metastases has a poor prognosis.

Epithelioid haemangioendothelioma: varying grade and outlook (CD 31 positive).

Others: rhabdomyosarcoma, fibrosarcoma, epithelioid sarcoma.

Lymphoma
— usually secondary to systemic disease.

Lymph Node Cancer

- Nodal Malignant Lymphoma (with comments on extranodal lymphoma and metastatic cancer)

Nodal Malignant Lymphoma
(with comments on extranodal lymphoma and metastatic cancer)

1. Gross description

Specimen

— fine needle aspirate/tru-cut needle biopsy core/ excisional biopsy/regional lymphadenectomy.

The preferred specimen for diagnosis, subtyping and grading of nodal malignant lymphoma is an excisional lymph node biopsy carefully taken by an experienced surgeon to ensure representation of disease and avoidance of traumatic artefact. Submission of the specimen fresh to the laboratory allows imprints to be made (to which a wide panel of immunohistochemical antibodies can be applied) and tissue harvested for molecular and genetic techniques. Morphological classification is generally based on well-fixed, thin slices, processed through to paraffin. Core biopsy may be the only option if the patient is unwell or the lesion relatively inaccessible, e.g. mediastinum. Allowances must be made in interpretation for sampling error and artefact; confirmation of lymphomatous (or other) malignancy is the prime objective and further comments on subtyping and grading given with care and only if definitely demonstrable. Tumour heterogeneity must also be borne in mind. The same principles apply to fine needle aspiration cytology, which is excellent at excluding inflammatory lymphadenopathy, e.g. abscess or sarcoidosis and non-lymphomatous cancer (e.g. metastatic squamous cell carcinoma, breast carcinoma or malignant melanoma) and reasonably robust at designating Hodgkin's and high-grade non-Hodgkin's lymphoma. Morphology must be complemented by confirmatory immunohistochemistry on the core or aspirate cytospin preparations; in addition, these techniques along with flow cytometry and molecular gene rearrangements are helpful in determining a diagnosis of low-grade lymphoma. These more limited sampling techniques can also be used in patients with a previous tissue biopsy-proven diagnosis of lymphoma and in whom recurrence is suspected. However, possible transformation of grade must be considered and even change of lymphoma type, e.g. small lymphocytic lymphoma to Hodgkin's lymphoma. A range of inflammatory nodal disease may also be encountered secondary to chemotherapy and immunosuppression, e.g. tuberculosis.

— size (cm) and weight (g)
— colour, consistency, necrosis.

2. Histological type and differentiation/grade

Non-Hodgkin's lymphoma

Non-Hodgkin's lymphoma (NHL) may be described using a combination of Kiel terminology and the REAL (Revised European American Lymphoma Classification) system, with reference also to the clinical prognostic categories of the IWF (International Working Formulation): low, intermediate and high grade (LG, IG, HG) – see Table 35.1 for comparison. The advantages of the REAL classification are that it defines each disease by its morphology, immunophenotype, genetic characteristics, proposed normal counterpart and clinical features, and is reproducible. The proposed new WHO classification is similar to REAL with only minor modification.

Hodgkin's lymphoma

RYE classification/REAL/WHO proposal

Lymphocyte and Histiocyte (L and H) predominant – multilobated "popcorn" cell.
— Nodular: a B cell lymphoma of low-grade indolent behaviour with a risk of diffuse large B cell change.
— Diffuse: a controversial category with overlap between lymphocyte-rich classic Hodgkin's disease, vaguely nodular lymphocyte predominant Hodgkin's and other entities such as T cell/histiocyte rich large B cell NHL.

Classic Hodgkin's disease includes nodular sclerosis, mixed cellularity and lymphocyte depletion categories:

Nodular sclerosis – lacunar cell.
— birefringent fibrous bands (capsule and intra-nodal septa) with mixed inflammatory cell nodules containing lacunar cells, or, cellular phase (rich in lacunar cells, scant fibrosis)

— *type 1.
— *type 2: lymphocyte depletion, pleomorphism of R-S (Reed-Sternberg) cells in more than 25% of nodules. An alternative descriptor is syncytial variant (sheets/clusters of R-S cells with central necrosis and a polymorph infiltrate).
*Grade 1/grade 2 British National Lymphoma Investigation (BNLI).

Mixed cellularity
— R-S cells of classic type in a mixed inflammatory background. A category of exclusion in that no specific features of other subtypes are present.

Lymphocyte depletion
— R-S cell ± pleomorphism; diffuse fibrosis (fibroblasts obscure scattered R-S cells) and reticular variants (cellular, pleomorphic R-S cells).

Other subtypes
— lymphocyte-rich classic Hodgkin's, follicular and interfollicular Hodgkin's, Hodgkin's with a high epithelioid cell content.
— R-S cells: classic mirror image, binucleated cell with prominent eosinophilic nucleolus characteristic of mixed cellularity and lymphocyte depleted. Mononuclear, polylobated and necrobiotic (mummified) forms are also common. Lacunar cells (nodular sclerosis) can be mono-, bi- or polylobated (± necrobiotic), with characteristic perinuclear artefactual cytoplasmic retraction and clarity.

In Hodgkin's disease the heterogeneous cellular background (comprising 90% of the tissue) is an important part of the diagnosis: small lymphocytes, eosinophils, neutrophils, fibroblasts, histiocytes and follicular dendritic cells. Note that this is also seen in T cell NHLs and T cell rich B cell NHLs. Other features are granulomas, necrosis and reactive follicular hyperplasia, all of which should prompt a careful search for R-S cells. Important non-malignant differential diagnoses for malignant lymphoma are drug-induced (e.g. phenytoin) and viral reactive hyperplasia with paracortical transformation (e.g. infectious mononucleosis), and necrotising and granulomatous lymphadenitis (Kikuchi's, toxoplasmosis).

3. Extent of local tumour spread

Part of node or whole of node.
Extracapsular into adjacent soft tissues or organ parenchyma.

Stage: Ann Arbor classification

I	Single lymph node region or localised extralymphatic site/organ
II	Two or more lymph node regions on same side of the diaphragm or single localised extralymphatic site/organ and its regional lymph nodes ± other lymph node regions on the same side of the diaphragm

Table 35.1. Classification of non-Hodgkin's lymphoma (NHL)

Revised European American Lymphoma classification	Updated Kiel classification	International Working Formulation
Precursor B-lymphoblastic leukaemia/lymphoma	B-lymphoblastic	Lymphoblastic, HG
B cell chronic lymphocytic leukaemia/prolymphocytic leukaemia/small lymphocytic lymphoma	B-lymphocytic, CLL B-lymphocytic, prolymphocytic leukaemia	Small lymphocytic, CLL, LG
Lymphoplasmacytoid lymphoma	Lymphoplasmacytoid immunocytoma	Small lymphocytic, plasmacytoid, LG
Mantle cell lymphoma	Centrocytic (mantle cell) Centroblastic, centrocytoid subtype	Diffuse, small cleaved, IG
Follicle centre lymphoma, follicular*		
Grade I	Centroblastic-centrocytic	Follicular, small cleaved cell, LG
Grade II	follicular	Follicular, mixed small cleaved and large cell, LG
Grade III	Centroblastic, follicular	Follicular, large cell, IG
Follicle centre lymphoma, diffuse, predominantly small cell (Provisional)	Centroblastic-centrocytic, diffuse	Diffuse, small cleaved and mixed small and large cell, IG
Extranodal marginal zone B cell lymphoma (low-grade B cell lymphoma of MALT type)	–	Small lymphocytic, or mixed small and large cell, LG
Nodal marginal zone B cell lymphoma (Provisional)	Monocytoid, including marginal zone Immunocytoma	
Splenic marginal zone B cell lymphoma (Provisional)	–	Small lymphocytic, LG
Hairy cell leukaemia	Hairy cell leukaemia	
Plasmacytoma/myeloma	Plasmacytic	Plasmacytoma
Diffuse large B cell lymphoma	Centroblastic (monomorphic, polymorphic and multilobated subtypes)	Diffuse large cell, IG
	B-immunoblastic B-large cell anaplastic	Large cell immunoblastic, HG
Primary mediastinal large B cell lymphoma	–	
Burkitt's lymphoma	Burkitt's lymphoma	Small noncleaved cell, Burkitt's, HG
High-grade B cell lymphoma, Burkitt-like (Provisional)	?	Small noncleaved cell, non-Burkitt's, HG

Precursor T lymphoblastic lymphoma/leukaemia	T lymphoblastic	Lymphoblastic, HG
T cell chronic lymphocytic leukaemia/prolymphocytic leukaemia	T lymphocytic, CLL type T lymphocytic, prolymphocytic leukaemia	Small lymphocytic, CLL type, LG
Large granular lymphocytic leukaemia T cell type NK cell type	T lymphocytic, CLL type –	Small lymphocytic, LG
Mycosis fungoides/Sézary syndrome	Small cell cerebriform (mycosis fungoides, Sézary syndrome)	Mycosis fungoides, LG
Peripheral T cell lymphomas, unspecified	T zone Lymphoepithelioid Pleomorphic, small T cell Pleomorphic, medium-size and large T cell T-immunoblastic	Diffuse small cleaved cell, IG Diffuse mixed small and large cell, IG Diffuse large cell, HG
Including subtype: subcutaneous panniculitic T cell lymphoma (Provisional)	–	
Hepatosplenic γδ T cell lymphoma (Provisional)		
Angioimmunoblastic T cell lymphoma	Angioimmunoblastic (AILD)	} Diffuse mixed small and large cell/ } large cell immunoblastic, IG/HG }
Angiocentric T cell lymphoma		
Intestinal T cell lymphoma		
Adult T cell lymphoma/leukaemia	Pleomorphic small T cell HTLVI+ Pleomorphic medium-sized and large T cell, HTLVI+	Diffuse, small cleaved cell, IG Diffuse, mixed small and large cell, IG
Anaplastic large cell lymphoma, T and null-cell types	T large cell anaplastic	Diffuse large cell immunoblastic, HG

LG, low grade; IG, intermediate grade; HG, high grade. *Follicular lymphoma – grade 1: 0–5, grade III: >15 centroblasts/high-power field
The proposed new WHO classification mirrors REAL with some terminological change: follicular lymphoma for follicle centre lymphoma, nasal T/NK lymphoma for angiocentric lymphoma, lymphoplasmacytic for lymphoplasmacytoid lymphoma. Anaplastic large cell lymphoma is subdivided into systemic and cutaneous forms; the provisional categories of nodal and splenic marginal zone lymphomas, subcutaneous panniculitic and hepatosplenic lymphoma are accepted. Burkitt's-like lymphoma is resolved into either Burkitt's or large B cell lymphoma. See Harris et al (2000)

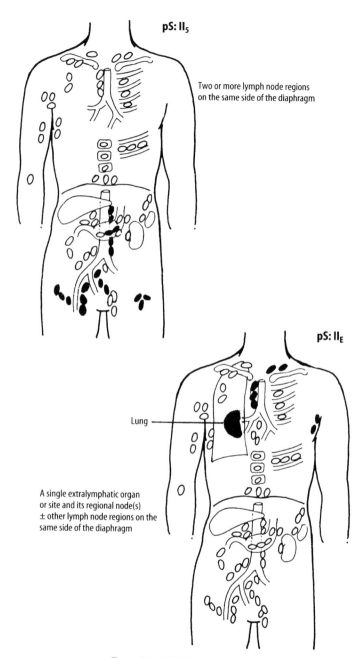

pS: II₅

Two or more lymph node regions on the same side of the diaphragm

pS: IIₑ

Lung

A single extralymphatic organ or site and its regional node(s) ± other lymph node regions on the same side of the diaphragm

Figures 126, 127. Malignant lymphoma.

Involvement of lymph node regions on both sides of the diaphragm (III) (Fig. 128)
which may also be accompanied by localised involvement of an associated extralymphatic
organ or site (III$_E$) (Fig. 129) or by involvement of the spleen (III$_S$), or both (III$_{E+S}$) (Fig. 130)

pS: III$_2$

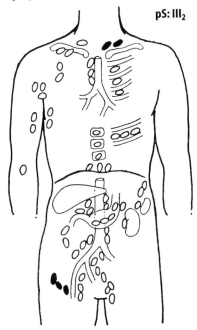

Figure 128. Malignant lymphoma.

III   Lymph node regions on both sides of the diaphragm ± a localised extra-lymphatic site/organ or spleen

IV   Disseminated (multifocal) involvement of one or more extralymphatic organs ± regional lymph node involvement, or single extralymphatic organ and non-regional nodes

    A   Without weight loss/fever/sweats

    B   With weight loss/fever/sweats:
        fever > 38.5 °C
        night sweats
        weight loss > 10% of body weight within the previous 6 months.

Subscripts e.g. III$_E$ denotes stage III with Extranodal disease
               III$_S$ denotes stage III with splenic involvement
               III$_3$ denotes stage III with involvement of 3 lymph node regions:
               > 2 is prognostically adverse.

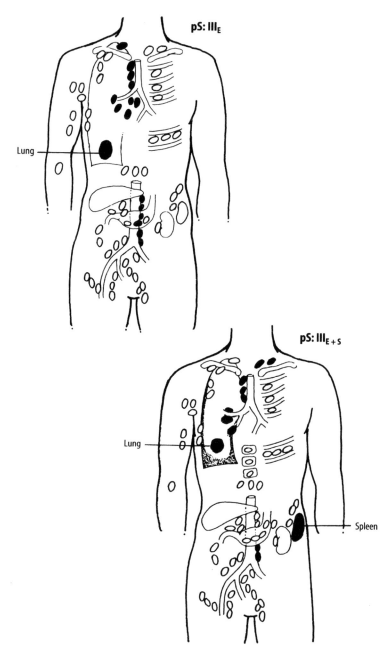

pS: III$_E$

Lung

pS: III$_{E+S}$

Lung

Spleen

Figures 129, 130. Malignant lymphoma.

Histopathology Reporting

Lymph node regions: head, neck, face
                              intrathoracic
                              intra-abdominal
                              axilla/arm
                              groin/leg
                              pelvis.

Once the primary tissue diagnosis has been made staging laparotomy has been largely replaced by assessment of clinical and radiological parameters. Bone marrow biopsy remains part of normal staging which is otherwise mostly clinical. Bone marrow or nodal granulomas per se are not sufficient for a positive diagnosis of involvement and diagnostic Hodgkin's cells are needed. Bone marrow involvement by NHL can be diffuse, nodular or focal and paratrabecular infiltration is a characteristic site.

4. Lymphovascular invasion

Present/absent.
Intra-/extratumoural.

Vessel wall invasion and destructive angiocentricity can be a useful indicator of malignancy in NHL and in specific subtypes, e.g. angiocentric T/NK cell lymphoma.

5. Markers

Markers are available for formalin-fixed paraffin-embedded sections. Examples are (Compton et al. 1999a,b):

Pan-lymphoid: CD 45 (CLA).
B cell: CD 20 (L26), CD 79a (pre-B), CD 75 (MB2).
T cell: CD 3, CD 45RO(UCHL1), CD 43 (MT1).
Hodgkin's: classic: CD 15 (Leu M1)/CD 30 (BerH$_2$) positive in 75%/90% of cases, EMA/CD45 negative.
                    L and H cells, nodular lymphocyte predominant: CD 45/CD 20/CD 79a/EMA/J chain positive, CD 15/30 negative.
Anaplastic large cell Ki 1 lymphoma:
                    CD 30, EMA ±, ALK-1 ±, CD 45 ±, t(2:5).
                    T (60%), B (10–20%) or null (20–30%) cell type: pleomorphic cells with plentiful cytoplasm and a solid sinusoidal growth pattern of infiltration. Systemic or cutaneous, primary or secondary to other lymphomas. Better prognosis is conferred by ALK-1 (anaplastic lymphoma kinase) positivity, and, CD 30 positivity in cutaneous ALCL.
Centrocytic/centroblastic (follicle centre) lymphoma:
                    bcl-2 t(14:18), CD 10 ±, CD 20.

Mantle cell lymphoma:

CD 5, bcl-1 (cyclin D1/PRAD1/t(11:14)), CD 20, CD 43.

Diffuse large cell lymphoma:

CD 20, CD 45, bcl-2 (30% of cases).

MALToma: CD 20, CD 43 positive, CD 5/CD 10/bcl-1 negative.

Lymphocytic lymphoma: CD 20, CD 5, CD 23, CD 43 positive.

Lymphoblastic lymphoma/leukaemia:

tdt (terminal deoxynucleotidyltransferase), CD 10, CD 99, CD 79a.

Burkitt's lymphoma: CD 10/20 positive, CD 99 negative, EBV 15–40% of cases, Ki-67 > 85%.

Hairy cell leukaemia: DBA44, antibody to tartrate resistant acid phosphatase, CD 20.

Myelomonocytic series:

CD 68, neutrophil elastase, lysozyme, myeloperoxidase, CD 15.

Cytotoxic T/natural killer (NK) cells:

CD 56 (granzyme): angiocentric sinonasal lymphoma (± CD 3 – also EBV positive).

Follicular dendritic cells:

CD 21.

Immunoglobulin heavy chain (IgG, M, D, A) and light chain (k, λ) restriction.

Immunoglobulin clonal heavy/light chain and T cell receptor molecular gene rearrangements using Southern blot analysis and polymerase chain techniques.

Aberrant B cell phenotypic expression, e.g. CD 43 and CD 5 positivity in small cell lymphoproliferative disorders.

In-situ hybridisation for EBV, e.g. positive in 40–60% of nodular sclerosis and mixed cellularity Hodgkin's disease, and light chain restriction.

MIB-1/Ki-67 (proliferation marker).

The evolution of new generation robust antibodies applicable to paraffin sections with unmasking of antigenic sites by antigen retrieval methods (microwave and pressure cooker techniques) has led to considerable reclassification of lymphomas with emergence of new entities. For example lymphocyte depleted and mixed cellularity Hodgkin's disease are diminishing as the full spectrum of NHL widens, viz. T cell NHL, anaplastic large cell Ki 1 NHL, T cell rich B cell lymphoma. Unusually composite (HD/NHL) and borderline (HD/ALCL) cases also occur. It is important that a panel of antibodies is used and markers assessed in combination, e.g. in the sometimes difficult differential diagnosis of florid reactive hyperplasia versus follicular lymphoma. Benign follicle centres are bcl-2 negative, CD 68 positive, and strongly Ki-67 positive whereas malignant follicles are diffusely bcl-2 positive with a low Ki-67 proliferation index (unless predominantly centroblastic) and absence of CD 68 positive macrophages. Thus morphology and immunohistochemistry are used in tandem supplemented by molecular immunoglobulin and gene rearrangement studies. It should also be noted that clonality does not always correlate with progression to lymphoma as has been demonstrated in some inflammatory skin, salivary and gastric biopsies.

Formalin fixation and high-quality, thin (4 μm) paraffin sections are adequate for morphological characterisation in most cases. Fixation should be sufficient (24–36 h) but not excessive as this may mask antigenic sites.

Progressive transformation of germinal centres will sometimes subsequently develop nodular lymphocyte predominant Hodgkin's disease characterised by the emergence of popcorn or diagnostic R-S cells.

The majority (60–70%) of NHLs are large B cell lymphomas and follicular lymphoma.

6. Extranodal lymphoma

Of NHLs, 25–40% are extranodal, defined as when a NHL presents with the main bulk of disease at an extranodal site usually necessitating the direction of treatment primarily to that site. In order of decreasing frequency sites of occurrence are:

— gastrointestinal tract (especially stomach then small intestine)
— skin
— Waldeyer's ring
— salivary gland
— thymus
— orbit
— thyroid
— lung
— testis
— breast
— bone.

A majority are aggressive large B cell lymphomas although T cell lesions also occur (cutaneous T cell lymphoma, enteropathy-associated T cell lymphoma, NK/T cell sinonasal lymphoma). Their incidence is rising partly due to increased recognition and abandonment of terms such as pseudolymphoma, but also because of aetiological factors, e.g. AIDS, immunosuppression after transplantation or chemotherapy, autoimmune diseases and infections (*H. pylorii*, EBV, hepatitis C virus).

Many are low-grade in character with indolent behaviour, remaining localised to the site of origin. However a significant proportion present as or undergo high-grade transformation and when they metastasise typically do so to other extranodal sites. This site homing can be explained by the embryological development and circulation of mucosa associated lymphoid tissue (MALT). The low-grade MALTomas often arise from a background of chronic antigenic stimulation:

gastric lymphoma	*H. pylorii* gastritis
thyroid lymphoma	Hashimoto's thyroiditis
salivary gland lymphoma	lympho(myo-)epithelial sialadenitis/Sjögren's syndrome.

Their classification does not strictly parallel that of nodal lymphoma but mirrors marginal zone or monocytoid B cell lymphoma. They normally comprise a sheeted or nodular infiltrate of centrocyte-like cells, destructive lymphoepithelial lesions and monotypic plasma cell immunoglobulin expression with interfollicular infiltration or follicular colonisation of reactive follicles by the neoplastic cells. There is often a component of blast cells and the immunophenotype is one of exclusion in that they are CD 5 and cyclin-D1 negative ruling out mantle cell lymphoma and other small B lymphocyte lymphoproliferative disorders. Other extranodal lymphomas have diverse morphology and immunophenotype correlating with the full spectrum of the REAL and Kiel classifications, although the node-based categories are not consistently transferable to extranodal sites.

Immunosuppressed post-transplant patients are prone to a wide spectrum of nodal/extranodal EBV associated polyclonal and monoclonal B cell lymphoproliferative disorders (PTLD). Three main categories exist: plasmacytic hyperplasia (low-grade PTLD), polymorphic B cell hyperplasia/polymorphic B cell lymphoma (intermediate-grade PTLD) and immunoblastic lymphoma/ multiple myeloma (high-grade PTLD). In these circumstances even what appears to be high-grade lymphoma may potentially regress if immunosuppressant therapy is decreased. Serum titres and/or tissue expression of EBV are ascertained and clinical response to alteration of immunotherapy assessed prior to use of chemotherapy. Similar findings can also be present in patients receiving chronic immunosuppression therapy for autoimmune and rheumatological disorders.

7. Prognosis

Radiotherapy and chemotherapy are the two principal treatment modalities for malignant lymphoma but surgical excision is often involved for definitive subtyping in primary nodal disease or for removal of a tumour mass and primary diagnosis of extranodal lymphoma, e.g. gastric lymphoma. Prognosis relates to lymphoma type (small cell and nodular are better than large cell and diffuse) and stage of disease. Low-grade or indolent nodal lymphomas have a high frequency (> 80% at presentation) of bone marrow and peripheral blood involvement but pursue a protracted time course and relapse at a late date (5–10 years) with potentially blast transformation (e.g. CLL: 23% risk at 8 years). High-grade or aggressive lymphomas develop bone marrow or peripheral involvement as an indication of advanced disease and are fatal within 1–2 years if left untreated. Prior to this the majority show good chemoresponsiveness with complete remission in 80% and potential cure in 60%. Overall, four broad prognostic categories are identified in NHL, although outlook does vary within individual types, e.g. grades I/II or III follicle centre (follicular) lymphoma:

NHL Type	5 year survival
1. anaplastic large cell/MALT/follicular	> 70%
2. nodal marginal zone/small lymphocytic/lymphoplasmacytoid	50–70%
3. mediastinal B cell/large B cell/Burkitt's	30–50%
4. T lymphoblastic/peripheral T cell/mantle cell	< 30%.

Hodgkin's disease is relatively radiotherapy and chemotherapy responsive; prognosis relates to histological category (e.g. type 2 nodular sclerosis is worse than type 1) and, more importantly, stage of disease. Average 5 year survival rates for Hodgkin's disease are 75% with worse outcome for older patients (> 40–50 years), disease of advanced stage (i.e. more than one anatomical site), involvement of the mediastinum, spleen or extranodal sites. Lymphocyte-depleted Hodgkin's disease is least favourable with the mixed cellularity category being of intermediate outlook. However, histological type is usually regarded as having prognostic value only in limited (stage I or II) disease. Hodgkin's disease has a bimodal age presentation (15–40 years, 60–70 years) with nodular sclerosis type in the head and neck of young people being the commonest (75% of cases). About 25% of patients have prognostically adverse B cell symptoms at presentation but the commonest complaint is painless cervical lymphadenopathy ± mediastinal disease. Disease usually involves contiguous, axial lymph node groups (neck, axilla, mediastinum, retroperitoneum, groin) with occasional extranodal involvement.

There is some evidence that early (confined to the mucosa), low-grade gastric MALToma is potentially reversible on removal of the ongoing antigenic stimulus ie. antibiotic treatment of *H. pylorii*. However, high-grade disease or low-grade lesions with deep submucosal or muscle invasion require surgical treatment supplemented by adjuvant therapy. Prognosis of MALT-derived NHL relates to the histological grade and stage of disease.

T cell lymphomas form a minority of NHL (10–15%) and tend to have a worse prognosis than B cell lesions. Their cytological features are not particularly reliable at defining disease entities or clinical course, which is more dependent on tumour site and clinical setting. Involvement of extranodal sites and relapse there is not infrequent with typically an aggressive disease course, e.g. enteropathy-associated T cell lymphoma and T/NK (angiocentric) sinonasal lymphoma. Cutaneous ALCL has a favourable prognosis while that of systemic ALCL with skin involvement is poor: 50% present with stage III/IV disease, there is a 65–85% 5 year survival rate but relapse is high (30–60%).

Similarly some B cell lymphomas have site-specific characteristics and clinical features, e.g. mantle cell lymphoma in the gut (lymphomatous polyposis) or diffuse mediastinal large B cell lymphoma – young females with a rapidly enlarging mediastinal mass associated with superior vena cava syndrome. A large (> 10 cm) mass and extramediastinal spread indicate poor prognosis. Generally adverse prognostic factors in NHL are:

— age > 60 years.
— male gender.
— systemic symptoms (fever>38.5 °C, weight loss > 10%, night sweats).
— poor performance status.
— elevated serum LDH.
— tumour bulk:
    5–10 cm (stage I/II); > 10 cm (stage III/IV)
    large mediastinal mass
    palpable abdominal mass
    combined paraortic and pelvic nodal disease.

8. Other malignancy

Carcinoma, germ cell tumours and malignant melanoma frequently metastasise to lymph nodes and are seen either in diagnostic biopsies (or fine needle aspiration cytology) in patients with lymphadenopathy or in regional lymph node resections in patients with known cancer. Spread of sarcoma to nodes is unusual although it does occur, e.g. epithelioid sarcoma, synovial sarcoma. Assessment is by routine morphology supplemented by ancillary techniques, e.g. immunohistochemistry and polymerase chain reaction methods, although it should be noted that the significance of nodal micrometastases in a number of cancers is still not resolved. Metastases are initially in the subcapsular sinus network expanding to partial or complete nodal effacement with potential for extracapsular spread. Anatomical site of involvement can be a clue as to the origin of the cancer, e.g. neck (cancer of the upper aerodigestive tract), axilla (breast cancer or malignant melanoma), groin (cancer of the perineum or perianal area) and retroperitoneum (germ cell tumour). The metastatic deposit may be necrotic or cystic (e.g. squamous cell carcinoma of the head and neck), resemble the primary lesion or be more or less well differentiated. Cell cohesion and plentiful cytoplasm favour non-lymphomatous neoplasia although this is not always the case, e.g. anaplastic large cell lymphoma. In this respect a broad but basic panel of antibodies is crucial for accurate designation (e.g. cytokeratins, CD 45, CD 30, S100, melan-A, chromogranin) supplemented by histochemistry (e.g. PAS diastase resistant mucin positivity, an organoid pattern of reticulin fibres). Some metastases also induce characteristic inflammatory responses, e.g. squamous cell carcinoma of head and neck, large cell lung cancer and nasopharyngeal carcinoma (lymphocytes, eosinophils, granulomas) even mimicking Hodgkin's disease. Some diagnostic clues are:

— malignant melanoma: cell nests, eosinophilic nucleolus, spindle/epithelioid cells, melanin pigment, S100, HMB-45, melan-A.

— germ cell tumour: midline (mediastinum or retroperitoneum), elevated serum βHCG or AFP (± tissue expression), PLAP (seminoma), cytokeratins (embryonal carcinoma).

— lobular breast cancer: sinusoidal infiltrate of sheeted, non-cohesive small cells, intracytoplasmic lumina, cytokeratins, GCDFP-15 and ER positive.

— small cell carcinoma: small (×2–4 the size of a lymphocyte), round to fusiform cells, granular chromatin, inconspicuous nucleolus, moulding, crush and DNA artefact, ± CAM 5.2 and chromogranin (Merkel cell tumour is CD 20 positive).

The reader is referred to the Introduction (Pages xxvi/xxvii) for further discussion of the use of immunohistochemistry.

Bone and Soft Tissue Cancer

- Sarcoma

Sarcoma

1. Gross description

Specimen

— fine needle aspirate/needle biopsy/open biopsy/ wide local excision/compartmentectomy/amputation (limb (below/above knee, etc.)/fore-/hind quarter).
— right or left.
— size (cm) and weight (g).

Tumour

Site

— osseous: paracortical; cortical; medullary (epiphysis/metaphysis/diaphysis); soft tissue extension.
— soft tissues: dermis/subcutaneous tissue/deep fascia/muscle/osseous extension/retroperitoneal.
— satellite nodules: size (cm) and distance (cm) from the main tumour.
— location: may be indicative, e.g. pelvis – Ewing's sarcoma; chest wall – Askin tumour, alveolar rhabdomyosarcoma.

Size

— length × width × depth (cm) or maximum dimension (cm).

Appearance

— solid/cystic/necrotic/lobulated/ fatty/myxoid/cartilaginous/osseous.

Edge

— circumscribed/irregular.

— relationship of tumour to vessels.

2. Histological type

Prior to histological evaluation of any bone or soft tissue sarcoma the pathologist must be aware of the patient's age, anatomical site of the lesion, subsite (e.g. epiphysis, metaphysis or diaphysis of bone) and crucially the radiological appearances. For example, a rapidly growing chest wall lesion in a young male may be nodular fasciitis rather than a sarcoma, peripheral chondroid lesions are benign whereas proximal are more likely to be malignant, and an epiphyseal lesion is likely to be a giant cell tumour (adult) or chondroblastoma (child) rather than an osteosarcoma (young/metaphysis). Age also closely correlates with type of soft tissue sarcoma: embryonal rhabdomyosarcoma (infants), synovial sarcoma (young adult), liposarcoma (middle age) and malignant fibrous histiocytoma (elderly). Close clinicopathological correlation is fundamental to the diagnosis.

Osteo-, chondro-, Ewing's, lipo-, synovial-, fibro-, rhabdo-, leiomyo-, angio-, neurosarcomas, malignant fibrous histiocytoma and variants are amongst the main categories of sarcoma and each comprises variable numbers of subtypes.

A panel of immunohistochemical antibodies to intermediate filaments and other markers (e.g. alkaline phosphatase on fresh tissue touch imprints for osteosarcoma), electron microscopy and cytogenetic analysis should be used as appropriate. This allows subclassification as to histogenetic type in the majority of lesions with, by exclusion, a minority designated malignant fibrous histiocytoma. Most soft tissue sarcomas arise from primitive multipotential mesenchymal cells which can differentiate along one of several lines resulting in histological overlap.

Metastatic carcinoma is the commonest malignant tumour of bone. It can be single or multiple, 70% affect the axial skeleton, and metaphysis is the preferred site.

3. Differentiation/grade

Well/moderate/poor.
Low-grade/high-grade. Some lesions define their own grade by way of their inherent clinical behaviour:

— high-grade: Ewing's sarcoma, rhabdomyosarcoma, angiosarcoma, pleomorphic liposarcoma, osteosarcoma (medullary).
— low-grade: well-differentiated liposarcoma, dermatofibrosarcoma protuberans, well differentiated chondrosarcoma.

Others are not graded but are potentially metastatic: synovial sarcoma, alveolar soft part sarcoma, epithelioid sarcoma.

Grading can be prognostically useful in spindle cell sarcomas: leiomyosarcoma, fibrosarcoma, malignant peripheral nerve sheath tumour.

Grading system, such as Coindre et al (1986):

	Scores
Differentiation	
well	1
moderate	2
poor	3
Necrosis	
none	1
< 50% tumour	2
> 50% tumour	3
Mitoses	
0–9/10 HPF	1
10–19/10 HPF	2
20+/10 HPF	3

HPF, high-power fields (×40 objective).

Grade 1 = ≤ 3
Grade 2 = 4 or 5
Grade 3 = ≥ 6

Histological differentiation or grade can be heterogeneous within a tumour, e.g. juxtaposition of well-differentiated and dedifferentiated chondrosarcoma or liposarcoma; the less differentiated component is chosen for grading purposes.

Preoperative adjuvant therapy can lead to quite extensive necrosis and changes in morphology potentially invalidating grading criteria on the resection specimen.

4. Extent of local tumour spread

Border: pushing/infiltrative.
Lymphocytic reaction: prominent/sparse.

Lymphatics/vessels/nerves including the proximal limit.

Single/more than one anatomical compartment.

Soft tissue sarcoma

pT1   tumour ≤ 5 cm in greatest dimension
    a. superficial
    b. deep
pT2   tumour > 5 cm in greatest dimension
    a. superficial
    b. deep

Superficial tumour is located exclusively above the superficial fascia. Deep tumour is located either exclusively beneath the superficial fascia or superficial

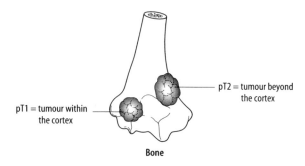

pT2 = tumour beyond
the cortex

pT1 = tumour within
the cortex

Bone

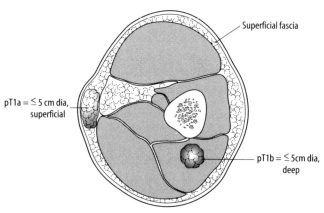

Superficial fascia

pT1a = ≤ 5 cm dia,
superficial

pT1b = ≤ 5cm dia,
deep

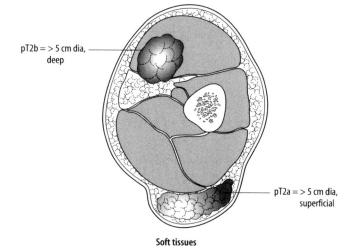

pT2b = > 5 cm dia,
deep

pT2a = > 5 cm dia,
superficial

Soft tissues

Figure 131. Sarcoma.

to the fascia with invasion of or through the fascia. Retroperitoneal, mediastinal and pelvic sarcomas are deep.

Bone sarcoma
pT1   tumour confined within cortex
pT2   tumour invades beyond cortex.

5. Lymphovascular invasion

Present/absent.
Intra-/extratumoural.

6. Lymph nodes

Site/number/size/number involved/limit node/extracapsular spread.
Regional nodes: those appropriate to the site of the primary tumour.

pN0   no regional lymph node involvement
pN1   metastases in regional node(s).

Lymph node metastases are unusual with the commonest mode of spread being haematogenous resulting in pulmonary secondaries. Some sarcomas, e.g. angiosarcoma, epithelioid sarcoma and synovial sarcoma, may show nodal spread.

7. Excision margins

Distance (mm) to the nearest painted excision margin.

A surgical margin clearance of less than 15–20 mm in soft tissue sarcoma has an increased risk of local recurrence unless further surgery or radiotherapy is given. This risk may be less if the margin is bound by a fascial plane.

8. Other pathology

Prosthesis allied to limb salvage surgery following wide local excision with preoperative neoadjuvant therapy.
    Radio-/chemotherapy changes: necrosis/inflammation and fibrosis in the primary tumour. Similar changes are seen in metastases and also tissue maturation, e.g. pulmonary metastases of osteosarcoma resulting in nodules of paucicellular osteoid.
    Paget's disease of bone, childhood chemotherapy and irradiation predispose to osteosarcoma.
    Fine needle aspiration cytology and needle core biopsy of sarcomas can allow categorisation into benign and malignant lesions in a majority of cases. They can also exclude diagnoses such as metastatic carcinoma, lymphoma and

malignant melanoma allowing a more focused approach to the diagnosis of sarcoma. However, the pathologist must be aware of the potential for sampling error with regard to heterogeneity in tumour type and grade; grade should only be commented on if it is high-grade. The use of preoperative needle biopsy with neoadjuvant treatment can impose limitations on the prognostic information in the resection, e.g. necrosis induced by adjuvant therapy invalidates traditional grading criteria.

Stage

Stage I	low-grade, T1, N0, M0
Stage II	low-grade, T2, N0, M0
Stage III	high-grade, T2, N0, M0
Stage IV	any grade, any T, N1 and/or M1

Markers

Immunohistochemical markers can be applied to formalin-fixed paraffin-embedded tissue to demonstrate a range of epithelial, neural, muscular, vascular and other mesenchymal antigens. None is totally specific or sensitive, indicating that an assimilation of results (including negative ones) from a panel of antibodies is necessary.

Antibody	*Use*
cytokeratin	synovial/epithelioid sarcoma
EMA	synovial/epithelioid sarcoma
myoglobin	rhabdomyosarcoma
desmin, sarcomeric actin	rhabdomyosarcoma, leiomyosarcoma
smooth muscle actin	leiomyosarcoma
S100 protein	malignant peripheral nerve sheath tumour, adipocytic and cartilaginous differentiation
MIC-2 (013 antibody) oncogene product	Ewing's sarcoma (plus PAS for glycogen)
Factor VIII, CD 31, CD 34	vascular markers
CD 34	dermatofibrosarcoma
HMB-45	clear cell sarcoma.

Chromosomal analysis

Chromosomal analysis is gaining increasing importance in classification, prognosis and choice of treatment for a range of sarcomas, e.g. Ewing's sarcoma, peripheral neuroectodermal tumours, liposarcoma, synovial sarcoma, rhabdomyosarcoma and desmoplastic small round cell tumour. Fresh tissue in a suitable transport medium is required for tissue culture although reverse transcriptase polymerase chain reaction (RT-PCR) techniques are being developed for use on paraffin-embedded tissue. For discussion see Graadt van Roggen et al. (1999).

Prognosis

Prognosis relates to:

— tumour size: > 5 cm diameter.
— grade: low versus high-grade.
— stage.
— histological type.
— site: superficial versus deep extremity versus retroperitoneum.
— age: > 50 years
— adequacy of surgery.

The importance of excision margins is emphasised in soft tissue sarcomas where negative and positive margins in low-grade lesions are associated with 5 year recurrence rates of 2% and 28% respectively. Current treatment of soft tissue sarcomas is wide monobloc resection with postoperative adjuvant radiotherapy to the operative site of high-grade lesions. With modern surgical techniques and adjuvant chemo-/radiotherapy average 5 year survival figures for soft tissue and bone based sarcomas are 70–80%. Prognosis varies with histological type, e.g. chondrosarcoma is better than osteosarcoma, and grade: grade I chondrosarcoma (78%) verus grade III (22%), myxoid liposarcoma (75%) versus round cell (28%). Surgical excision of pulmonary metastases (20% of sarcomas) is also helpful.

9. Other malignancy

Metastatic carcinoma, malignant melanoma, lymphoma (primary or secondary) and leukaemia can all mimic soft tissue or bone sarcoma and immunohistochemical markers will be required to make these distinctions. Lymphoma is usually of high-grade B cell type, solitary but occasionally multifocal. The cells are CD 20 (L26) positive with large irregular, multilobated nuclei. Fibrosis is present in 50% of cases giving spindle cell (mimicking sarcoma) or compartmentalised (mimicking metastatic carcinoma) appearances. A minority are CD 30 positive with cytological features of anaplastic lymphoma and aggressive behaviour. Metastatic carcinoma to bone may be osteolytic (breast, lung, thyroid, renal) leading to pathological fracture or osteoblastic (prostate) in character. It can be focal or diffuse resulting in a leucoerythroblastic blood picture and extramedullary haemopoiesis. Rarely the bone marrow can show a granulomatous response as an indicator of micrometastasis (e.g. infiltrating lobular carcinoma of breast) which can be demonstrated by immunohistochemistry. Certain carcinomas tend to a preferred pattern of bone metastases, e.g. thyroid carcinoma goes to shoulder girdle, skull, ribs and sternum.

Carcinoma
— cytokeratins, CEA, EMA.

Malignant melanoma

— S100, HMB-45, melan-A.

Leukaemia

— CD68, chloroacetate esterase, tdt.

Specific markers

— thyroglobulin (thyroid), PSA (prostate), CA125 (ovary), ER/PR/GCDFP-15 (breast), PLAP/AFP/βHCG (germ cell tumour).

Ophthalmic Cancer

Intraocular Malignancy

Extraocular Malignancy

Intraocular Malignancy

1. Gross description

Specimen

— fine needle aspirate/local resection/enucleation/ evisceration.
— weight (g).
— anteroposterior, horizontal and vertical dimensions (cm).
— length of optic nerve (mm).

Tumour

Site

— bulbar conjunctiva/sclera/cornea: malignant melanoma, lymphoma, squamous carcinoma.
— iris/ciliary body/choroid: uveal melanoma.
— retina/optic nerve: retinoblastoma.
— anterior chamber/posterior chamber: posterior; equatorial – superior, inferior, lateral.

Size

— length × width × depth (mm) but in particular maximum tumour dimension (mm).

Appearance

— nodular/plaque/pigmented/non-pigmented/haemorrhage/necrosis.

Edge

— circumscribed/irregular.

2. Histological type

Malignant melanoma
— 80% in the choroid; the commonest intraocular malignancy in adults.

Retinoblastoma
— < 3 years of age; 40% familial of which 90% bilateral; retinoblastoma suppressor gene 13q14 deletion.

Metastatic carcinoma
— breast, lung, gastrointestinal tract (stomach).
— 10% incidence at autopsy in carcinomatosis.
— posterior choroid is the commonest site.

Leukaemia/lymphoma
— 50% of leukaemia patients at autopsy (infiltration and/or haemorrhage).
— lymphoma is usually secondary to extraocular disease.

Rare
— medulloepithelioma, glioma, meningioma of optic nerve.

3. Differentiation

Malignant melanoma
— epithelioid   worse prognosis
— mixed (50%)
— spindle cell   better prognosis
— nucleolar enlargement (spindle cell type B) is an adverse prognostic sign.
— S100, HMB-45, melan-A positive.

Retinoblastoma
— well differentiated: Homer Wright rosettes.
— poorly differentiated: vascular pseudo-palisading necrosis, mitoses.
— S100, NSE, synaptophysin, GFAP positive.

4. Extent of local tumour spread

Border: pushing/infiltrative.
Lymphocytic reaction: prominent/sparse.
Intraocular: ciliary body, iris, anterior chamber.
Transscleral/extrascleral spread: depth (mm).
Optic nerve invasion.

pT3   Tumour more than 15 mm in greatest dimension or with an elevation more than 5 mm (Fig. 132)
pT4   Tumour with extraocular extension (Fig. 133)

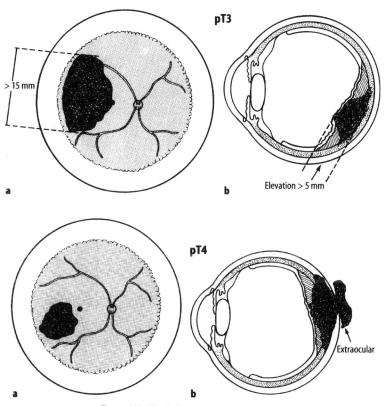

Figures 132, 133. Malignant melanoma of choroid.

Uveal melanoma of choroid

pT1   ≤ 10 mm greatest dimension, ≤ 3 mm elevation
      a. ≤ 7 mm, ≤ 2 mm
      b. > 7 to 10 mm, > 2 to 3 mm
pT2   > 10 to 15 mm greatest dimension, > 3 to 5 mm elevation
pT3   > 15 mm greatest dimension or > 5 mm elevation
pT4   extraocular extension.

There is a tendency for spread along the optic nerve with metastases to liver, lung, bone and skin.

Retinoblastoma

— endophytic, exophytic (subretinal) or retinal spread.

pT2   Tumour(s) involve(s) more than 25% but not more than 50% of the retina (Fig. 134)
pT3   Tumour(s) involve(s) more than 50% of the retina and/or invade(s) beyond the retina
        but remain(s) intraocular
        3a Tumour(s) involve(s) more than 50% of the retina and/or tumour cells in the
        vitreous body (Fig. 135)

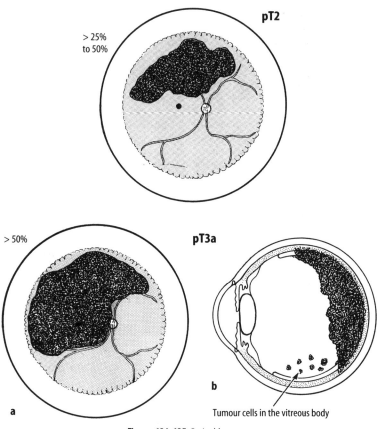

Figures 134, 135. Retinoblastoma.

pT1   ≤ 25% of retina
pT2   > 25% to 50% of retina
pT3   > 50% of retina and/or intraocular beyond retina
       a. and/or cells in vitreous
       b. optic nerve to lamina cribrosa
       c. anterior chamber and/or uvea and/or intrascleral
pT4   extraocular
       a. beyond lamina cribrosa, not at resection line
       b. other extraocular and/or at resection line.

3b   Tumour(s) involve(s) optic disc (Fig. 136)
3c   Tumour(s) involve(s) anterior chamber and/or uvea (Fig. 137)

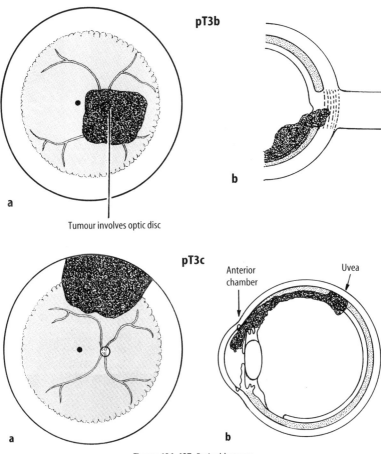

Figures 136, 137. Retinoblastoma.

There is a tendency for spread along the optic nerve into subarachnoid fluid and brain with metastases to the cranial vault and skeleton.

5. Lymphovascular invasion

Present/absent.
Intra-/extratumoural.
Schlemm's canal of ciliary body.
Vortex veins: adverse prognostic sign.

pT4   Tumour with extraocular invasion (Figs. 138, 139)
    4a   Tumour invades retrobulbar optic nerve (Fig. 138)
    4b   Extraocular extension other than invasion of optic nerve and/or tumour at resection
          line of optic nerve (Fig. 139)

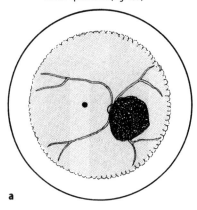

a

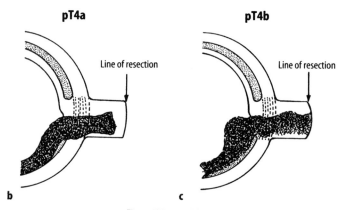

pT4a   **pT4b**

Line of resection   Line of resection

b   c

Figure 138. Retinoblastoma.

6. Lymph nodes

Site/number/size/number involved/limit node/extracapsular spread.
Regional nodes: pre-auricular, submandibular, cervical.

pN0   no regional lymph node metastasis
pN1   metastasis in regional lymph node(s).

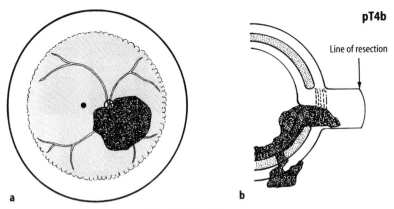

pT4b

Line of resection

a b

Figure 139. Retinoblastoma.

7. Excision margins

Distances (mm) to the nearest painted resection margin of the optic nerve or edge of the evisceration.

8. Other pathology

Tumour necrosis
— spontaneous or secondary to aspiration cytology or irradiation/cryotherapy/photocoagulation.

Glaucoma
— invasion of Schlemm's canal or secondary to aspiration cytology.

Metastatic malignant melanoma
— jaundice, hepatomegaly due to secondary deposits and a glass eye.

Prognosis

Malignant melanoma has a 15 year mortality rate of 50%, but 66% at 5 years for those with extrascleral extension. Maximum tumour dimension is the strongest prognostic indicator. Cell type is influential as 5 year survival rates are lower in epithelioid (25–35%) than spindle cell B lesions (66–75%). Therefore a small (< 7 mm) pure spindle cell A melanoma has a 5 year survival ≥ 95%. Retinoblastoma has a 5 year survival of 90%; the hereditary form is slightly worse and 6–20% of patients develop a second malignancy after 10–15 years, e.g. osteosarcoma, rhabdomyosarcoma. Localised resection of malignant melanoma may be considered if it is small (maximum dimension<1 cm) and anterior or equatorial in location. Enucleation is indicated for posterior melanoma, irrespective of its size, due to its interference with visual acuity. Sporadic retinoblastoma is treated by enucleation (unless early, when radiation is used) and familial cases by enucleation and selective radiotherapy to the contralateral eye to treat any early metachronous lesions. Irradiation and systemic chemotherapy are reserved for cases with involvement of the surgical margins.

Adverse prognostic indicators are:

— tumour maximum dimension.
— epithelioid cell type/nucleolar enlargement in melanoma.
— invasion of the ciliary body, anterior chamber, optic nerve, sclera, vortex veins.

Extraocular Malignancy

1. Gross description

Specimen

— fine needle aspirate/excision biopsy/exenteration.
— size (cm) and weight (g).

Tumour

Site

— ocular adnexae: eyelid
                                conjunctiva
                                lacrimal apparatus.
— orbit/retro-orbital tissues.

Size

— length × width × depth (cm) or maximum dimension (cm).

Appearance

— exophytic/verrucous/sessile/ulcerated/fleshy/infiltrative/pigmented.

Edge

— circumscribed/irregular.

2. Histological type

Adnexae

— basal cell carcinoma: most common, >80%.
— squamous cell carcinoma:<5%.
— lacrimal gland carcinoma: e.g. adenoid cystic carcinoma.

- sebaceous carcinoma: epithelioma/carcinoma.
- Merkel cell tumour: NSE/chromogranin/cytokeratin (CAM 5.2, CK20) positive; aggressive.
- malignant melanoma: primary (origin in conjunctival naevus) or secondary.
- lymphoma: low-grade MALToma with indolent behaviour.
- metastatic carcinoma: breast, gut, lung.

Orbit – children
- embryonal (less commonly alveolar) rhabdomyosarcoma, Burkitt's lymphoma.

Orbit – adults
- lymphoma – (MALToma): the presence of lymphoid tissue in the orbit (not usual) is suspicious of neoplasia and up to 50% are part of systemic disease.
- fibro-/osteo-/chondro-/liposarcoma, malignant fibrous histiocytoma, alveolar soft part sarcoma, malignant teratoma – all rare but fibrosarcoma/ malignant fibrous histiocytoma is the commonest orbital sarcoma of adulthood.
- glioma or meningioma of optic nerve origin.
- myeloma/leukaemia.
- metastatic carcinoma
  15–30% of orbital tumours.
  direct spread: retinoblastoma; uveal melanoma; paranasal sinus carcinoma.
  distant spread: neuroblastoma; embryonal rhabdomyosarcoma; breast, lung, kidney, prostatic carcinoma, carcinoid tumour of lung or small bowel.
- malignant melanoma: direct or distant spread.

3. Differentiation

Well/moderate/poor.
- carcinoma.
Low-grade/high-grade.
- lymphoma and sarcoma.

4. Extent of local tumour spread

Border: pushing/infiltrative.
Lymphocytic reaction: prominent/sparse.
- TNM varies according to exact anatomical site and tumour type.

Adnexae, e.g. carcinoma of eyelid
pT1   tumour of any size not in tarsal plate, or, at lid margin ≤ 5 mm maximum dimension
pT2   tumour invades tarsal plate, or, at lid margin > 5 mm but ≤ 10 mm maximum dimension

pT1　Tumour of any size, not invading the tarsal plate; or at eyelid margin, 5 mm or less in greatest dimension (Fig. 140)

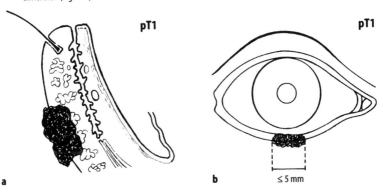

pT1

pT1

a

b　≤ 5 mm

pT2　Tumour invades tarsal plate; or at eyelid margin, more than 5 mm but not more than 10 mm in greatest dimension (Fig. 141)

pT3　Tumour involves full eyelid thickness; or at eyelid margin, more than 10 mm in greatest dimension (Fig. 142)

pT4　Tumour invades adjacent structures (Fig. 143)

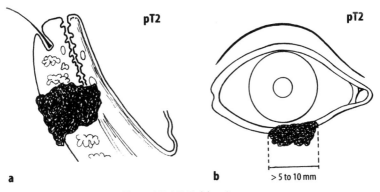

pT2

pT2

a

b　> 5 to 10 mm

Figures 140, 141. Eyelid carcinoma.

pT3　tumour involves full eyelid thickness, or, at lid margin > 10 mm maximum dimension

pT4　tumour invades adjacent structures.

Orbit

pT1　tumour ≤ 15 mm maximum dimension

pT2　tumour > 15 mm maximum dimension

pT3　tumour of any size, diffuse invasion of orbital tissues and/or bony walls

pT4　tumour invades beyond the orbit to adjacent sinuses/cranium.

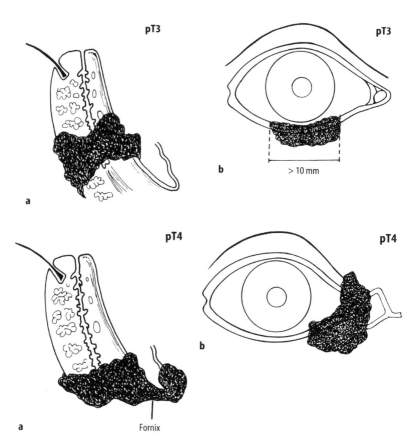

Figures 142, 143. Eyelid carcinoma.

5. Lymphovascular invasion

Present/absent.
Intra-/extratumoural.

6. Lymph nodes

Site/number/size/number involved/limit node/extracapsular spread.
Regional nodes: pre-auricular, submandibular, cervical.

pN0   no regional lymph node metastasis
pN1   metastasis in regional lymph node(s).

7. Excision margins

Distances (mm) to the nearest painted excision margins.

8. Other pathology

Mikulicz's disease (the pathology of which is similar to Sjögren's syndrome) is characterised by benign lymphoepithelial lesion (syn. lympho(myo-)epithelial sialadenitis) and in 10–15% progresses to develop low-grade lymphoma of MALT type.

Sun exposure, actinic keratosis and Bowen's disease are predisposing factors in carcinoma of the eyelid and conjunctiva.

The commonest indications for exenteration are malignant tumours of the eyelid such as basal cell, squamous cell or sebaceous carcinomas.

Prognosis

Orbital tumours present with unilateral proptosis, the commonest types being malignant lymphoma and metastatic carcinoma. Rhabdomyosarcoma occurs in childhood, embryonal variants being of better prognosis than the alveolar type; a 50% survival is achieved with chemo-/radiotherapy and resection is reserved for non-responsive cases. Malignant fibrosarcoma/fibrous histiocytoma is the commonest type of sarcoma in adulthood with a 10 year survival rate of 20–25%; it is treated by radiotherapy. Note that an orbital tumour may be the first presentation of an ocular tumour due to direct spread, e.g. retinoblastoma or malignant melanoma.

The tissues behind the orbital septum are normally devoid of lymphatics and lymphoid tissue. The presence of any lymphoid tissue at this site is therefore suspicious of malignancy. Prognosis, which can be unpredictable, relates to the grade and stage of disease but is generally reasonably good (80% survival). Malignant lymphoma is the commonest adult orbital malignancy. Tissues anterior to the septum show a wider range of antigen-driven reactive and low-grade neoplastic lymphoid proliferation. Treatment of malignant lymphoma is radio-/chemotherapy depending on the stage and grade of disease.

Markers
— malignant melanoma: S100, HMB-45, melan-A.
— malignant lymphoma: CD45, CD20, CD3; κ/λ light chain restriction; heavy/light chain immunoglobulin and T cell receptor gene rearrangements.
— carcinoma: cytokeratins, EMA (nb plasma cells can also be EMA positive).
— rhabdomyosarcoma: desmin, myoglobin, sarcomeric actin.

Bibliography

General

Chetty R, O'Leary JJ, Gatter KC. Immunocytochemistry as a diagnostic tool. Curr Diagn Pathol 1995;2:38–45

Cross SS. Grading and scoring in histopathology. Histopathology 1998;33:99–106

Domizio P, Lowe D. Reporting histopathology sections. London: Chapman and Hall, 1997

Expert Advisory Group on Cancer to the Chief Medical Officers of England and Wales. A policy framework for commissioning cancer services. London: Department of Health, 1995 (EL (95) 51)

Eyden B. Electron microscopy in tumour diagnosis: continuing to complement other diagnostic techniques. Histopathology 1999;35:102–108

Fletcher CDM (ed). Diagnostic histopathology of tumours. Edinburgh: Churchill Livingstone, 1995

Fletcher JA. DNA In situ hybridization as an adjunct in tumor diagnosis. Am J Clin Pathol 1999;112 (Suppl 1):S11–S18

Geradts J. Immunohistochemical prognostic and predictive markers in common tumours. CPD Bulletin Cellular Pathology 1999; 1(4):144–148

Hamilton PW, Allen DC (eds). Quantitative clinical pathology. Oxford: Blackwell Scientific, 1995

Hammar SP. Metastatic adenocarcinoma of unknown primary origin. Hum Pathol 1998;29:1393–1402

Hermanek P, Hutter RVP, Sobin LH, Wagner G, Wittekind Ch (eds). TNM atlas: illustrated guide to the TNM/pTNM classification of malignant tumours . UICC. 4th edn. Berlin Heidelberg New York: Springer, 1997

Liefers GJ, Tollenaar RAEM, Cleton-Jansen AM. Molecular detection of minimal residual disease in colorectal and breast cancer. Histopathology 1999;34:385–390

McNicol AM, Richmond JA. Optimising immunohistochemistry: antigen retrieval and signal amplification. Histopathology 1998;32:97–103

O'Leary JJ, Engels K, Dada MA. The polymerase chain reaction in pathology. J Clin Pathol 1997;50:805–810

Rosai J. Ackerman's Surgical pathology. 8th edn. St Louis: Mosby, 1996

Silverberg SG (ed). Principles and practice of surgical pathology. 2nd edn. New York: Churchill Livingstone, 1990

Sobin L H, Wittekind Ch (eds). TNM Classification of malignant tumours. UICC. 5th edn. New York: Wiley-Liss, 1997

Solcia E. Histological typing of endocrine tumours. 2nd edn. WHO: International histological classification of tumours. Berlin Heidelberg New York: Springer, 1999

Squire JA, Perlikowski S. Molecular cytogenetics in modern pathology. In: Kirkham N, Lemoine NR (eds). Progress in pathology 4. Edinburgh: Churchill Livingstone, 1998:1–17

Stephenson TJ. Criteria for malignancy in endocrine tumours. In: Anthony PP, MacSween RNM (eds). Recent advances in histopathology 17. Edinburgh: Churchill Livingstone, 1997:93–111

Van Dam PA, Tjalma WAA. Clinical applications of flow cytometry. In: Lowe DG, Underwood JCE (eds). Recent advances in histopathology 18. Edinburgh: Churchill Livingstone, 1999:131–145

Williams GR. Unravelling the unknown primary. CPD Bulletin Cellular Pathology 1999; 1(4):140–143

Gastrointestinal cancer

Abe K, Sasano H, Itakura Y, Nishihira T, Mori S, Nagura H. Basaloid-squamous carcinoma of the oesophagus. Am J Surg Pathol 1996;20:453–461

Albores-Saavedra J, Heffess C, Hruban RH, Klimstra D. Longnecker D. Recommendations for the reporting of pancreatic specimens containing malignant tumors. Am J Clin Pathol 1999;111:304–307

Albores-Saavedra J, Henson DE, Sobin LH. Histological typing of tumours of the gall-bladder and extrahepatic bile ducts. 2nd edn. WHO: International histological classification of tumours. Berlin Heidelberg New York: Springer, 1991

Association of Directors of Anatomic and Surgical Pathology. Recommendations for the reporting of resected large intestinal carcinomas. Hum Pathol 1996;27:5–8

Birbeck KF, Quirke P. Reporting protocols in colorectal cancer. CPD Bulletin Cellular Pathology 1999;1(2):58–64

Bogomeletz WV. Early squamous cell carcinoma of oesophagus. Curr Diagn Pathol 1994;1:212–215

Bull AD, Biffin AHB, Mella J, Radcliffe AG, Stamatakis JD, Steele RJC, Williams GT. Colorectal cancer pathology reporting: a regional audit. J Clin Pathol 1997;50:138–142

Capella C, Heitz PU, Höfler H, Solcia E, Klöppel G. Revised classification of neuroendocrine tumours of the lung, pancreas and gut. Virchows Arch 1995;425:547–560

Carneiro F. Classification of gastric carcinomas. Curr Diagn Pathol 1997;4:51–59

Carr NJ, McCarthy WF, Sobin LH. Epithelial and noncarcinoid tumors and tumor-like lesions of the appendix. Cancer 1995;75:757–768

Cooper HS, Deppisch LM, Kahn EI, Lev R, Manley PN, Pascal RR, Qizilbash AH, Rickert R R, Silverman JF, Wirman JA. Pathology of the malignant colorectal polyp. Hum Pathol 1998;29:15–26

Day DW, Dixon MF. Biopsy pathology of the oesophagus, stomach and duodenum. 2nd edn. London: Chapman and Hall Medical, 1995

Dixon MF, Martin IG, Sue-Ling HM, Wyatt, JI, Quirke P, Johnston D. Goseki grading in gastric cancer: comparison with existing systems of grading and its reproducibility. Histopathology 1994;25:309–316

Domizio P, Owen RA, Shepherd NA, Talbot IC, Norton AJ. Primary lymphoma of the small intestine. A clinicopathological study of 119 cases. Am J Surg Pathol 1993;17: 429–442

Dukes CE, Bussey HJR. The spread of rectal cancer and its effect on prognosis. Br J Cancer 1958;12:309–320

Emory TS, Sobin LH, Lukes L, Lee DH, O'Leary TJ. Prognosis of gastrointestinal smooth-muscle (stromal tumors): dependence on anatomic site. Am J Surg Pathol 1999;23:82–87

Foulis AK. Neuroendocrine tumours of the pancreas. Association of Clinical Pathologists Yearbook 1998:58–60

Goldblum JR, Hart WR. Perianal Paget's disease. A histologic and immunohistochemical study of 11 cases with and without associated rectal adenocarcinoma. Am J Surg Pathol 1998;22:170–179

Goldman H. Gastrointestinal mucosal biopsy. New York: Churchill Livingstone, 1996

Goldstein NS, Hart J. Histologic features associated with lymph node metastasis in stage T1 and superficial T2 rectal adenocarcinomas in abdominoperineal resection specimens. Am J Clin Pathol 1999;111:51–58

Haggitt RC, Glotzbach RE, Soffer EE, Wruble LD. Prognostic factors in colorectal carcinomas arising in adenomas: implications for lesions removed by endoscopic polypectomy. Gastroenterology 1985;89:328–336

Ibrahim NBN. Guidelines for handling oesophageal biopsies and resection specimens and their reporting. J Clin Pathol 2000; 53: 89–9

Isaacson PG. Gastrointestinal lymphoma. Hum Pathol 1994;25:1020–1029

Ishak KG, Anthony PP, Sobin LH. Histological typing of tumours of the liver. 2nd edn. WHO: International histological classification of tumours. Berlin Heidelberg New York: Springer, 1994

Jass JR. Diagnosis of hereditary non-polyposis colorectal cancer. Histopathology 1998;32:491–497

Jass JR, Love SB, Northover JMA. A new prognostic classification of rectal cancer. Lancet 1987;i:1303–1306

Jass JR, Sobin LH. Histological typing of intestinal tumours. 2nd edn. WHO: International Histological classification of tumours. Berlin Heidelberg New York: Springer, 1988

Klöppel G, Solcia E, Longnecker DS, Capella C, Sobin LH. Histological typing of tumours of the exocrine pancreas. 2nd edn. WHO: International histological classification of tumours. Berlin Heidelberg New York: Springer, 1996

Konishi F, Morson BC. Pathology of colorectal adenomas: a colonoscopic survey. J Clin Pathol 1982;35:830–841

Lewin KJ, Appelman HD. Tumors of the esophagus and stomach. Atlas of tumor pathology. 3rd series. Fascicle 18. Washington: AFIP, 1996

Lioe TF, Biggart JD. Primary adenocarcinoma of the jejunum and ileum: clinicopathological review of 25 cases. J Clin Pathol 1990:43:533–536

MacSween RNM, Anthony PP, Scheuer PJ, Burt AD, Portmann BC (eds). Pathology of the liver. 3rd edn. Edinburgh: Churchill Livingstone, 1994

Mapstone N. A minimum data set for reporting oesophageal carcinoma. CPD Bulletin Cellular Pathology 1999;1(2):44–46

Morson BC, Dawson P, Day DW, Jass JR, Price AB, Williams GT. Morson and Dawson's gastrointestinal pathology. 3rd edn. Oxford: Blackwell Scientific, 1990

Newman PL, Wadden C, Fletcher CDM. Gastrointestinal stromal tumours:correlation of immunophenotype with histological features. J Pathol 1991;164:107–111

Paraf F, Fléjou J-F, Pignon J-P, Fékété F, Potet F. Surgical pathology of adenocarcinoma arising in Barrett's esophagus. Am J Surg Pathol 1995;19:183–191

Quirke P, Durdey P, Dixon MF, Williams NS. Local recurrence of rectal adenocarcinoma due to inadequate surgical resection. Histopathological study of lateral tumour spread and surgical excision. Lancet 1986;ii:996–998

Quirke P. The pathologist, the surgeon and colorectal cancer: get it right because it matters. In: Kirkham N, Lemoine N R (eds). Progress in pathology 4. Edinburgh: Churchill Livingstone, 1998:201–213

Riddell RH, Iwafuchi M. Problems arising from Eastern and Western classification systems for gastrointestinal dysplasia and carcinoma: are they resolvable. Histopathology 1998;33:197–202

Ronnett BM, Kurman RJ, Shmookler BM, Sugarbaker PH, Young RH. The morphologic spectrum of ovarian metastases of appendiceal adenocarcinomas. Am J Surg Pathol 1997;21:1144–1155

Seidal T, Edvardsson H. Expression of c-kit (CD117) and Ki67 provides information about the possible cell of origin and clinical course of gastrointestinal stromal tumours. Histopathology 1999;34:416–424

Shepherd NA, Baxter KJ, Love SB. Influence of local peritoneal involvement on pelvic recurrence and prognosis in rectal cancer. J Clin Pathol 1995;48:849–855

Shepherd NA. Pathological prognostic factors in colorectal cancer. In:Kirkham N, Lemoine N R (eds). Progress in pathology 2. Edinburgh: Churchill Livingstone, 1995:115–141

Shepherd NA. Polyps and polyposis syndromes of the intestines. Curr Diagn Pathol 1997;4:222–238

Shepherd NA, Biddlestone LR. The histopathology and cytopathology of Barrett's oesophagus. CPD Bulletin Cellular Pathology 1999;1(2):39–43

Sircar K, Hewlett BR, Huizinga JD, Chorneyko K, Berezin I, Riddell RH. Interstitial cells of Cajal as precursors of gastrointestinal stromal tumors. Am J Surg Pathol 1999;23:377–389

Solcia E, Capella C, Klöppel G. Tumors of the pancreas. Atlas of tumour pathology. 3rd series. Fascicle 20. Washington: AFIP, 1997

Sutherland F, Haine L, Quirke P. Molecular approaches to colorectal cancer: a review. Curr Diagn Pathol 1998;5:34–43

Talbot IC, Ritchie S, Leighton M, Hughes AO, Bussey HJR, Morson BC. Invasion of veins by carcinoma of rectum: method of detection, histological features and significance. Histopathology 1981;5:141–163

The Royal College of Pathologists. Minimum dataset for colorectal cancer histopathology reports. London: RCP, July 1998

The Royal College of Pathologists. Minimum dataset for oesophageal carcinoma histopathology reports. London: RCP, November 1998

Tworek JA, Goldblum JR, Weiss SW, Greenson JK, Appelman HD. Stromal tumors of the abdominal colon. A clinicopathologic study of 20 cases. Am J Surg Pathol 1999a;23: 937–945

Tworek JA, Goldblum JR, Weiss SW, Greenson JK, Appelman HD. Stromal tumors of the anorectum. A clinicopathologic study of 22 cases. Am J Surg Pathol 1999b;23:946–954

UK Co-ordinating Committee on Cancer Research. Handbook for the clinico-pathological assessment and staging of colorectal cancer. 2nd edn. London: UKCCR, April 1997

Warren BF. Gastrointestinal polyps. CPD Bulletin Cellular Pathology 1999;1(2):65–67

Watanabe H, Jass JR, Sobin LH. Histological typing of oesophageal and gastric tumours. 2nd edn. WHO: International histological classification of tumours. Berlin Heidelberg New York: Springer, 1990

Whitehead R (ed). Gastrointestinal and oesophageal pathology. 2nd edn. Edinburgh: Churchill Livingstone, 1995

Williams GR, Sheffield JP, Love SB, Talbot IC. Morphology of anal carcinoma: a reappraisal. Curr Diagn Pathol 1995;2:32–37

Williams GR, Talbot IC. Anal carcinoma: a histological review. Histopathology 1994;25: 507–516

Williams GT. Neuroendocrine tumours of the gastrointestinal tract. Association of Clinical Pathologists Yearbook 1998:54–55

Williams GT, Maynard N. Early gastric cancer. CPD Bulletin Cellular Pathology 1999;1(2); 56–57

Head and neck cancer

Delellis RA. Tumors of the parathyroid gland. Atlas of tumor pathology. 3rd series. Fascicle 6. Washington: AFIP, 1993

Ellis GL, Auclair PL. Gnepp DR. Surgical pathology of the salivary glands. MPP 25. Philadelphia: Saunders, 1991

Ellis G , Auclair P . Tumors of the salivary glands. Atlas of tumor pathology. 3rd series. Fascicle 17. Washington: AFIP, 1996

Friedmann I (ed). Nose, throat and ears. Systemic pathology. 3rd edn. Vol 1. Edinburgh: Churchill Livingstone, 1986

Gnepp DR, Barnes L, Crissman J, Zarbo R. Recommendations for the reporting of larynx specimens containing laryngeal neoplasms. Am J Clin Pathol 1998;110:137–139

Hedinger C. Histological typing of thyroid tumours. 2nd edn. WHO: International histological classification of tumours. Berlin Heidelberg New York: Springer, 1988

MacDonald DG, Browne, RM. Tumours of odontogenic epithelium. In:Anthony PP Macsween RNM (eds). Recent advances in histopathology 17. Edinburgh: Churchill Livingstone, 1997;139–166

Nishida T, Katayama S, Tsujimoto M, Nakamura J, Matsuda H. Clinicopathological significance of poorly differentiated thyroid carcinoma. Am J Surg Pathol 1999; 23:205–211

Orell SR, Sterrett GF, Walters MN-I, Whitaker D. Fine needle aspiration cytology. 2nd edn. Edinburgh: Churchill Livingstone, 1992

Pindborg JJ, Reichart PA, Smith CJ, Van der Waal I. Histological typing of cancer and precancer of the oral mucosa. 2nd edn. WHO: International histological classification of tumours. Berlin Heidelberg New York: Springer, 1997

Rosai J, Carcangiu ML, Delellis RA. Tumors of the thyroid gland. Atlas of tumor pathology. 3rd series. Fascicle 5. Washington: AFIP, 1992

Seifert G. Histological typing of salivary gland tumours. 2nd edn. WHO: International histological classification of tumours. Berlin Heidelberg New York: Springer, 1991

Shanmugaratnam K. Histological typing of tumours of the upper respiratory tract and ear. 2nd edn. WHO: International histological classification of tumours. Berlin Heidelberg New York: Springer, 1991

Simpson RHW. Salivary gland tumours. In:Anthony PP, MacSween RNM (eds). Recent advances in histopathology 17. Edinburgh: Churchill Livingstone, 1997;167–190

Simpson RHW, Sarsfield PTL. Benign and malignant lymphoid lesions of the salivary glands. Curr Diagn Pathol 1997;4:91–99

Sneed DC. Protocol for the examination of specimens from patients with malignant tumors of the thyroid gland, exclusive of lymphomas. Arch Pathol Lab Med 1999; 123:45–49

Sobrinho-Simoes M, Fonseca E. Recently described tumours of the thyroid. In: Anthony P P, MacSween R N M (eds). Recent Advances in Histopathology 16. Edinburgh: Churchill Livingstone, 1994;213–229

Sobrinho-Simoes M. Tumours of thyroid: a brief overview with emphasis on the most controversial issues. Curr Diagn Pathol 1995;2:15–22

Speight PM, Farthing PM, Bouquot JE. The pathology of oral cancer and precancer. Curr Diagn Pathol 1996;3:165–176

The Royal College of Pathologists. Minimum dataset for head and neck carcinoma histopathology reports. London: RCP, November 1998

Young JA. Diagnostic problems in fine needle aspiration cytopathology of the salivary glands. J Clin Pathol 1994;47:193–198

Respiratory and mediastinal cancer

Association of Directors of Anatomic and Surgical Pathology. Recommendations for the reporting of resected primary lung carcinomas. Hum Pathol 1995;26:937–939

Battifora H, McCaughey WT. Tumors of the serosal membranes. Atlas of tumor pathology. 3rd series. Fascicle 15. Washington: AFIP, 1995

Burnett RA, Swanson Beck J, Howatson SR, Lee FD, Lessells AM, McLaren KM, Ogston S, Robertson AJ, Simpson JG, Smith GD, Tavadia HB, Walker F. Observer variability in histopathological reporting of malignant bronchial biopsy specimens. J Clin Pathol 1994;47:711–713

Colby TV, Koss MN. Tumors of the lower respiratory tract. Atlas of tumor pathology. 3rd series. Fascicle 13. Washington: AFIP, 1995

Corrin B. Neuroendocrine neoplasms of the lung. Curr Diagn Pathol 1997;4:239–250

Corrin B (ed). Pathology of Lung Tumours. New York. Churchill Livingstone, 1997

Corrin B (ed). The lungs. Systemic pathology. 3rd edn. Vol 5. Edinburgh: Churchill Livingstone, 1990

Gosney JR. Endocrine pathology of the lung. In: Anthony PP, MacSween RNM (eds). Recent advances in histopathology 16. Edinburgh: Churchill Livingstone, 1994;147–165

Hasleton PS, Hammar SP. Malignant mesothelioma. Curr Diagn Pathol 1996;3:153–164

Herbert A. Cytology of metastatic neoplasia in the lung. In: Lowe D G, Underwood J C E (eds). Recent advances in histopathology 18. Edinburgh: Churchill Livingstone, 1999;109–116.

Kitamura H, Kameda Y, Ito T, Hayashi H. Atypical adenomatous hyperplasia of the lung. Implications for the pathogenesis of peripheral lung adenocarcinoma. Am J Clin Pathol 1999;111:610–622

Müller-Hermelink HK, Marx A, Kirchner Th. Advances in the diagnosis and classification of thymic epithelial tumours. In: Anthony PP, MacSween RNM (eds). Recent advances in histopathology 16. Edinburgh: Churchill Livingstone, 1994;49–72

Nash G, Otis CN. Protocol for the examination of specimens from patients with malignant pleural mesothelioma. Arch Pathol Lab Med 1999;123:39–44

Nicholson AG. The role of immunohistochemistry in differentiating tumours presenting in the pleura. CPD Bulletin Cellular Pathology 1999; 1(4):149–153

Nicholson AG, Corrin B. Pulmonary lymphoproliferative disorders. In: Anthony PP, MacSween RNM (eds). Recent advances in histopathology 17. Edinburgh: Churchill Livingstone, 1997:47–68

Olszewski W. Aspiration biopsy of intrathoracic lesions. Curr Diagn Pathol 1995; 2:146–152

Ordonez NG. Role of imunohistochemistry in differentiating epithelial mesothelioma from adenocarcinoma. Am J Clin Pathol 1999;112:75–89

Rosai J. Histological typing of tumours of the thymus. 2nd edn. WHO: International histological classification of tumours. Berlin Heidelberg New York: Springer, 1999

The Royal College of Pathologists. Minimum dataset for lung cancer histopathology reports. London: RCP, November 1998

Travis WD, Colby TV, Corrin B, Shimosato Y, Brambilla E. Histological typing of lung and pleural tumours. 3rd edn. WHO: International histological classification of tumours. Berlin Heidelberg New York: Springer, 1999

Skin cancer

Blessing K. Benign atypical naevi: diagnostic difficulties and continued controversy. Histopathology 1999;34:189–198

Cerroni L, Kerl H, Gatter K. An illustrated guide to skin lymphoma. Oxford: Blackwell Scientific, 1998

Cochran AJ, Bailly C, Cook M, Crotty K, Mihm M, Mooi W, Sagebiel R. Recommendations for the reporting of tissues removed as part of the surgical treatment of cutaneous melanoma. Hum Pathol 1997;28:1123–1125

Cook MG. Problems in the histological assessment of melanoma emphasising the importance of the vertical/nodular component. Curr Diagn Pathol 1994;1:98–104

Cook MG. A practical approach to spindle cell melanocytic lesions. CPD Bulletin Cellular Pathology 1999;1(3):101–104

Cook MG, Clarke TJ, Humphreys S, Fletcher A , McLaren KM, Smith NP, Stevens A, Theaker JM, Melia J. The evaluation of diagnostic and prognostic criteria and the terminology of thin cutaneous malignant melanoma by the CRC Melanoma Pathology Panel. Histopathology 1996;28:497–512

Elder DE, Murphy GF. Melanocytic tumors of the skin. Atlas of tumor pathology. 3rd series. Fascicle 2. Washington: AFIP, 1991

Heenan PJ, Elder D, Sobin LH. Histological typing of skin tumours. 2nd edn. WHO: International histological classification of tumours. Berlin Heidelberg New York: Springer, 1996

Hollowood K. The diagnosis of sweat gland carcinomas: a practical approach. CPD Bulletin Cellular Pathology 1999;1(3):105–110

Kirkham N. Malignant melanoma: progress in diagnosis and prognosis. In: Kirkham N, Lemoine NR (eds). Progress in pathology 4. Edinburgh: Churchill Livingstone, 1998:241–253

Lever WF, Schaumburg-Lever G. Histopathology of the skin. 7th edn. Philadelphia: Lippincott, 1990

McKee PH. Pathology of the skin with clinical correlations. 2nd edn. London: Mosby-Wolfe, 1996

Mooi WJ. The dysplastic naevus. J Clin Pathol 1997;50:711–715

Murphy GF, Elder DE. Non-melanocytic tumors of the skin. Atlas of tumor pathology. 3rd series. Fascicle 1. Washington: AFIP, 1991

Robson A. Primary cutaneous B cell lymphoma: an overview. CPD Bulletin Cellular Pathology 1999;1 (3):111–115

Sanders DSA, Blessing K. Guidelines on reporting cutaneous malignant melanoma. CPD Bulletin Cellular Pathology 1999;1(3):97–100

Spatz A, Shaw HM, Crotty KA, Thompson JF, McCarthy SW. Analysis of histopathological factors associated with prolonged survival of 10 years or more for patients with thick melanomas (> 5 mm). Histopathology 1998;33:406–413

Willemze R, Meijer CJLM. Classification of cutaneous lymphomas: crosstalk between pathologist and clinician. Curr Diagn Pathol 1998;5:23–33

Breast cancer

Al-Nafussi A. Spindle cell tumours of the breast: practical approach to diagnosis. Histopathology 1999;35:1–13

Anderson TJ, Page DL. Risk assessment in breast cancer. In: Anthony PP, MacSween RNM (eds). Recent advances in histopathology 17. Edinburgh: Churchill Livingstone, 1997:69–91

Dahlstrom JE, Sutton S, Jain S. Histological precision of stereotactic core biopsy in diagnosis of malignant and premalignant breast lesions. Histopathology 1996;29:537–541

Douglas-Jones AG, Gupta SK, Attanoos RL, Morgan JM, Mansel RE. A critical appraisal of six modern classifications of ductal carcinoma in situ of the breast (DCIS): correlation with grade of associated invasive carcinoma. Histopathology 1996;29:397–409

Elston CW, Ellis IO (eds). The breast. Systemic pathology. 3rd edn. Vol 13. Edinburgh: Churchill Livingstone, 1998

Histological types of breast tumours. 2nd edn. WHO: International histological classification of tumours. Geneva: WHO, 1981

Moffat CJC, Pinder SE, Dixon AR, Elston CW, Blamey RW, Ellis IO. Phyllodes tumours of the breast: a clinicopathological review of thirty-two cases. Histopathology 1995;27:205–218

National Coordinating Group for Breast Screening Pathology. Pathology reporting in breast cancer screening. NHSBSP Publication No 3 April, 1995

Page DL, Anderson TJ. Diagnostic histopathology of the breast. Edinburgh: Churchill Livingstone, 1987

Pinder SE, Ellis IO, Elston CW. Prognostic factors in primary breast carcinoma. J Clin Pathol 1995;48:981–983

Pinder SE, Elston CW, Ellis IO. The role of the pre-operative diagnosis in breast cancer. Histopathology 1996;28:563–566

Rosen PP. Rosen's breast pathology. Philadelphia: Lippincott-Raven, 1997

Rosen PP. Breast pathology: diagnosis by needle core biopsy. Philadelphia: Lippincott Williams and Wilkins, 1999

Rosen PP, Oberman HA. Tumors of the mammary gland. Atlas of tumor pathology. 3rd series. Fascicle 7. Washington: AFIP, 1993

Sousha S. Diagnosis of "early", "minimal" and impalpable breast carcinoma. Curr Diagn Pathol, 1994;1:90–97

The Royal College of Pathologists. Minimum dataset for breast cancer histopathology reports. London: July, 1998

Turner RR, Ollila DW, Stern S, Giulano A. Optimal histopathologic examination of the sentinel lymph node for breast carcinoma staging. Am J Surg Pathol 1999;23:263–267

UK National Coordinating Group for Breast Screening Pathology. Consistency of histopathological reporting of breast lesions detected by screening: findings of the UK National external quality assessment (EQA) scheme. Eur J Cancer 1994;30:1414–1419

Gynaecological cancer

Arends MJ, Buckley CH, Wells M. Aetiology, pathogenesis, and pathology of cervical neoplasia. J Clin Pathol 1998;51:96–103

Bell SW, Kempson RL, Hendrickson MR. Problematic uterine smooth muscle neoplasms. Am J Surg Pathol 1994;18:535–558

Buckley CH, Fox H. Biopsy pathology of the endometrium. London: Chapman and Hall Medical, 1989

Burton JL, Wells M. Recent advances in the histopathology and molecular pathology of carcinoma of the endometrium. Histopathology 1998;33:297–303

Coleman DV, Evans DMD. Biopsy pathology and cytology of the cervix. 2nd edn. London: Arnold, 1999

Eichorn JH, Bell DA, Young RH, Scully RE. Ovarian serous borderline tumours with micropapillary and cribriform patterns. A study of 40 cases and comparison with 44 cases without these patterns. Am J Surg Pathol 1999;23:397–409

Fox H. Primary neoplasia of the female peritoneum. Histopathology 1993;23:103–110

Fox H. Endometrial hyperplasia. Curr Diag Pathol 1994;1:151–157

Fox H. Ovarian tumours of borderline malignancy: time for a reappraisal? Curr Diagn Pathol 1996;3:143–151

Fox H. Trophoblastic disease. In: Kirkham N, Lemoine NR (eds). Progress in pathology 3. New York: Churchill Livingstone, 1997:86–101

Fox H, Wells M (eds). Haines and Taylor's obstetrical and gynaecological pathology. 4th edn. New York: Churchill Livingstone, 1995

Ismail S M. Gynaecological effects of Tamoxifen. J Clin Pathol 1999;52:83–88

Kasprzak L, Foulkes WD, Shelling AN. Hereditary ovarian carcinoma. BMJ 1999;318:786–789

Kennedy MM, Manek S. The endometrium and hormonal manipulation: morphological features and review. CPD Bulletin Cellular Pathology 1998;1(1):15–18

Kurian K, Al-Nafussi A. Relation of cervical glandular intraepithelial neoplasia to microinvasive and invasive adenocarcinoma of the uterine cervix: a study of 121 cases. J Clin Pathol 1999;52:112–117

Kurman RJ, Amin MB. Protocol for the examination of specimens from patients with carcinomas of the cervix. Arch Pathol Lab Med 1999;123:55–61

Kurman RJ, Norris HJ, Wilkinson EJ. Tumors of the cervix, vagina and vulva. Atlas of tumor pathology. 3rd series. Fascicle 4. Washington: AFIP, 1992

Lage JM. Protocol for the examination of specimens from patients with gestational trophoblastic malignancies. Arch Pathol Lab Med 1999;123:50–54

Lagendijk JH, Mullink H, van Diest PJ, Meijer GA, Meijer CJLM. Immunohistochemical differentiation between primary adenocarcinoma of the ovary and ovarian metastases of colonic and breast origin. Comparison between a statistical and an intuitive approach. J Clin Pathol 1999;52:283–290

Lowe DG, Buckley CH, Fox H. Advances in gynaecological pathology. In: Anthony PP, MacSween RNM (eds). Recent advances in histopathology 17. Edinburgh: Churchill Livingstone, 1997:113–137

Manek S, Wells M. Borderline ovarian tumours. CPD Bulletin Cellular Pathology 1998;1(1):11–14

Manek S. Immunohistochemistry in gynaecological diseases. CPD Bulletin Cellular Pathology 1999; 1(4):162–166

Paradinas FJ. The histological diagnosis of hydatidiform moles. Curr Diagn Pathol 1994;1:24–31

Paradinas FJ. The differential diagnosis of choriocarcinoma and placental site tumour. Curr Diagn Pathol 1998;5:93–101

Riopel MA, Ronnett BM, Kurman RJ. Evaluation of diagnostic criteria and behaviour of ovarian intestinal-type mucinous tumors. Atypical proliferative (borderline) tumors and intraepithelial, microinvasive, invasive and metastatic carcinomas. Am J Surg Pathol 1999;23:617–635

Rollason TP. Aspects of ovarian pathology. In: Anthony PP, MacSween RNM (eds). Recent advances in histopathology 15. Edinburgh: Churchill Livingstone, 1992:195–218

Rollason TP. Epithelial lesions of the endocervix. In: Kirkham N, Lemoine NR (eds). Progress in pathology 4. Edinburgh: Churchill Livingstone, 1998:179–199

Rollason TP. Recent advances in vulvar pathology. CPD Bulletin Cellular Pathology 1998;1(1):19–25

Russell P, Farnsworth A. Surgical pathology of the ovaries. 2nd edn. New York. Churchill Livingstone, 1997

Scully R. Histological typing of ovarian tumours. 2nd edn. WHO: International histological classification of tumours. Berlin Heidelberg New York: Springer, 1999

Scully RE. Protocol for the examination of specimens from patients with carcinoma of the vagina. Arch Pathol Lab Med 1999;123:62–67

Scully RE, Bonfiglio TA, Kurman RJ, Silverberg SG, Wilkinson EJ. Histological typing of female genital tract tumours. 2nd edn. WHO: International histological classification of tumours. Berlin Heidelberg New York: Springer, 1994

Scully RE, Young RH, Clement PB. Tumors of the ovary, maldeveloped gonads, fallopian tube, and broad ligament. Atlas of tumor pathology. 3rd series. Fascicle 23. Washington: AFIP, 1998

Silverberg SG. Protocol for the examination of specimens from patients with carcinomas of the endometrium. Arch Pathol Lab Med, 1999;123:28–32

Silverberg SG, Kurman RJ. Tumors of the uterine corpus and gestational trophoblastic disease. Atlas of tumor pathology. 3rd series. Fascicle 3. Washington: AFIP, 1992

Wilkinson N. Recent advances in mesenchymal lesions of the uterus. CPD Bulletin Cellular Pathology 1998;1(1):26–27

Young RH, Clement PB (eds). Recent advances in gynaecological pathology. Hum Pathol 1991;22:737–806, 847–891

Young RH. New and unusual aspects of ovarian germ cell tumours. Am J Surg Pathol 1993;17:1210–1224

Urological cancer

Association of Directors of Anatomic and Surgical Pathology. Recommendations for the reporting of resected prostate carcinomas. Hum Pathol 1996;27:321–323

Association of Directors of Anatomic and Surgical Pathology. Recommendations for the reporting of resected neoplasms of the kidney. Hum Pathol 1996;20:1005–1007

Bostwick DG, Dundore PA. Biopsy pathology of the prostate. London: Chapman and Hall Medical, 1997

Bostwick DG, Eble JN (eds). Urological surgical pathology. St Louis: Mosby, 1997

Cheng L, Cheville JC, Neumann RM, Bostwick DG. Natural history of urothelial dysplasia of the bladder. Am J Surg Pathol 1999;23:443–447

Epstein JI, Amin MB, Reuter VR, Mostofi FH and the Bladder Consensus Conference Committee. The World Health Organization/International Society of Urological Pathology consensus classification of urothelial (transitional cell) neoplasms of the urinary bladder. Am J Surg Pathol 1998;22:1435–1448

Farrow G, Amin MB. Protocol for the examination of specimens from patients with carcinomas of renal tubular origin, exclusive of Wilms tumor and tumors of urothelial origin. Arch Pathol Lab Med 1999;123:23–27

Ferry JA, Young RH. Malignant lymphoma of the genitourinry tract. Curr Diagn Pathol 1997;4:145–169

Fuhrman SA, Lasky LC, Limas C. Prognostic significance of morphologic parameters in renal cell carcinoma. Am J Surg Pathol 1982;6:655–663

Grigor KM. Germ cell tumours of the testis. In: Anthony PP, MacSween RNM (eds). Recent advances in histopathology 15. Edinburgh: Churchill Livingstone, 1992:177–194

Harnden P, Parkinson MC. Transitional cell carcinoma of the bladder: diagnosis and prognosis. Curr Diagn Pathol 1996;3:109–121

Montironi R, Schulman CC. Pathological changes in prostate lesions after androgen manipulation. J Clin Pathol 1998;51:5–12

Montironi R, Thompson D, Bartels PH. Premalignant lesions of the prostate. In: Lowe DG, Underwood JCE (eds). Recent advances in histopathology 18. Edinburgh: Churchill Livingstone, 1999:147–172

Mostofi FK, Davis CJ, Sesterhenn IA. Histological typing of kidney tumours. 2nd edn. WHO: International histological classification of tumours. Berlin Heidelberg New York: Springer, 1998

Mostofi FK, Sesterhenn IA. Histological typing of testis tumours. 2nd edn. WHO: International histological classification of tumours. Berlin Heidelberg New York: Springer, 1998

Mostofi FK, Davis CJ, Sesterhenn IA. Histological typing of urinary bladder tumours. 2nd edn. WHO: International histological classification of tumours. Berlin Heidelberg New York: Springer, 1999

Murphy WM, Beckwith JB, Farrow GM. Tumors of the kidney, bladder and related urinary structures. Atlas of tumor pathology. 3rd series. Fascicle 11. Washington: AFIP, 1994

Parkinson MC. Pre-neoplastic lesions of the prostate. Histopathology 1995;27:301–311

Petersen RO. Urologic pathology. 2nd edn. Philadelphia: Lippincott, 1992

Pugh RCB (ed). Pathology of the testis. Blackwell Scientific, Oxford, 1976

Renshaw AA, Richie JP. Subtypes of renal cell carcinoma. Different onset and sites of metastatic disease. Am J Clin Pathol 1999;111:539–543

Ulbright TM. Protocol for the examination of specimens from patients with malignant germ cell and sex cord-stromal tumors of the testis, exclusive of paratesticular malignancies. Arch Pathol Lab Med 1999;123:14–19

Ulbright TM, Amin MB, Young RH. Tumors of the testis, adnexa, spermatic cord, and scrotum. Atlas of tumor pathology. 3rd series. Fascicle 25. Washington: AFIP, 1999.

Vargas SO, Jiroutek M, Welch WR, Nucci MR, D'Amico AV, Renshaw AA. Perineural invasion in prostate needle biopsy specimens. Correlation with extraprostatic extension at resection. Am J Clin Pathol 1999;111:223–228

Webb JN. Aspects of tumours of the urinary bladder and prostate gland. In: Anthony PP, MacSween RNM (eds). Recent advances in histopathology 15. Edinburgh: Churchill Livingstone, 1992:157–176

Weiss LM, Gelb AB, Medeiros LJ. Adult renal epithelial neoplasms. Am J Clin Pathol 1995;103:624–635

Young RH (ed). Pathology of the urinary bladder. New York. Churchill Livingstone, 1989

Lymph node cancer

Bagg A, Kallakury BVS. Molecular pathology of leukaemia and lymphoma. Am J Clin Pathol 1999;112 (Suppl 1):S76–S92

Bain BJ, Clark DM, Lampert IA. Bone marrow pathology. Oxford: Blackwell Scientific, 1992

Buley ID. Cytology of metastatic neoplasms in lymph nodes. In: Lowe DG, Underwood JCE (eds). Recent advances in histopathology 18. Edinburgh: Church Livingstone, 1999:116–118

Chan JKC, Banks PM, Cleary ML, Delsol G, de Wolf-Peters C, Falini B, Gatter KC, Grogan TM, Harris NL, Isaacson PG, Jaffe ES, Knowles DM, Mason DY, Müller-Hermelink HK, Pileri SA, Piris MA, Ralfkiaer E, Stein H, Warnke RA. A proposal for classification of lymphoid neoplasms (by the International Lymphoma Study Group). Histopathology 1994;25:517–536

Compton CC, Harris NL, Ross DW. Protocol for the examination of specimens from patients with non-Hodgkin's lymphoma. Arch Pathol Lab Med 1999a;123:68–74

Compton CC, Ferry JA, Ross DW. Protocol for the examination of specimens from patients with Hodgkin's disease. Arch Pathol Lab Med 1999b;123:75–80

Diebold J, Jungman P, Molina T, Audouin J. Recent advances in Hodgkin's disease: an overview and review of the literature. Curr Diagn Pathol 1995;2:153–162

Extranodal hematopoietic/lymphoid disorders. Pathology patterns. Am J Clin Pathol 1999;111 (Suppl 1):S1–S152

Gatter K, Brown D. An illustrated guide to bone marrow diagnosis. Oxford: Blackwell Scientific 1997

Harris NL, Jaffe ES, Diebold J, Flandrin G, Muller-Hermelink HK, Vardiman J, Lister TA, Bloomfield CD. The World Health Organization classification of neoplastic diseases of the haemopoietic and lymphoid tissues: report of the clinical advisory committee meeting, Airlie House, Virginia, November 1997. Histopathology 2000; 36:69–87

Isaacson PG, Norton AJ. Extranodal lymphomas. Edinburgh: Churchill Livingstone, 1994

Lauder I. T-cell malignant lymphomas. In: Anthony PP, MacSween RNM (eds). Recent advances in histopathology 15. Edinburgh: Churchill Livingstone, 1992:93–112

Lee FD. Unusual sites and types of lymphoma. In: Anthony PP, MacSween RNM (eds). Recent advances in histopathology 16. Edinburgh: Churchill Livingstone, 1994:73–93

Mason D, Gatter K. Lymphoma classification. Glostrup, Denmark: DAKO, 1999

Müller-Hermelink H K, Marx A, Kirchner Th. Advances in the diagnosis and classification of thymic epithelial tumours. In: Anthony PP, MacSween RNM (eds). Recent advances in histopathology 16. Edinburgh: Churchill Livingstone, 1994:49–72

Pileri SA, Sabattini E. A rational approach to immunohistochemical analysis of malignant lymphomas on paraffin wax sections. J Clin Pathol 1997;50:2–4

Shimosato Y, Mukai K. Tumors of the mediastinum. Altas of tumor pathology. 3rd series. Fascicle 21. Washington: AFIP, 1997

Stansfeld AG, d'Ardenne AJ (eds). Lymph node biopsy interpretation. 2nd edn. Edinburgh: Churchill Livingstone, 1992

Stevenson SK, Wright DH. Hodgkin's disease and immunoglobulin genetics. In: Kirkham N, Lemoine NR (eds). Progress in pathology 4. Edinburgh: Churchill Livingstone, 1998:99–111

Strauchen JA. Diagnostic histopathology of the lymph node. Oxford: Oxford University Press, 1998

Swerdlow SH. Post-transplant lymphoproliferative disorders: a working classification. Curr Diagn Pathol 1997;4:28–35

Warnke RA, Weiss LM, Chan JKC, Cleary ML, Dorfman RF. Tumors of the lymph nodes and spleen. Atlas of tumor pathology. 3rd series. Fascicle 14. Washington: AFIP, 1995

Wotherspoon AC. Immunocytochemistry of low grade B cell lymphomas. CPD Bulletin Cellular Pathology 1999; 1(4):158–161

Wright D, McKeever P, Carter R. Childhood non-Hodgkin's lymphomas in the United Kingdom: findings from the UK Children's Cancer Study Group. J Clin Pathol 1997;50:128–134

Bone and soft tissue cancer

Association of Directors of Anatomic and Surgical Pathology. Recommendations for the reporting of soft tissue sarcomas. Hum Pathol 1999;30:3–7

Bullough PG. Bullough and Vigorita's orthopaedic pathology. 3rd edn. London: Mosby-Wolfe, 1997

Enzinger FM, Weiss SW. Soft tissue tumours. 3rd edn. St Louis: Mosby, 1995

Goodlad JR, Fletcher CDM. Recent developments in soft tissue tumours. Histopathology 1995;27:103–120

Graadt van Roggen JF, Bovée JVMG, Morreau J, Hogendoorn PCW. Diagnostic and prognostic implications of the unfolding molecular biology of bone and soft tissue tumours. J Clin Pathol 1999;52:481–489

Guillou L, Fletcher CDM. Newer entities in soft tissue tumours. Curr Diagn Pathol 1997;4:210–221

Jones D, Kraus MD, Dorfman DM. Lymphoma presenting as a solitary bone lesion. Am J Clin Pathol 1999;111:171–178

Malone M. Soft tissue tumours in childhood. Histopathology 1993;23:203–216

Mentzel T, Fletcher CDM. Recent advances in soft tissue tumor diagnosis. Am J Clin Pathol 1998;110:660–670

Pringle JAS. Osteosarcoma: the experiences of a specialist unit. Curr Diagn Pathol 1996;3:127–136

Schajowicz F. Histological typing of bone tumours. 2nd edn. WHO: International histological classification of tumours. Berlin Heidelberg New York: Springer, 1993

Weiss SW. Histological Typing of soft tissue tumours, 2nd edn. WHO: International histological classification of tumours. Berlin Heidelberg New York: Springer, 1994

Wijnaendts LCD, van der Linden JC, van Unnick AJM, Voûte PA, Meijer CJLM. Rhabdomyosarcoma: results of a Dutch unicenter study. Curr Diagn Pathol 1996;3:137–142

Ophthalmic cancer

Campbell RJ. Histological typing of tumours of the eye and its adnexa. 2nd edn. WHO: International histological classification of tumours. Berlin Heidelberg New York: Springer, 1998

Lee WR. Ophthalmic histopathology. London: Springer-Verlag, 1993

McLean IW, Burnier MN, Zimmerman LE, Jakobiec FA. Tumors of the eye and ocular adnexa. Atlas of tumor pathology. 3rd series. Fascicle 12. Washington: AFIP, 1994

Index

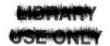